A NOTE ON THE EXERCISE INSTRUCTIONS

Repetitions

Unless otherwise stated, assume that for the majority of exercises, a suitable number of repetitions to perform would be around ten. For beginners, it is more likely to be around six repetitions, or whatever the body can handle, so long as technique is not compromised. For the advanced student, two sets of ten repetitions may be appropriate, provided ability allows on certain exercises.

Target muscles

This is a broad overview of the prime muscles involved in any particular exercise. It is not an exhaustive list by any means. Often, muscles are grouped together to make the list more compact. For example, scapula stabilizers often appear under this category. When broken down, this includes the lower trapezius and serratus anterior muscles. Below is a short list of grouped muscles that are broken down into their component parts for future reference.

Contra-Indications

Some exercises may not be appropriate for certain medical conditions or physical problems, since it may aggravate or exacerbate pre-existing conditions. At the end of each exercise is a list (not exhaustive) of contra-indications to that particular exercise. This is a general guideline only, which may or may not apply to each individual student. For example, it may state that the exercise is unsuitable for certain disc-related back problems. It is up to the individual instructor to help the student ascertain whether that broad guideline actually applies to them. Suitability for the exercise would depend upon several factors. Age, ability, severity of the disc problem, any other problems (related or not) as well as the level of core strength, would all be factors to take into consideration when attempting a contra-indicated exercise. A student who is young and active, with a reasonable amount of core strength may well be able to attempt the exercise without any problems or side effects. Conversely, an elderly student with a severe back problem, who has relatively poor core strength, may find that the exercise makes their condition worse. That is not to say that they will never be able to perform a certain exercise that initially was too difficult or painful. It is often the case that when a certain level of core strength has been built up over a period of time from regular Pilates practice, the same exercise may be attempted further down the line without any adverse effects.

There will be some exercises that will always remain contra-indicated no matter what factors are taken into consideration. Students with osteoporosis in the spine should never attempt forward flexion since it will always exacerbate the condition, regardless of core strength. However, mild osteoporosis in any other bones and joints would not affect forward flexion of the spine. It is likely that if osteoporosis is present in the bones, then it is more than likely to be present in the spine also and any exercise involving forward bending would therefore be unsuitable.

There will be certain exercises that are completely unsuitable for pregnant women. These exercises are not listed here, since this is not a manual for pregnancy. Pregnant ladies should seek the advice of a medical practitioner or professional exercise instructor before attempting any exercise. There are many pregnancy related exercise manuals and DVD's available but the advice given in this instructional manual does not cater for the needs of pregnant women and is therefore unsuitable.

PILATES BASICS

Relaxation Position

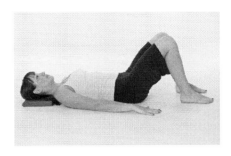

Aim

To relax the body and mind and release tension

Starting Position

Lie supine with the knees bent and the feet flat on the floor. The middle of the hip should be in alignment with the middle of the knee, down to the second toe of the foot. The feet face forwards. The arms rest down by the sides of the body with the palms facing the floor. A small head cushion may be placed underneath the skull in order to place the cervical spine in its natural position.

Action

Become aware of the points of contact between the body and the floor. The back of the skull and the floor, the shoulder blades, elbows, hands, pelvis, buttocks and feet. Try to allow the body to feel heavy, almost as if the floor is made of sand and the body is sinking into it.

Now work your way through the body from head to toe, relaxing each body part. Try to visualize each body part as you work your way down. Start by releasing tension in the facial muscles; chin; jaw and throat. Then allow the neck and shoulders to relax. Feel the collarbones opening and widening. The scapula and spine release. Allow the abdomen, hips, buttocks and pelvis to feel heavy and grounded. Finally dissolve any tension in the legs, feet and toes.

Once you have worked your way through the body, observe the natural breathing rhythm. On the inhalation the abdomen rises and on the exhalation the abdomen falls. Allow the mind and body to release. Ask yourself this question. "How easy or how difficult is it for you to relax?" Does it come naturally with minimal effort? Or, do you fight the relaxation? Is your mind busy and does your body want to fidget? Can you let go easily and just "be"? Observe without judgment. The more you practice relaxation, the easier relaxation comes to you.

Emma Newham's

Power Ring Workout

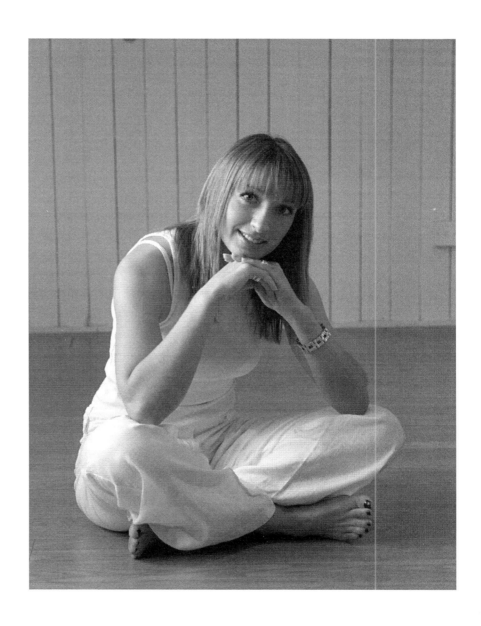

By Emma Newham

Published in the United Kingdom by

Pilates Union UK
Station Road
East Boldon
Tyne & Wear
NE36 0LE
www.pilatesunion.co.uk

ISBN – 978-0-9565285-4-4

Emma Newham – Author

Printed in the UK by Jasprint

Neutral Pelvis

Aim

To find the natural curve of the lumbar spine so that we can learn correct placement of the spine for future exercises

Starting Position

Lie supine in the relaxation position with the knees bent and the feet flat on the floor, hip distance apart. A small head cushion may be placed underneath the skull in order to place the cervical spine in its natural position.

Action

North Position of the Pelvis

Inhale to prepare. As you exhale, gently tilt the pelvis backwards into a posterior tilt. The pubic bone will point up to the ceiling. The pubic bone will be higher than the hipbones resulting in the lumbar spine being lengthened towards flexion. The lower back will press down into the floor.

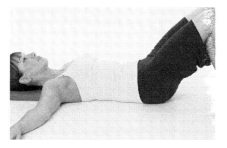

South Position of the Pelvis

Inhale to prepare. As you exhale, gently tilt the pelvis forwards into an anterior tilt. The pubic bone will point down to the floor. The hipbones will now be higher than the pubic bone, resulting in the lumbar spine being in an extended position. The lower back will arch away from the floor.

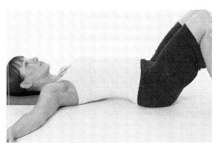

Action

Tilt the pelvis gently north, then centre and then south and return to the centre a few times and come to rest half way between the two points. The true definition of a neutral pelvis is when the anterior superior iliac spine (ASIS) is level with the pubic symphysis (i.e. if you got a spirit level between each hip bone and the pubic bone, all bones would be level at the same plane and height). Ideally this neutral pelvis should feel natural but because of different postural types, this may not be the case. A neutral position should not be forced if it feels uncomfortable in any way. If it does not happen naturally initially, then it is something to work towards as the body gets stronger.

Watchpoints

- Try not to grip in the hip flexors and glutes.
- Maintain good alignment with the hip, knee and second toe.
- Ensure that the back of the neck stays long and the shoulders stay away from the ears.

Contra-Indications

Certain back problems may feel uncomfortable with the flexion and extension of the lumbar spine. In this case, keep the range of movement to a minimum or avoid the position that causes discomfort.

Breathing

Joseph Pilates stated, "Even if you follow no other instructions, learn to breathe correctly". He likened the lungs to bellows, using them to pump air fully in and out of the body. Pilates believed in enriching the blood with oxygen so that it could awaken all the cells in the body and eliminate stale air and the wastes related to fatigue. He believed that forced exhalation was the key to a full inhalation.

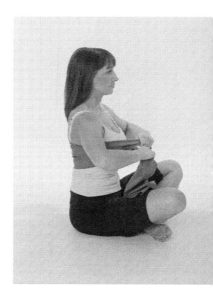

Every movement in Pilates has a specific breath pattern. Together with the timing of the breath, it enhances effective muscle use. Generally speaking, we tend to exhale on the effort (or exertion) as this helps prevent the body from creating tension. Effective breathing can help to lengthen the abdomen, broaden the upper back and helps train the correct muscle recruitment for everyday core strength. The lungs need to open to the front, back and sides. If we can successfully do this, then our oxygen uptake also increases and therefore our lung capacity. Unfortunately, most of us only open the front lungs, using the upper lobes, since sedentary lives lead to shallow breathing. Many people often hold their breath during exercise, particularly when new to Pilates, due to the concentrated effort of co-coordinating a difficult task. Muscles can tense up when we hold our breath, which can exacerbate poor posture.

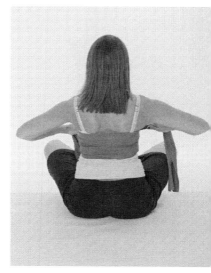

Proper breathing will assist in flowing movements and it is an integral part of the technique and one of the key principles. Pilates encourages deep breathing, using the lower and upper lobes of the lungs. Benefits of correct breathing allow the blood to be enriched with oxygen, which nourishes all the cells in our body, whilst expelling stale air. Our circulation increases and we feel rejuvenated. More oxygen in the muscles helps them to relax and therefore reduces tension. It also assists in concentration and control whilst exercising. We use the breath to initiate and support movement.

Thoracic or lateral breathing allows us to keep the abdominal muscles pulled in whilst inhaling and exhaling. This protects the spine whilst exercising. The aim is to keep the abdominals contracted whilst we breathe laterally, so that we have maximum support during movement. The focus is to breathe into the lower lobes of the lungs, all the way down the spine and into the pelvic basin, trying to expand the breath into the sides and back of the ribs. There is more efficient gaseous exchange in the lower lobes. Exhaling deeply encourages the engagement of the deep core muscles. The combination of correct breathing and stabilization needs to occur before movement for safe and effective technique.

To practice thoracic breathing, you may use a stretch band wrapped around the mid back. As you inhale, allow the ribs to expand and therefore stretch the band but avoid lifting the breastbone too high. On the exhalation, the abdomen should hollow and the pelvic floor should be engaged, lending to lumbar and pelvic stability. The goal is to keep these muscles engaged on the inhalation and the exhalation to a low level of contraction (around 30%). As you practice lateral breathing, you will find that you are able to perform Pilates exercises with greater ease. Whilst lateral breathing is the technique to use when you want to keep your abdominals engaged during exercise, we do not want to walk around with our abdominals contracted all of the time. Diaphragmatic breathing, with a natural extension of the belly on an inhalation, is the healthiest way to breathe regularly.

Pelvic Stability

The combination of the transversus abdominis, a deep back muscle known as the multifidus and also the pelvic floor muscles make up our core. The correct engagement of these core muscles will hold our pelvis in the safe neutral position whilst we are performing our exercises. This helps to prevent any tilting or arching of the lumbar spine, causing potential stress to the lower back. We call this pelvic stability.

Transversus Abdominis

We shall learn how to engage the transversus abdominus in 4 different positions. Remember we only need to recruit this muscle by about 30%. The reasons that we recruit at a low level is that we need to try to isolate these muscles in order to prevent other stronger muscles helping out and doing the job of the core. Also, the core muscles should be working for the whole of our Pilates class and if they are engaged too much then they will fatigue very quickly. We need them for endurance so a low level of recruitment will make them last longer. "Less is more" – the less you contract, the more you will be able to isolate. The harder you contract, the less you will be able to isolate.

Position One – Relaxation Position

Starting Position

Lie supine in the relaxation position with the knees bent and the feet hip distance apart. A small head cushion may be placed underneath the skull in order to place the cervical spine in its natural position. Find the neutral position of the pelvis. You may like to slide the fingertips of one hand underneath the natural lumbar curve in order to check that the pelvis remains in a neutral position. Ensure that the body does not move an inch as you slide the fingertips under. Check that there is an even pressure on the fingers throughout the exercise (i.e. no decrease in pressure if the pelvis tilts south and no increase in pressure if the pelvis tilts north). You may place the opposite hand on top of the belly.

Action

Inhale to prepare. Exhale and gently draw in the navel back down towards the spine. Try to achieve around 30% contraction. If you are unsure what 30% feels like then contact the navel as hard as you can (i.e. 100%). Then release the contraction by half (i.e. 50%). Then release by half again and that will be around 25% contraction.

Watchpoints

- Watch out for any tension in the body, particularly around the neck and shoulders
- Keep the length between ears and shoulders and the back of the neck long
- Ensure that there is not change in pressure on the hand that is under the pelvis as you engage the transversus abdominus
- Try not to grip around the hip flexors, buttocks or legs

Position Two – Lying Prone

Starting Position

Lie face down on the floor with the legs together. The elbows are bent and the hands rest under the forehead, palms facing down.

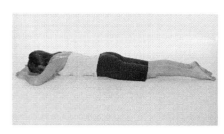

Action

As you inhale, imagine the abdomen and waistline are expanding, almost like a balloon filling with air. Exhale and pull the navel in back towards the spine against gravity. Imagine you have a precious egg underneath the abdomen and you are gently taking the pressure off it. You could almost slide a piece of paper under the belly.

Watchpoints

- As you pull in the navel ensure that the buttocks do not engage or the pelvis move
- Maintain the distance between ears and shoulders

Contra-Indications

If lying prone feels uncomfortable initially for certain back problems, then place a small cushion underneath the hipbones.

Position Three – Kneeling on all fours

Starting Position

Come to an all fours position with the knees bent directly under the hips and place the hands on the floor directly under the shoulders. The elbows are soft and the fingers are pointing forwards. Ensure that there is equal weight between the hands and feet and between right and left sides of the body by gently rocking the body forward and back and from side to side a little. Allow the body weight to come to rest between all four limbs equally. Keep a good length between the ears and shoulders. The back of the neck should follow the natural cervical curves.

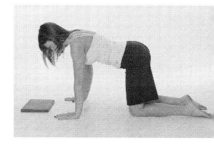

Action

Find the neutral pelvis by tilting the pelvis north and south and coming to rest half way in between. Inhale to prepare. As you exhale, gently pull in the navel back towards the spine against gravity. Imagine there is a scalding hot cup of tea balancing on the pelvis and lumbar spine so that as the navel is pulled in, the tea does not spill.

Watchpoints

- As the navel is pulled in, ensure that the back does not arch
- Maintain the gap between the ears and the shoulders
- Do not allow the shoulder blades to collapse together. Pull the shoulder blades apart on the ribcage using the serratus anterior muscle.
- There is a tendency for the head to start to drop downwards. Ensure that the back of the neck stays long with the back of the skull pushing up towards the ceiling.
- Ensure that the elbows do not lock out as the joint should stay soft

Contra-Indications

This position places extra stress on the wrist and knee joints and may be unsuitable for clients with problems in these joints.

Pelvic Floor

Most people have a vague idea of where the pelvic floor muscles are located and what they do but they may not be aware of all of the different openings from front to back. These are the muscles that stop us from "going to the toilet". Women have three openings and men have two. You will be shown how to isolate each opening of the pelvic floor separately in order to be familiar with each section. Then, when each component part has been felt, you can engage the entire area as one whole.

Together with the transversus abdominus muscle, the pelvic floor forms what we refer to as the "core", so they are very important.

When we are learning to isolate each opening, the amount of contraction is very small indeed. This is because the openings are very close together and if you engage one opening too much, the other openings will also contract.

It is impossible to tell if somebody is performing pelvic floor correctly, since no movement in the body can be detected. However, you can tell if somebody is doing it incorrectly, since external movement can be seen. Common mistakes include gripping in the glutes and hip flexors or tilting the pelvis or tensing the legs. It is not always obvious when you engage the contraction, whether you have managed to isolate a particular opening or not. It is more obvious as the contraction is released. You may think to yourself "Ah, I felt my buttocks relax there". In which case, the glutes have engaged as well as the pelvic floor but you may not have realised that when you contracted the muscles. So, it is easier to tell when you let go of the contraction, since you will sense other parts also release. If this is the case, then remember, "Less is more". The less you contract, the more you will be able to isolate. So next time, contract a little less. These kegel exercises are best done with the eyes closed. With the eyes open, the brain tends to take in visual stimulus from around the room. When the eyes are closed, the brain is free to concentrate on the internal environment and becomes more sensitive to different sensations within the body (i.e. you can "feel"more).

The relaxation position is the preferred position in which to practice pelvic floor contractions although it may be done in any position such as side lying, sitting upright, standing or on all fours. The relaxation position has been chosen since it is a comfortable position within which to work as the body is relaxed and the mind therefore free to concentrate.

Pelvic floor isolation - Starting Position

Lie supine in the relaxation position with the knees bent and the feet flat on the floor, hip distance apart.   A small head cushion may be placed underneath the skull in order to place the cervical spine in its natural position. You may like to slide the fingertips of one hand underneath the natural lumbar curve in order to check that the pelvis remains in a neutral position.

<u>The back passage opening – The sphincter muscle</u>
Action

Inhale to prepare. As you exhale, gently and slowly start to contract your back passage (your bottom hole) by drawing it inwards and upwards. This is your sphincter muscle and the sensation you want to achieve is that you are stopping yourself from passing wind. It is very tempting to squeeze the cheeks of the bottom here so be aware. Hold the contraction for around 5 seconds, continuing to exhale as you hold the contraction. Then inhale to release the contraction and see if you are able to tell if you managed to isolate the sphincter muscle.

<u>The front passage opening –</u>
Action

Inhale to prepare. As you exhale, gently and slowly start to contract the front passage (this is the muscle that you pee out of) by drawing it inwards and upwards. The sensation you need to achieve here is that you are stopping or lessening the flow of urine mid flow. Try not to grip around the hip flexors or legs here and ensure that the pelvis does not tilt. Hold the contraction for 5 seconds whilst exhaling and inhale to release and see if you were able to isolate again.

<u>The middle passage – The vagina (women only!!)</u>
Action

Inhale to prepare. As you exhale slowly and gently contract the walls of the vagina by drawing the muscle inwards and upwards. Imagine an elevator in your mind. Visualise the elevator doors closing. The walls of the vagina have to come together in a similar way, almost like drawing a pair of curtains together. You may also like to imagine a drawstring bag or purse. When the string is pulled, the gap tightens together. Then the walls of the vagina need to lift upwards to the first floor (towards the navel) and then continue lifting up to the second floor (towards the ribs).   So the action is to draw the curtains first and then lift up to the various floors after. Hold the contraction for 5 seconds whilst exhaling and inhale to release and see if you were able to isolate again.

<u>Men only!!</u>

In addition to the front and back passage, it may be helpful to feel like you are lifting up "the family jewels".

Sliding the leg away

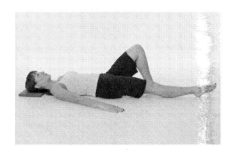

Aim

Now that we have learned how to engage the key core muscles, we will test the theory of pelvic stability. Sliding the leg away without the recruitment of the core abdominals will result in the pelvis tilting south. The weight of the leg acts as a lever, pulling the pelvis into an anterior tilt. The activation of the core abdominals will ensure that the pelvis stays in a safe neutral position against the resistance of the leg.

Starting Position

Lie supine in the relaxation position with the knees bent and the feet flat on the floor, hip distance apart. A small head cushion may be placed underneath the skull in order to place the cervical spine in its natural position. You may like to slide the fingertips of one hand underneath the natural lumbar curve in order to check that the pelvis remains in a neutral position.

Action

Inhale to prepare. As you exhale engage the pelvic floor openings first, followed by the transversus abdominus. It is almost like pulling up a zip on your jeans. Start low with the pelvic floor and work your way up to the transversus. Once these core muscles are correctly engaged, continue exhaling and gently slide one leg along the floor, away from the body until it is fully straight. Inhale, continuing to keep the abdominals engaged and gently use the core muscles to bend the knee and draw the leg back in towards the body.

The pelvis should not have moved if the core muscles have been recruited correctly.

Watchpoints

•   You may notice that, as the leg slides away, it weighs more as it travels further. The significance of this is that you will need to engage the core a little more against the increasing resistance of the leg.

•   Ensure that the heel remains in contact with the floor the whole time. It is only the toes that lose contact with the floor.

•   Only push the leg as far as a neutral pelvis allows

•   Once you have finished the exercise, relax the body. Notice if there is any change in the pelvis as you relax. Does it fall into its natural position? If so, then there must have been some movement north or south during the course of the exercise. The pelvis should not move as you relax, as it should have been held in the natural position all along.

•   Keep the back of the neck long and the shoulders away from the ears. The collar bones should be wide.

Ribcage closure

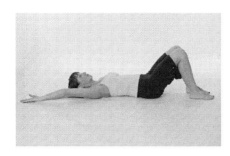

We have seen how to stabilize the lumbar spine and pelvis in a neutral position, using the combination of transversus abdominus and pelvic floor. This is essential when there is a leg movement, which can potentially pull on the lower back. However, when there is an arm movement involved, it is a different story. As the arm rises above the head, it can potentially pull on the ribs, making them flare outwards. Since the ribs are attached to the thoracic spine, this arm movement can potentially pull the upper back out of the neutral position. We therefore need to engage the oblique abdominal muscles to draw down the ribcage to stop it from flaring.

Sliding the arm away

Aim

To learn how to draw down the ribs using the oblique abdominals when moving an arm away (to prevent the ribcage from flaring thereby allowing the back to arch).

Starting Position

Lie supine on the floor in the relaxation position with knees bent and feet are hip width apart. Place the right hand flat against the left rib whilst the left arm is down by the side of the body. Initially just raise the left arm up in the air and back behind the head without engaging the abdominals. Feel just how much the ribcage actually moves as this happens. Some peoples ribs move a little whilst others move a lot. Leave the arm behind the head with the ribs flared. Take a breath in and then have a very loud, deep and prolonged "cough". Feel what happens to the ribs as you cough! They literally close down and lock. Every time you cough, sneeze, laugh and even vomit, the ribcage closes. You do not think to yourself "I am going to cough so I had better lock my ribs". It is an automatic, involuntary, reflex reaction. We now need to learn to draw down the ribs under conscious, voluntary control since when the ribs are flared, the spine is vulnerable.

Action

Inhale to prepare. Exhale to engage the oblique abdominals to draw down the ribcage and raise the right arm upwards to the ceiling and back overhead as far as flexibility allows, without forcing the arm back. Exhale to raise the arm back to the start.

Target Muscles

Core abdominals, pectorals, anterior deltoid, scapula stabilisers

Watchpoints

- Ensure the back of the neck stays long and the shoulders stay away from the ears
- Ensure good oblique engagement to avoid the ribs flaring when the arm goes back
- Do not force the arm backwards, stay within a good range of movement
- Ensure good alignment of the shoulder, elbow and wrist to avoid the tendency to bend the elbow or flick the wrist in order to get the backward arm closer to the floor

Neutral Spine

So far, you have learned that the combination of the transversus abdominus and pelvic floor muscles stabilise the lumbar spine and pelvis into a neutral position. This is important when there is a leg movement involved, which can potentially pull on the lower back. In addition, the oblique muscles prevent the ribcage from flaring out, thereby pulling the upper back out of a neutral position, particularly when there is an arm movement involved. This next exercise involves sliding the leg and opposite arm away from the body. Therefore you will need to engage all three areas in order to stabilise the entire spine (not just the pelvis or upper back on their own) into a neutral position. The three areas should be engaged in the following order; pelvic floor, transversus abdominus and obiques.

Here, you will have the weight of two limbs potentially pulling the spine out of a neutral position. However, t is not necessarily the weight of the limbs that will make the back arch – it is the brain instead! When learning a new skill, the brain tends to focus on one thing at a time. Up until now, it has only had one limb to contend with and it was therefore easier to move a single limb whilst holding onto the core muscles. Now the brain has two limbs to think about, so the element of co-ordination has entered into the equation. The brain now has the breathing, the core engagement and the co-ordination of opposite limbs to negotiate. Initially, it is unlikely that all these elements will be correctly activated at once. For example, you may have perfect breathing and perfect co-ordination but the pelvic floor may be relaxed. If any part of the core abdominals is not engaged, then you are not practicing safe and effective technique and not doing Pilates correctly. Don't worry initially if your co-ordination is poor or if the breathing is not quite right. It is more important to have the core engaged correctly over the co-ordination or breathing since the back is vulnerable to stress if these muscles are not working properly. Get the core right first and then the breathing and co-ordination will follow.

Starfish

To learn how to maintain a neutral spine, whilst moving two limbs away from the body

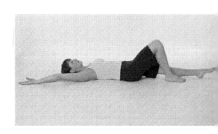

Starting Position

Lie supine in the relaxation position with the knees bent and the feet flat on the floor, hip distance apart.   A small head cushion may be placed underneath the skull in order to place the cervical spine in its natural position. The arms are down by the sides of the body.

Action

Inhale to prepare. Exhale engage the pelvic floor openings first, followed by the transversus abdominus and finally the obliques. It is almost like pulling up a zip on your jeans. Start low with the pelvic floor and work your way up to the transverses, then draw down the ribcage. Once these core muscles are correctly engaged, continue exhaling and gently slide one leg along the floor, away from the body until it is straight. Simultaneously raise the opposite arm upwards to the ceiling and overhead as far as flexibility allows, without forcing the arm back. Inhale, continuing to keep the abdominals engaged and gently use the core muscles to bend the knee and draw the leg and arm back in towards the body.

Watchpoints

Only push the arm and leg as far as a neutral spine allows

The collar bones should be wide, the neck long and the shoulders away from the ears

Do not force the arm back, stay within a good range of movement so as not to compromise technique

Ensure that the shoulder, elbow and wrist stay in alignment (don't bend the elbow or flick the wrist)

Opposition

This is the principle of lengthening whilst strengthening. Think of energy lines in the body and try to push the limbs in opposing directions along these lines, whilst maintaining a strong centre. In order to experience this, try the following exercise firstly without opposition and then using opposition.

Lie on your side with the arm outstretched and the head resting on the shoulder. The underneath leg is bent forwards and the top leg is outstretched straight along the floor in alignment with the spine. Relax the body and do not stretch the leg. Perform the exercise in a lazy way in order to feel the difference between the two methods. Just raise the top leg up off the floor a few inches until the foot is just above hip height. Ask yourself two questions. "Where do you feel the muscle contraction?' and "How intense is the workload?". Give it a mark out of 10 for effort (1 being minimal, easy effort and 10 being hard, maximal effort). The answer to the first question should be; outer thigh. The workload is usually fairly low, generally below 5 out of 10 depending upon ability. Now try the same exercise using opposition.

Lie on your side with the arm outstretched and the head resting on the shoulder. Walk the fingers of this hand along the floor so that the arm is really lengthening. Feel energy coming out of the crown of the head, almost like the head is being pulled by a piece of string attached to it, so that it too lengthens along the arm. Think of the 3 body spaces. The gap between the ear and shoulder is wide. Also the gap between the last rib and the iliac crest (i.e. the waist) is long. Finally, make space in the hip joint (i.e. lengthen the femur out of the hip socket). The top arm is bent in front of the body and the hand is pressing downwards into the floor whilst the elbow is reaching upwards to the ceiling in opposition.

The underneath leg is bent forwards and the top leg is outstretched straight along the floor in alignment with the spine. Lengthen the toes of the top leg along the floor to achieve a long leg. Pull up the knee-cap so that the thighs are firm. The whole body from the fingers to the toes should now be long. Imagine that your body is on an old fashioned rack, being pulled apart in two different directions. The head and underneath arm are lengthening northwards, whilst the waist and top leg are lengthening southwards. Watch you don't buckle in the middle!! A strong centre is needed to prevent the spine from arching. Make good use of the full powerhouse here in order to keep a neutral spine whilst lengthening.

Raise the leg as before but don't just lift and lower the leg, keep lengthening it the whole time.

Now ask yourself the same two questions. The answer to question one should still be "outer thigh" but in addition, the whole body is involved. Before, the rest of the body may have been relaxed and so the effort was just felt in one area. With opposition, the outer thigh is the primary muscle working but the whole body is lengthening and working as well in order to maintain the length. The intensity should therefore be well above a 5 out of 10 now. See how much effort lengthening the body involves? It takes a lot of energy to work in this way. The results, however, speak for themselves. It is the length rather than any height in the leg that makes this exercise (or any exercise for that matter) much harder. This sets Pilates apart from a normal body conditioning class. It is "how" you do it. Quality of movement over quantity, or number of repetitions. Try the Star exercise where all four limbs are stretched out. Here, you have 4 energy lines pulling in 4 opposing directions. The right arm is reaching forwards to the right hand corner of the room whilst the left arm is reaching forwards to the left hand corner of the room. In addition the right leg is reaching backwards to the back right hand corner of the room, whilst the left leg is reaching backwards to the back left hand corner of the room. Whenever you are working, keep thinking about the energy lines in the body and try to create as much length as possible, whilst keeping a strong centre.

Segmental Control

This is the ability to move the spine segment by segment, sequentially one vertebra at a time. It is particularly used in the spine curls, roll downs and full curl up exercises.

In the spine curls exercise the spine is lifted off the floor one vertebra at a time. It is helpful to visualise a bike chain on the floor when performing this exercise. The chain lifts link by link and that is exactly the movement we want to achieve in the spine. The vertebrae do not lump together and lift as a whole. The segmental and controlled movement will ensure that the spine stays mobile and flexible.

Scapula Stability

The shoulder blades have no direct boney connection to the rib cage, which means that there is a lot of potential for mobility and often instability here. Learning the correct placement of the scapula is essential for good movement patterns. They should not be hiking up to our ears or winging out to the side. Nor do we want to pull them down forcibly. By using a combination of the mid back muscles and in particular the lower trapezius and serratus anterior, we can anchor the shoulder blades down in the back which places them in the best possible position for movement.

THE STRETCHES

SPINE STRETCH FORWARD

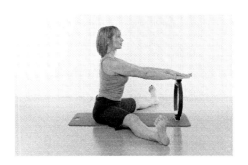

Aim

To stretch the back muscles and achieve segmental control of the spine

Starting Position

Sit upright with the legs apart and the ring on the floor in front of you in between the legs. The ring is upright and place one hand on top of the other on the top of the ring.

Action

Inhale - to prepare and lengthen tall.

Exhale - engage the core abdominals and lightly press down on the ring as you curve the upper back, one vertebra at a time. The ring will tilt away from you as you reach forwards.

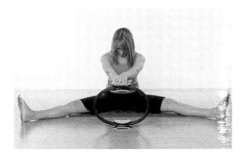

Inhale - to return to the starting position, one vertebra at a time.

Target Muscles

Neck flexors and spinal flexors and adductors

Watchpoints

- Try to ensure an even curve throughout the spine
- Do not over flex the cervical or thoracic spine
- Ensure correct segmental control of each vertebra
- Try not to collapse – think of lengthening up and over a large beach ball
- Ensure the scapula are stabilised

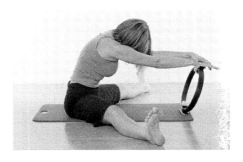

Contra-Indications

Forward flexion of the spine may be unsuitable for osteoporosis

Take care when working with clients who have disc related problems

THE SAW

Aim

To stretch the inner thighs whilst maintaining an upright spine

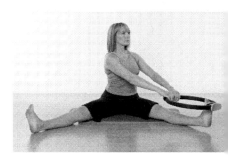

Starting Position

Sit upright with legs apart and place the ring behind one foot. The ring is held in both hands.

Action

Inhale - to prepare and lengthen the body.

Exhale - engage the core abdominals and pull the body forwards towards the foot. As you reach forward, the elbows will bend.

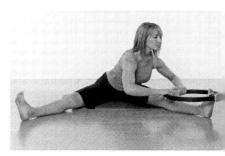

Inhale - to return to the start position and repeat to the opposite side.

Target Muscles

Adductors, Latissimus Dorsi and Hamstrings

Watchpoints

- Ensure the spine stays long
- Avoid any hiking of the ear towards the shoulder
- Ensure the legs, knees and feet stay aligned to prevent the legs or feet rolling in or out

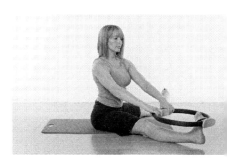

- Lean forwards from the waist to avoid the movement coming from the thoracic spine
- Try to maintain equal length in both sides of the waist

Variation One (Adaptation)

If hamstrings or lower back are tight, then a small cushion may be placed under the buttocks to make it easier.

HAMSTRING STRETCH

Aim

To stretch the hamstrings whilst maintaining a neutral pelvis

Starting Position

Lie supine on the floor with both knees bent. Bend one knee in towards the chest and place the ring behind the foot. The ring is held in both hands although it can be held in one hand if preferred.

Action

Inhale - to straighten the bent leg away from the body.

Exhale - and gently bring the straightened leg towards the chest. Try to keep the knee as straight as possible with the foot softly pointed.

Target Muscles

Hamstrings

Watchpoints

- Ensure that the tailbone remains in contact with the floor so that a neutral pelvis is maintained
- The waist should remain long on both sides to avoid any hip hitching
- Keep shoulders relaxed away from the ears
- Ensure the spine stays in neutral with the head on the floor
- Keep the neck long

Variation One (Adaptation)

The knee may be kept bent as an alternative stretch for those with tight hamstrings. This means that the leg may come closer to the body and the pelvis still remain in a neutral position

Variation Two

The foot may flex in order to obtain a nerve stretch

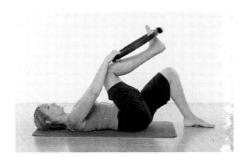

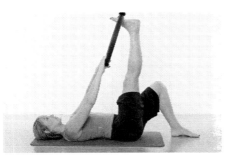

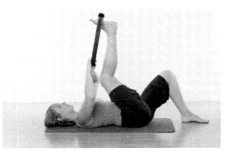

Variation One

4

SCIATIC STRETCH

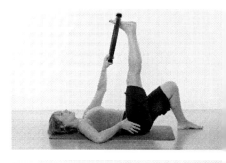

Aim

To stretch the sciatic nerve

Starting Position

Lie supine on the floor with both knees bent. Bend right knee in towards the chest and place the ring behind the foot. The ring is held in the opposite hand to the foot (i.e. left hand). Extend the right leg until the leg is as straight as possible and bring it in towards the chest (i.e. hamstring stretch)

Action

Inhale - to prepare.

Exhale - guide the right leg across the body towards the left side, using the ring to pull it gently over to the opposite side. Simultaneously bring the left bent knee also towards the opposite right side ensuring that the foot stays on the floor. Effectively the legs criss-cross each other. There are two actions for the straight leg here; the leg comes towards the chest; the leg comes across the body. Use the right hand to press down on the right hip so that it does not lift away from the floor as the leg comes across the body.

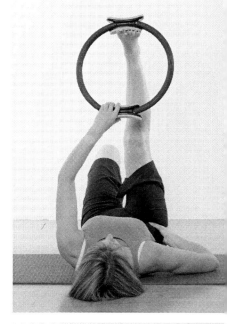

Target Muscles

Sciatic Nerve, hamstrings

Watchpoints

- Ensure that the hip of the straight leg stays on the floor and does not lift
- Keep the waist long and equal on both sides to avoid hip hitching
- Keep the foot flexed to ensure a nerve stretch is obtained
- The knee must be as straight as possible or the stretch will not be felt as much
- This is a rather unpleasant stretch so be careful not to go too far and overstretch
- Ensure the spine stays in neutral with the head on the floor
- Keep the neck long

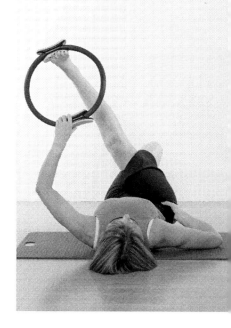

ADDUCTOR STRETCH

Aim
To stretch the inner thighs

Starting Position
Lie supine with one knee bent and foot on the floor. The other leg is straight up in the air (as for hamstring stretch) with the ring placed behind the ball of the foot. Hold the ring with the same hand as the leg that is in the air (i.e. when the left leg is held in the air, hold the ring with the left hand).

Action
Inhale - to prepare.

Exhale - and guide the leg out to the side and away from the body trying to keep the knee straight until a stretch is felt in the inner thigh muscles. Keep the leg as close to the chest as possible as it is guided out to the side.

Target Muscles
Adductors

Watchpoints
- Ensure the hipbones remain level to ensure a neutral pelvis and avoid any rolling or tilting of the pelvis as the leg is taken out to the side.
- Try to keep the knee as straight as possible
- Keep the shoulders relaxed and away from the ears
- Ensure the spine stays in neutral with the head on the floor
- Keep the neck long

Variation One
The bent leg may reach out in the opposite direction to the straight leg to help balance the pelvis and possibly increase the stretch by stretching the opposite side simultaneously

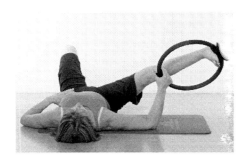

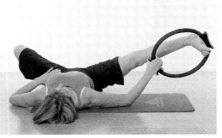

Variation One

ROLLING LIKE A BALL

Aim

To massage the spine and work the abdominals

Starting Position

Sit upright with the knees bent and place the ring in between the ankles. Hold the hands on the outside of the ankles. Lift the feet a few inches from the floor to balance just back of the sit bones. Tuck in the chin and maintain a C-curve in the spine.

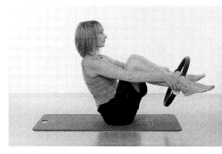

Action

Inhale - and allow the body to roll back (maintaining spinal flexion) without allowing the head to touch the floor.

Exhale - to roll back up to the starting position without allowing the feet to touch the floor. A certain degree of momentum plus abdominal strength will be employed here to ensure a successful roll. Try to pause and balance before going into the next roll.

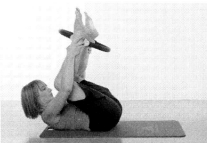

Target Muscles

Core abdominal muscles are working and the spinal muscles are stretching and receiving a nice massage

Watchpoints

- Try to maintain a ball position with the body throughout (i.e. distance between the knees and chest as well as the distance between the heels and buttocks should remain the same)
- Keep chin tucked in to avoid throwing the head back

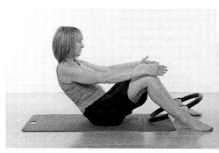

Variation One

Variation One (Adaptation)

Roll part way back slowly and under control with the feet remaining on floor

Variation Two

Hold the ring in the hands

Variation Three

Place the ring in between the knees

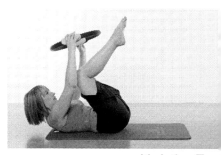

Variation Two

Contra-Indications

This may be unsuitable for certain back problems

This may be unsuitable for osteoporosis

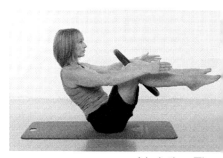

Variation Three

OPEN LEG ROCKER

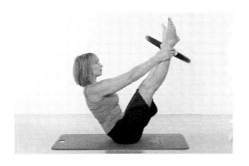

Aim

To stretch the hamstrings, challenge the abdominals further and massage the spine.

Starting Position

Sit upright with two straight legs in the air and apart, balancing just back of the sit bones. Place the ring in between the ankles and hold onto the outside of the ankles with the hands.

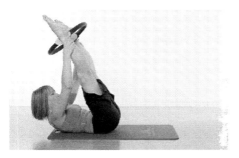

Action

Inhale - and allow the body to roll back without allowing the head to touch the floor.

Exhale - to roll back up to the starting position without allowing the feet to touch the floor. A certain degree of momentum plus abdominal strength will be employed here to ensure a successful roll. Try to pause and balance before going into the next roll. This is a much more challenging position than the previous Rolling Like a Ball exercise.

Target Muscles

Core abdominal muscles are working and the spinal muscles are stretching and receiving a nice massage

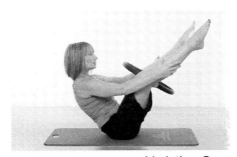

Variation One

Watchpoints

- Keep the chin tucked in to avoid throwing back the head
- Maintain an equal distance between the knees and chest throughout
- Keep the shoulders away from the ears

Variation One (Adaptation)

To make this exercise easier, place the ring between the knees and have the knees slightly bent (but not as bent as for Rolling Like a Ball)

Variation Two (Adaptation)

Hold onto the calves or behind the thighs instead of the ankles as the higher up the leg towards the pubic bone you hold, the easier it makes the exercise

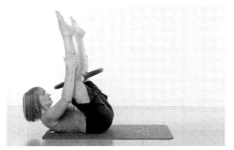

Contra-Indications

This may be unsuitable for certain back problems

This may be unsuitable for osteoporosis

Variation Two

LEG WORK

STANDING PLIES

Aim

To work the adductors whilst maintaining an upright posture

Starting Position

Stand in Pilates stance, with the legs turned out from the hip socket (heels together and toes apart). Your knees will be bent in the starting position since the ring will be in between the knees forcing them apart.

Action

Inhale - to prepare and lengthen the body.

Exhale - engage the core abdominals and try to straighten the legs as much as possible thereby squeezing the ring.

Inhale - to bend the knees again, keeping the abdominals hollowed.

Target Muscles

This will strengthen the quadriceps, adductors, buttocks and external rotators.

Watchpoints

- For the starting position, if the heels do not touch, then get them as close together as possible
- If the ring is uncomfortable in between the knees then a small, squashy ball may be used instead.
- Try not to stick out the buttocks as you bend the knees. Ensure the tailbone stays tucked under
- Try to keep the knees aligned with the second toe so that they don't roll inwards
- Ensure the weight is spread evenly on the feet to avoid any rolling in on the ankle

Variation One (Progression)

A heel raise may be added in between plies for extra challenge

Contra-Indications

The turned out position of the leg may be unsuitable for sciatica

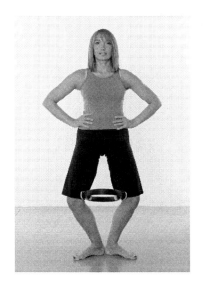

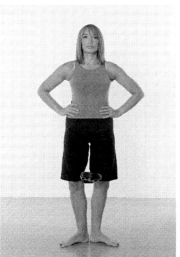

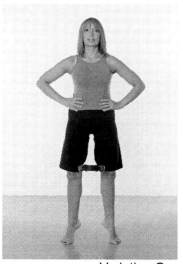

Variation One

HAMSTRING PRESS

Aim

To strengthen the hamstrings whilst maintaining an upright posture

Starting Position

Sit upright with the legs outstretched straight in front. Place the ring under the lower calf of the right leg (the ring is standing upright on the floor). The arms are straight behind you, propping you up with the hands on the floor.

Action

Inhale - to prepare.

Exhale - engage the core abdominals and depress the ring with the right leg, keeping the knee soft or slightly bent.

Inhale - to return to the starting position.

Repeat with the opposite leg.

Target Muscles

Hamstrings, scapula stabilisers

Watchpoints

- Ensure the knee does not lock as the ring is depressed
- Ensure the elbows stay soft throughout
- Keep the shoulders away from the ears
- Maintain an even length in both sides of the waist
- Keep both sit bones firmly in contact with the floor

Variation One (Adaptation)

For wrist problems, the exercise may be performed resting on the elbows

Contra-Indications

This may be unsuitable for those with wrist problems (choose variation one instead)

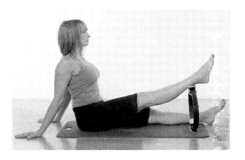

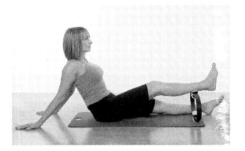

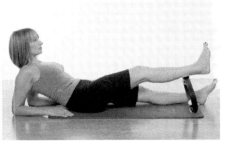

Variation One

OUTER THIGH RAISE

Aim

To strengthen the abductors whilst maintaining a neutral spine

Starting Position

Lie on the right side of the body, with two straight legs outstretched. Ensure good alignment of feet, knees and hips with all joints stacked on top of each other. The right arm is outstretched above the head and the head rests on the right shoulder. Place the ring upright on its side and put the two straight legs inside the ring with the ring just above the ankles.

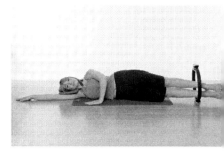

Action

Inhale - to prepare.

Exhale - engage the core abdominals and raise the top left leg upwards to push against the ring. The bottom leg remains on the floor. As you push upwards, the ring will elongate.

Inhale - to return to the start position. Turn over and repeat with the opposite leg.

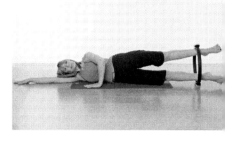

Target Muscles

Abductors, core abdominals

Watchpoints

- Keep the abdominals engaged throughout to ensure a neutral spine so that the back does not over arch or over flex
- Ensure the pelvis does not roll forward or back
- Keep the waist long and even on both sides
- Ensure the shoulder stays away from the ear

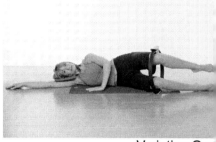

Variation One

Variation One (Adaptation)

The ring may be placed higher up above the knees with the knees bent as for oyster. Lift the top bent leg

Variation Two

The leg may be slightly medially rotated

Contra-Indications

Certain back problems may experience discomfort on one side of the spine whilst performing this exercise. This discomfort may only be present whilst lying on a particular side (not necessarily both sides). If any discomfort is felt in one side of the back, then discontinue the exercise.

SIDE LYING INNER THIGH SQUEEZE

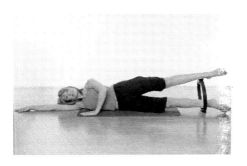

Aim

To strengthen the inner thighs

Starting Position

Lie on the right side of the body, with two straight legs outstretched. Ensure alignment of feet, knees and hips with all joints stacked on top of each other. The right arm is outstretched above the head and the head rests on the right shoulder. Place the right leg on the inside of the ring with the ring standing upright on its side on the floor. Place the left leg resting on the outside of the ring, just above the ankle

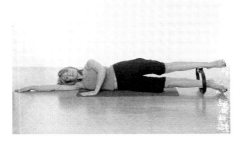

Action

Inhale - to prepare.

Exhale - engage the core abdominals and depress the ring with the left leg. Inhale to return to the starting position. Repeat with the opposite leg.

Target Muscles

Adductors

Watchpoints

- Keep the abdominals engaged throughout to ensure a neutral spine so that the back does not over arch or over flex
- Ensure the pelvis does not roll forward or back
- Keep the waist long and even on both sides
- Ensure the shoulders stay away from the ears
- Try to keep the leg straight

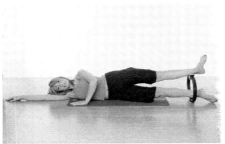

Variation Three

Variation One (Adaptation)

The ring may be placed in between the knees with the knees bent. Depress the ring with the top bent leg

Variation Two

The leg may be slightly medially rotated

Variation Three

The leg may be slightly laterally rotated

Contra-Indications

Clients with certain back problems or those with weak postural muscles and poor core abdominals may feel this on one side of the spine. In this case this exercise is unsuitable for them at this stage.

SUPINE INNER THIGH SQUEEZE

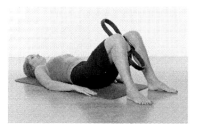

Aim

To strengthen the inner thighs whilst maintaining a neutral spine

Starting Position

Lie supine with the knees bent and the feet on the floor in the relaxation position. Place the ring in between the knees.

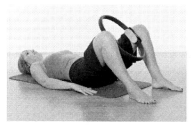

Action

Inhale - to prepare.

Exhale - engage the core abdominals and squeeze the ring.

Inhale - to return to the starting position.

Target Muscles

Adductors

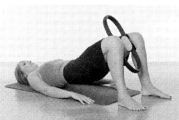

Watchpoints

- Maintain a neutral pelvis and spine throughout to avoid the tendency to tilt the pelvis posteriorly
- Try not to grip the hip flexors
- Keep the neck long
- Ensure the shoulders stay away from the ears

Variation One

Variation One (Progression)

Lift the buttocks in the air as for spine curl. This will target the hamstrings and gluteals also.

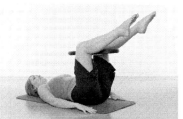

Variation Two (Progression)

Legs in the air with the feet off the floor.

Variation Three (Progression)

Legs in the air with the feet off the floor and the legs straight. The ring is placed between the ankles.

Variation Two

Variation Four (Progression)

With any of these variations a chest press may be added at the same time (with ring in between hands at shoulder height for variation and challenge). Two rings will be needed.

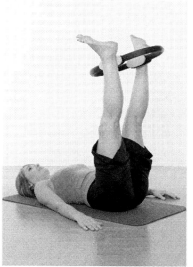

Variation Five (Progression)

With any of these variations an abdominal curl-up may be added

Contra-Indications

No contra-indications with the normal version. Some lumbar discomfort may be experienced with some of the variations. In this case, the normal version should be done

Variation Three

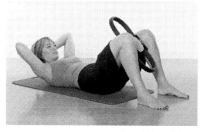

Variation Five

GLUTE PRESS

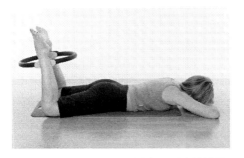

Aim

To strengthen the abductors, adductors and hamstrings whilst maintaining a neutral lumbar spine

Starting Position

Lie prone with the knees bent at 90 degrees. Place the ring in between the ankles.

Action

Inhale - to prepare.

Exhale - engage the core abdominals and push the pubic bone into the floor to prevent the lower back from arching. This will engage the gluteals. Squeeze the ring.

Inhale - to return to the starting position.

Target Muscles

Gluteals, hamstrings and adductors

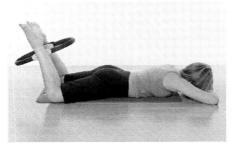

Watchpoints

- As you squeeze the ring, keep the pubic bone pressed down to avoid the tendency to over arch the lumbar spine
- Try to keep the angle at the knee joint even throughout (knees above ankles)
- Ensure the neck stays long and the shoulders stay away from the ears
- Keep the abdominals engaged
- Try to squeeze evenly from both sides. If the ring twists to one side, it is because one leg is pressing harder than the other
- Maintain an equal length on both sides of the waist

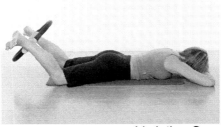

Variation One

Variation One

As you squeeze, you may push the ring towards the floor, thereby changing the joint angle at the knee

Variation Two (Progression)

As you squeeze the ring, you may lift the thighs off the floor challenging the gluteals further (N.B. This variation places more stress on the lumbar spine so may not be suitable for certain back problems)

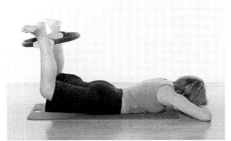

Variation Two

Variation Three (Progression)

As you squeeze, you may add in a small back extension to work the upper body

Contra-Indications

No contra-indications are usually experienced with the normal version except in the case of excessive lordosis. In this case, a small cushion may be placed under the hipbones to lessen any discomfort. Some lumbar discomfort may be experienced with some of the variations. In this case, the normal version should be performed.

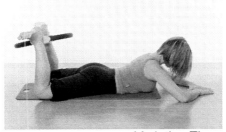

Variation Three

TORPEDO

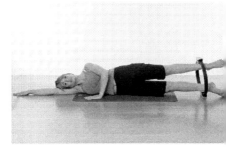

Aim

To strengthen the inner and outer thighs whilst maintaining a neutral spine

Starting Position

Lie on your right side with two straight legs outstretched. Ensure good alignment of feet, knees and hips with all joints stacked on top of each other. The right arm is outstretched above the head and the head rests on the right shoulder. Place the ring upright on its side and put the two straight legs inside the ring with the ring just above the ankles.

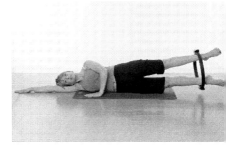

Action

Inhale - to prepare.

Exhale - engage the core abdominals and raise two straight legs. The legs will be pulling in opposite directions (i.e. the top leg pushes upwards whilst the bottom leg pushes downwards) in order to maintain contact with the ring throughout. The ring should be stretched in two opposing directions.

Inhale - to return to the starting position.

Target Muscles

Core abdominals, obliques, abductors and adductors

Watchpoints

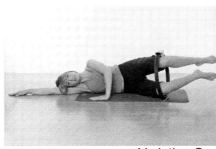

- Keep abdominals engaged throughout to ensure a neutral spine so that the back does not over arch or over flex
- Ensure the pelvis does not roll forward or back
- Keep the waist long
- Ensure the shoulder stays away from the ear
- Try to get a sense of opposition in the body

Variation One

Variation One (Adaptation)

This may be performed with bent knees and the ring placed on the outside of the knees rather than ankles

Variation Two (Progression)

As the legs are lifted, the head and upper body may also lift slightly. Here the top arm will be placed on the top thigh and as the upper body is raised, the hand will slide down the thigh

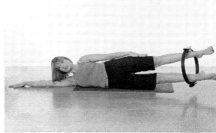

Contra-Indications

If discomfort is felt in one side of the spine, then discontinue the exercise.

Variation Two

ABDOMINAL EXERCISES

HALF CURL UPS

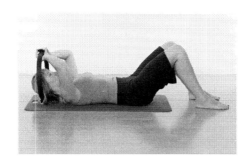

Aim
Learn how to curl up whilst maintaining length in the spine and a neutral pelvis.

Starting Position
Lie supine in the relaxation position with the knees bent and the feet flat on the floor. Place the head inside the ring with the back of the skull touching the inner rim and place the hands on the inside of the inner rim opposite the forehead

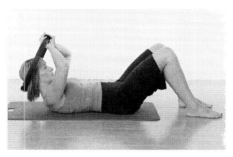

Action
Inhale - to prepare.

Exhale - to engage the core abdominals, tuck in the chin and lift the head and torso off the floor.

Inhale - to return to the starting position.

Target Muscles
Rectus abdominis, transversus abdominis

Watchpoints
- Only lift as high as a neutral pelvis can be maintained
- Keep the chin tucked in to the chest to avoid shortening the back of the neck
- Imagine a ripe peach between the chin and the chest – maintain a gap there to avoid pulling on the back of the neck (thereby breaking the delicate skin)
- Ensure the shoulders stay away from the ears
- Try not to grip around the hip flexors or buttocks
- Try to maintain length in the spine. Imagine a piece of sellotape between the sternum and the pubic bone. Try to keep the tape as flat as possible.

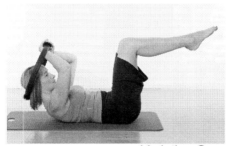

Variation One

Variation One (Progression)
This exercise may be performed with the legs in the air, bent at 90 degrees above the hips

Contra-Indications
Curl-ups may be unsuitable for certain disc-related back problems. Forward flexion of the spine may be unsuitable for osteoporosis

OBLIQUE HALF CURL UPS

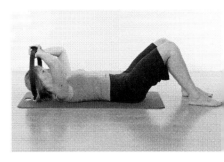

Aim
Learn how to curl up and rotate, whilst maintaining length in the spine and a neutral pelvis.

Starting Position
Lie supine in the relaxation position with the knees bent and the feet flat on the floor. Place the head inside the ring with the back of the skull touching the inner rim and place the hands on the inside of the inner rim opposite the skull

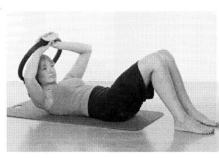

Action
Inhale - to prepare.

Exhale - to engage the core abdominals, tuck in the chin, oblique twist to the right as you lift the head and torso off the floor. The left shoulder blade will be higher than the right shoulder blade.

Inhale - to return to the starting position. Repeat to the opposite side.

Target Muscles
Rectus abdominis, transversus abdominis, oblique abdominals

Watchpoints

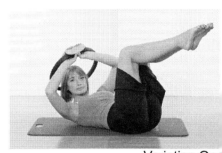

Variation One

- Only lift as high as a neutral pelvis can be maintained
- Keep the chin tucked in to the chest to avoid shortening the back of the neck
- Imagine a ripe peach between the chin and the chest – maintain a gap there to avoid pulling on the back of the neck (thereby breaking the delicate skin)
- Ensure the shoulders stay away from the ears
- Try not to grip around the hip flexors
- Ensure the lift comes from the "steering wheel" (i.e. the ribcage) and not from twisting the head or shoulders
- Try not to over twist otherwise one side of the pelvis will lift off the floor (i.e. will tilt from east to west or vice versa depending upon which way the body is twisting)
- Ensure the relationship between the elbows, shoulders and ears remains the same to avoid turning the head or moving one elbow inwards
- Think of the rib lifting towards the opposite hip bone therefore the movement comes from the ribs and not from the head or elbows

Variation One (Adaptation)
This exercise may be performed with the legs in the air, bent at 90 degrees above the hips

Variation Two (Adaptation)
This exercise may be performed without twisting the upper torso. Perform an abdominal half curl up (see previous exercise). The legs are twisted to one side (i.e. the feet are on the floor and twist the legs to the right so that the feet, knees and hips are stacked on top of one another). Repeat with the legs to the opposite side.

Contra-Indications
Curl-ups combined with rotation may be unsuitable for certain disc-related back problems. Forward flexion of the spine may be unsuitable for osteoporosis

LEAN BACKS WITH SWEEPING ARMS AND OBLIQUE TWIST

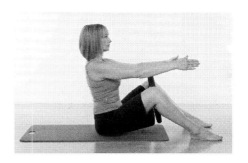

Aim

To work the core abdominals and obliques

Starting Position

Sit upright with the knees bent and the feet flat on the floor. Place the ring in between the knees and raise the arms straight out to shoulder height directly in front of the chest

Action

Inhale - to prepare.

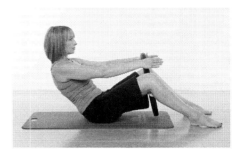

Exhale - engage the core abdominals and squeeze the ring. Simultaneously tuck the pelvis into a posterior tilt and lean back with an oblique twist to the right, keeping a C-curve in the spine. The right arm sweeps down to touch the floor as you lean back.

Inhale - to return the starting position. Repeat to the opposite side.

Target Muscles

Core abdominals, obliques

Watchpoints

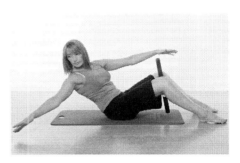

- As you lean back, ensure the lumbar spine stays in flexion.
- Ensure that the twist comes from the 'steering wheel' (ribcage) therefore using the oblique muscles only in order to avoid the rotation coming from either the head or arms
- Keep neck long (do not over flex)
- Ensure an even curve throughout the spine (do not over flex thoracic spine)
- Keep the shoulders away from the ears and avoid hiking
- Keep the waist long and even on both sides

Variation One (Progression)

Arms lift above the head to add extra weight and more challenge

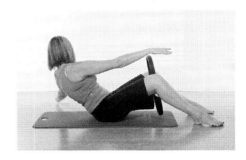

Contra-Indications

Lean backs may not be suitable for certain disc-related back problems

OBLIQUE TWIST

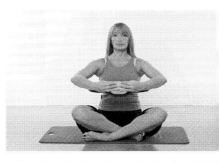

Aim

To work the oblique abdominals whilst maintaining a neutral spine

Starting Position

Sit upright, cross-legged and place the ring against the breastbone. Wrap the arms around the outside of the ring and clasp hands together in the middle in front of the breastbone.

Action

Inhale - to prepare.

Exhale - engage the core abdominals and oblique twist to the right keeping the ring in contact with the breastbone throughout.

Inhale - to return to the starting position. Repeat to the left.

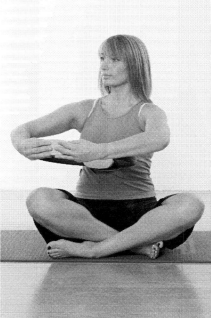

Target Muscles

Core abdominals and obliques

Watchpoints

- Ensure that the twist comes from the 'steering wheel' (ribcage) therefore using the oblique muscles only in order to avoid the rotation coming from either the head or arms
- Try to maintain alignment of the nose and breastbone throughout.
- Keep the shoulders level and away from the ears
- Keep waist long and even on both sides
- Maintain an equal weight on both sit bones

Variation One (Progression)

Arms above the head holding the ring in between the hands to add weight and challenge

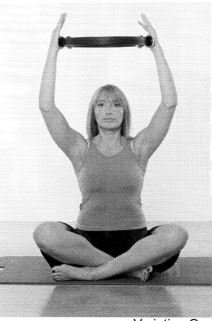

Variation One

FULL CURL UPS

Aim
To work the abdominals whilst achieving segmental control of the spine

Starting Position
Lie supine in the relaxation position with the knees bent and the feet flat on the floor. Place the head inside the ring with the back of the skull touching the inner rim and place the hands on the inside of the inner rim opposite the forehead

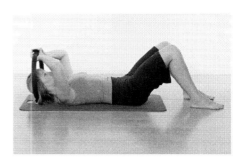

Action
Inhale - to prepare.

Exhale - to engage the core abdominals, tuck in the chin and lift the head and torso off the floor, peeling off one vertebra at a time until fully sitting upright.

Inhale - to prepare

Exhale - to slowly reverse the movement to return to the starting position.

Target Muscles
Rectus abdominis, transversus abdominis

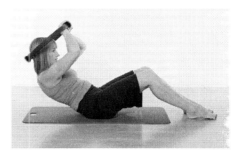

Watchpoints
- Keep the chin tucked in as if holding a small apple between the chin and the chest
- Ensure the shoulders stay away from the ears
- Try not to grip around the hip flexors
- Try to move sequentially through each vertebra, one at a time

Variation One (Adaptation)
Half curl up as for previous exercise

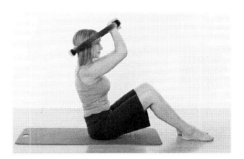

Variation Two (Adaptation)
Roll back exercise – Sitting upright with the ring behind the skull. Perform a posterior pelvic tilt and start to roll back on an exhalation, maintaining a C-curve in the spine. Roll back only as far as is comfortable and then inhale to return to the starting position.

Contra-Indications
Full curl-ups may be unsuitable for certain back problems. Forward flexion of the spine may be unsuitable for osteoporosis

FULL CURL UPS WITH OBLIQUE TWIST

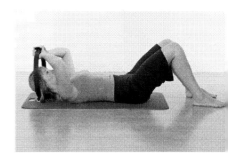

Aim
To work the oblique abdominals whilst achieving segmental control of the spine

Starting Position
Lie supine in the relaxation position with the knees bent and the feet flat on the floor. Place the head inside the ring with the back of the skull touching the inner rim and place the hands on the inside of the inner rim opposite the forehead

Action
Inhale - to prepare.

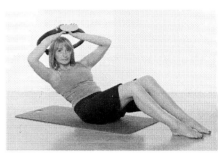

Exhale - to engage the core abdominals, tuck in the chin and oblique twist to the right as you lift the head and torso off the floor, one vertebra at a time until fully sitting upright.

Inhale - at the top and exhale to slowly return to the starting position, maintaining the oblique twist to the right. Repeat to the opposite side.

Target Muscles
Rectus abdominis, transverses abdominis, oblique abdominals

Watchpoints

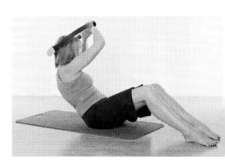

- Keep the chin tucked in as if holding a small apple between the chin and the chest
- Ensure the shoulders stay away from the ears
- Try not to grip around the hip flexors
- Try to move sequentially through each vertebra, one at a time
- Ensure the lift comes from the "steering wheel" (i.e. the ribcage) and not from twisting the head or shoulders

Contra-Indications
Full curl-ups, particularly combined with rotation, may be unsuitable for certain back problems. Forward flexion of the spine may be unsuitable for osteoporosis

AROUND THE GLOBE

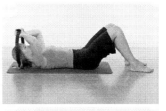

Aim

To work the oblique abdominals whilst achieving segmental control of the spine

Starting Position

Lie supine in the relaxation position with the knees bent and the feet flat on the floor. Place the head inside the ring with the back of the skull touching the inner rim and place the hands on the inside of the inner rim opposite the forehead

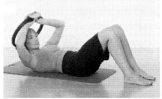

Action

Inhale - to prepare.

Exhale - to engage the core abdominals, tuck in the chin and oblique twist to the right as you lift the head and torso off the floor, one vertebra at a time until fully sitting upright.

Inhale - at the top and oblique twist to the left

Exhale - to slowly return to the starting position, maintaining the oblique twist to the left. Repeat to the opposite direction.

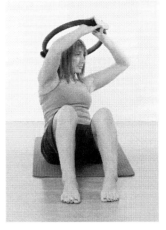

Target Muscles

Rectus abdominis, transversus abdominis, oblique abdominals

Watchpoints

- Keep the chin tucked in as if holding a small apple between the chin and the chest
- Ensure the shoulders stay away from the ears
- Try not to grip around the hip flexors
- Try to move segmentally through each vertebra, one at a time
- Ensure the lift comes from the "steering wheel" (i.e. the ribcage) and not from twisting the head or shoulders

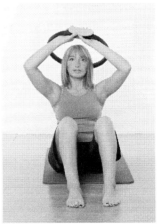

Contra-Indications

Full curl-ups, particularly combined with rotation, may be unsuitable for certain back problems. Forward flexion of the spine may be unsuitable for osteoporosis

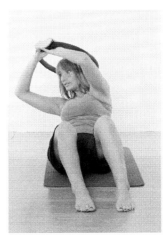

FULL CURL UPS WITH STRAIGHT LEGS INTO HAMSTRING STRETCH

Aim
To work the abdominals whilst achieving segmental control of the spine and to stretch the hamstrings

Starting Position
Lie supine with straight legs together and adducted and arms outstretched straight behind the head. Place the ring in between the ankles.

Action
Inhale - to prepare.

Exhale - engage the core abdominals, tuck in the chin and raise the arms off the floor. When the fingertips are pointing directly up to the ceiling, lift the head off the floor and continue peeling the spine, vertebra by vertebra until the body is in a fully upright sitting position. Continue forward flexion of the spine and fold the body forward until a hamstring stretch is achieved. The arms reach forward aiming to touch the ring.

Inhale – to sit upright

Exhale – to roll back down to the floor, one vertebra at a time

Target muscles
Rectus abdominis, core abdominals, hamstring stretch

Watchpoints

- Keep the chin tucked in as if holding a small apple between the chin and the chest to avoid the tendency to shorten the back of the neck
- Ensure the shoulders stay away from the ears
- Try not to grip around the hip flexors
- Try to move segmentally through each vertebra, one at a time
- When reaching forward into the stretch, try to maintain an even curve in the spine and avoid the tendency to over flex the thoracic spine (stretch should be initiated from the lumbar spine)

Variation One
Place the ring in between the hands instead of the feet

Variation Two (Progression)
Hands are clasped behind the head (Neck Pull exercise) instead of arms outstretched. This is a much more challenging position

Contra-Indications
Full curl-ups may be unsuitable for certain back problems. Forward flexion of the spine may be unsuitable for osteoporosis

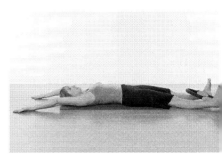

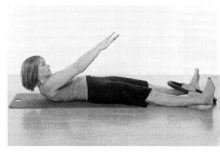

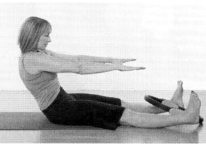

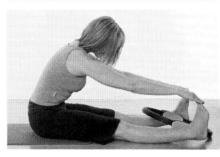

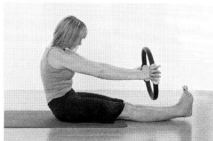

Variation One

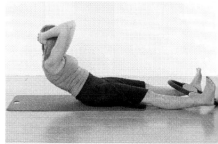

Variation Two

THE HUNDRED

Aim

To work the core abdominals, whilst practising thoracic breathing. The brisk beating of the arms warms up the body, whilst the scapula stabilisers assist in good shoulder movement

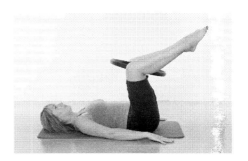

Starting Position

Lie supine in the relaxation position. Inhale to prepare and as you exhale, engage the core abdominals to raise one leg off the floor at a time until the knees are bent at 90 degrees above the hips with the toes softly pointed. Place the ring in between knees.

Action

Inhale - to lift the head, torso and arms off the floor until the arms are just above hip height.

Exhale - for a count of five breaths whilst beating the arms up and down a few inches.

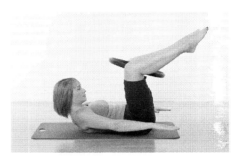

Inhale - for a count of five breaths continuing to briskly beat the arms up and down. Continue inhaling and exhaling for counts of five whilst beating the arms until a count of 100 has been reached. Finish the counting on an inhalation.

Exhale - keep the abdominals engaged and remove the ring. Put the head and arms back down on the floor and place one foot back down on the floor at a time.

Target Muscles

Rectus abdominis, core abdominals, scapula stabilisers

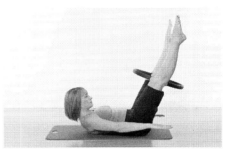

Watchpoints

- Ensure the scapula are stabilised to avoid hiking the shoulders up to the ears whilst beating the arms

Variation One

- The beating comes from the shoulder joint, not the elbow or wrist so maintain alignment of shoulder, elbow and wrist
- If inhaling for 5 breaths proves difficult initially, the counting may be done as follows: inhaling for 4 breaths and exhaling for 6 breaths or inhaling for 3 breaths and exhaling for 7 breaths
- Keep chin tucked in with eyes focused down towards the pelvis so that the back of the neck stays long to minimise neck strain
- Maintain good engagement of the core abdominals, particularly on the inhalation to avoid any popping or bulging of the abdominals

Variation One (Progression)

Extend the legs for five breaths and bend the knees for five breaths.

Variation Two (Progression)

Add an inner thigh squeeze on the exhalation and release on the inhalation

PLOUGH

Aim

To work the core, achieve segmental control of the spine and stretch the back and neck

Starting Position

Lie supine in the relaxation position with the knees bent. Inhale to prepare. As you exhale, engage the core abdominals and lift one leg up at a time until the legs are bent at 90 degrees above the hips. Place the ring between the ankles. Straighten the legs as much as possible ensuring that the knees stay directly above the hips. The arms are down by the sides of the body with the hands pressing down into the floor lightly.

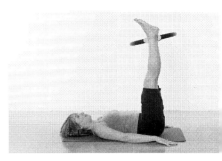

Action

Inhale - to prepare.

Exhale - engage the core abdominals and tilt the pelvis, lifting the tailbone, sacrum and lumbar spine off the floor. Continue peeling the spine off the floor, aiming to get the legs behind the head with the feet on the floor. Keep lightly squeezing the ring throughout. **Inhale** - to prepare

Exhale - slowly reverse the movement to return back to the starting position. Use the hands to act as a brake by lightly pressing the palms into the floor.

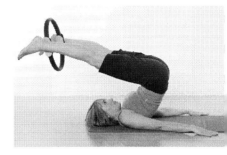

Target Muscles

Core abdominals, spinal flexors, neck flexors, hamstrings

Watchpoints

- As you come back to the starting position on the returning phase of the movement, ensure that the head stays on the floor
- Try to keep the shoulders away from the ears
- Try to move sequentially, one vertebra at a time throughout the movement
- Keep the core engaged, particularly on the returning phase
- If the hamstrings or lower back muscles are tight, then bend the legs as necessary
- The feet may not touch the floor, depending upon flexibility
- On the returning phase of the movement, the closer the legs are to the body, the easier the abdominal work. Therefore, to increase abdominal workload, lift the legs away from the body before attempting the descent

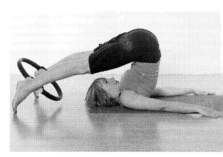

Variation One (Adaptation)

If lifting the spine off the floor proves difficult, then just perform a posterior pelvic tilt and lift as much of the tailbone and sacrum off the floor as the body allows. To make it easier bend the knees as you come out of the plough position.

Contra-Indications

This exercise may be unsuitable for neck problems due to increased pressure on the cervical vertebra. This is unsuitable for osteoporosis.

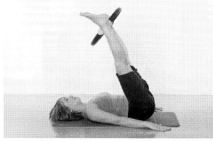

Variation One

DOUBLE LEG PRESS

Aim
To work the abdominals whilst maintaining a neutral pelvis

Starting Position
Lie supine in the relaxation position with the knees bent. Inhale to prepare. Exhale, engage the core abdominals and lift one leg up off the floor at a time until the legs are bent at 90 degrees above the hips. Place the ring in between the ankles. Straighten the legs as much as possible ensuring that the knees stay directly above the hips. For tight hamstrings, the knees may be bent slightly. The arms are down by the sides of the body.

Action
Inhale - to prepare.

Exhale - engage the core abdominals and push the legs away from the chest as far as a neutral pelvis can be maintained.

Inhale - to return to the starting position.

Target Muscles
Core abdominals, adductors, gluteals

Watchpoints
- Ensure the neck stays long and the shoulders stay away from the ears
- Keep the abdominals hollowed and only move the legs as far as a neutral pelvis can be maintained
- For tight hamstrings or to make the exercise easier, the knees may stay bent as is necessary

Variation One
The ring may be placed in between the knees rather than the ankles

Variation Two
This exercise may be performed with the head off the floor throughout. The hands are clasped behind head.

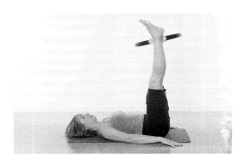

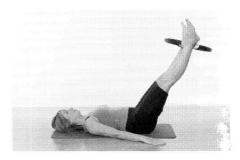

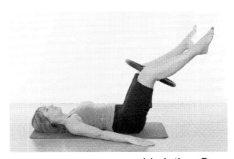

Variation One

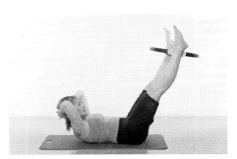

Variation Two

PLOUGH INTO DOUBLE LEG PRESS
(combination of the previous two exercises)

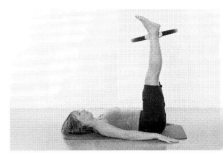

Starting Position

Lie supine in the relaxation position with the knees bent. Inhale to prepare. Exhale, engage the core abdominals and lift one leg up at a time until the legs are bent at 90 degrees above the hips. Place the ring in between the ankles. Straighten the legs as much as possible ensuring that the knees stay directly above the hips. The arms are down by the sides of the body with the hands pressing down into the floor lightly.

Action

Inhale - to prepare.

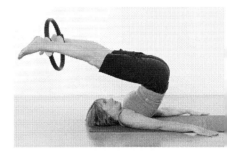

Exhale - engage the core abdominals and tilt the pelvis, lifting the tailbone, sacrum and lumbar spine off the floor. Continue peeling the spine off the floor, aiming to get the legs behind the head with the feet on the floor. Keep lightly squeezing the ring throughout.

Inhale - to prepare

Exhale - slowly reverse the movement to return back to the starting position. Use the hands to act as a brake by lightly pressing the palms into the floor.

Inhale - to prepare.

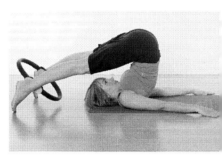

Exhale - engage the core abdominals and push the legs away from the chest as far as a neutral pelvis can be maintained. Inhale to return to the starting position.

Target Muscles

Core abdominals, spinal flexors, neck flexors, hamstrings, gluteals

Watchpoints

- As you come back to the starting position on the returning phase of the movement, ensue that the head stays on the floor

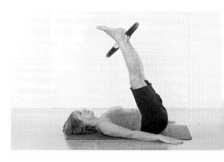

- Try to keep the shoulders away from the ears
- Try to move sequentially, one vertebra at a time throughout the movement
- Keep the core engaged, particularly on the returning phase where more abdominal work is required
- If the hamstrings or lower back muscles are tight, then bend the legs as necessary
- The feet may not touch the floor, depending upon flexibility

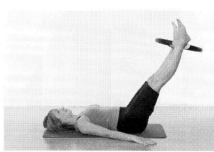

- On the returning phase of the movement, the closer the legs are to the body, the easier the abdominal work. Therefore, to increase abdominal workload, lift the legs away from the body before attempting the descent
- Keep the abdominals hollowed when performing the double leg press and only move the legs as far as a neutral pelvis can be maintained

Contra-Indications

This exercise may be unsuitable for neck problems due to increased pressure on the cervical vertebra. This exercise is unsuitable for osteoporosis.

SINGLE LEG STRETCH

Aim

To work the core abdominals in order to maintain a neutral pelvis and to challenge co-ordination

Starting Position

Lie supine in the relaxation position with the knees bent. Inhale to prepare. Exhale, engage the core abdominals and lift one leg up at a time until the legs are bent at 90 degrees above the hips. The arms are raised directly above the shoulders, holding the ring in the hands.

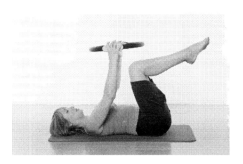

Action

Inhale - to tuck the chin in and raise the head and shoulders off the floor. The arms will move forwards and lower until the hands are above the shins. Elbows stay soft.

Exhale - as the right leg straightens.

Inhale - to prepare and exhale to swap legs (i.e. right leg returns as the left leg straightens). Repeat with the opposite leg, alternating legs each time.

(To finish) **inhale** - to return the head to the floor

Exhale - to return the bent legs to the floor one at a time, keeping the abdominals hollowed. Gently squeeze the ring each time the leg changes.

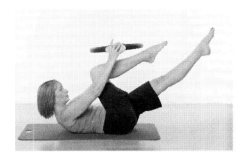

Target Muscles

Rectus abdominis, core abdominals, hip flexors, scapula stabilisers, pectorals

Watchpoints

- Keep the chin tucked in and the eyes focused down towards the pelvis to minimise neck strain
- Keep the abominals hollowed throughout to avoid any bulging or popping
- Keep the scapula stabilising muscles working to avoid any shoulder hiking
- Only move the straight leg as far away from the body as a neutral pelvis can be maintained
- The lower the straight leg moves towards the floor, the more challenging the exercise
- Try to maintain an even height in the torso throughout to avoid the body dropping back down towards the floor

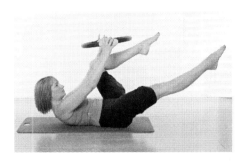

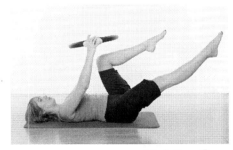

Variation One

Variation One (Adaptation)

This exercise may be performed with the head on the floor for neck problems or place the ring behind the skull, holding it in the hands to support the neck

Variation Two (Progression)

Reverse bicycle – The same leg action as for single leg stretch but the legs move in a circular motion as if riding a bike, lightly tapping the floor with the foot as you circle. This can be done clockwise or anti-clockwise

Contra-Indications – This exercise may be unsuitable for those suffering certain neck problems. The alternative is to perform variation one with the head on the floor. Forward flexion of the spine is unsuitable for osteoporosis. A half curl up position may be unsuitable for certain disc related back problems.

SINGLE LEG STRETCH WITH OBLIQUE TWIST

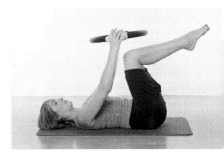

Aim

To work the oblique abdominals in order to maintain a neutral pelvis and to challenge co-ordination

Starting Position

Lie supine in the relaxation position with the knees bent. Inhale to prepare. Exhale, engage the core abdominals and lift one leg up at a time until the legs are bent at 90 degrees above the hips. The arms are raised directly above the shoulders, holding the ring in the hands

Action

Inhale - to tuck the chin in and raise the head and shoulders off the floor. The arms will move forwards and lower until the hands are above the shins. The elbows stay soft.

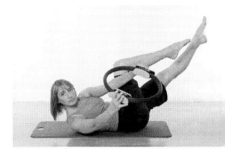

Exhale - as the right leg straightens and simultaneously oblique twist the torso to the left, aiming to place the ring on the outside edge of the left knee.

Inhale to prepare

Exhale - to swap legs (i.e. right leg returns as the left leg straightens and oblique twist to the right, aiming to place the ring on the outside edge of the right knee). Continue to alternate each leg.

(To finish) - **Inhale** - to return the head to the floor and exhale to return the bent legs to the floor one at a time, keeping the abdominals hollowed. Gently squeeze the ring each time the leg changes.

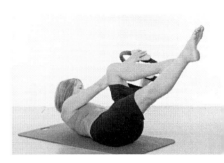

Target Muscles

Rectus abdominis, core abdominals, oblique abdominals, hip flexors, pectorals

Watchpoints

- Keep the chin tucked in with the eyes focused down towards the pelvis to minimise neck strain
- Keep the abominals hollowed throughout to avoid any bulging or popping
- Keep the scapula stabilising muscles working to avoid any shoulder hiking
- Only move the straight leg as far away from the body as a neutral pelvis can be maintained
- The lower the straight leg moves towards the floor, the more challenging the exercise
- Try to maintain an even height in the torso throughout to avoid the body dropping back down towards the floor, particularly as you transition between sides
- Ensure the lift comes from the "steering wheel" (i.e. the ribcage) and not from twisting the head or shoulders
- Try not to over twist or one side of the pelvis will lift off the floor (i.e. will tilt from east to west or vice versa depending upon which way the body is twisting)

Contra-Indications – This exercise may be unsuitable for those suffering certain neck problems. This exercise is unsuitable for those with osteoporosis

SCISSORS

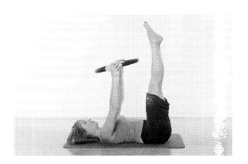

Aim

To strengthen the core abdominals whilst maintaining pelvic stability and to stretch the hamstrings

Starting Position

Lie supine in the relaxation position with the knees bent. Inhale to prepare. Exhale, engage the core abdominals and lift one leg up at a time until the legs are straight above the hips at 90 degrees. Straighten the legs as much as possible ensuring that the knees stay directly above the hips. For tight hamstrings, the knees may be bent as necessary. Hold the ring in the hands with the arms straight up in the air directly above the shoulders.

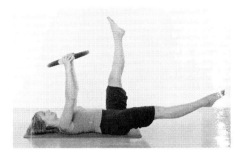

Action

Inhale - to prepare.

Exhale - engage the core abdominals and push the right leg away from the chest as far as a neutral pelvis can be maintained. Lightly squeeze the ring as the leg pushes away.

Inhale - to return to the starting position, keeping abdominals hollowed. Repeat with the opposite leg.

Target Muscles

Core abdominals, hip flexors, hamstrings, pectorals

Watchpoints

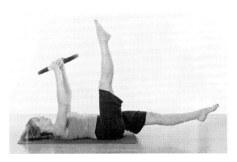

- Ensure the neck stays long and the shoulders are away from the ears
- Keep the abdominals hollowed and only move the legs as far as a neutral pelvis can be maintained
- For tight hamstrings or to make the exercise easier, the knees may stay as bent as is necessary

Variation One (Progression)

This exercise may be performed at a faster pace. As the right leg returns, simultaneously push the left leg away, so the legs literally "scissor" each other. Bring the leg towards the chest as far as possible in order to stretch the hamstrings and pulse it three times inwards before changing legs

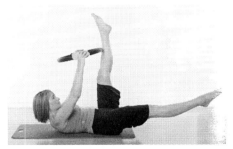

Variation Two (Progression)

This exercise may be performed with the head and shoulders off the floor provided there are no neck problems

Variation One

DOUBLE LEG STRETCH – Variation One

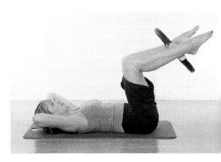

Aim

To work the deep and superficial abdominals whilst maintaining stability in the pelvis

Starting Position

Lie supine in the relaxation position with the knees bent. Inhale to prepare. As you exhale, engage the core abdominals and lift one leg up at a time until the legs are bent at 90 degrees above the hips. Place the ring in between the ankles and clasp the hands behind the head

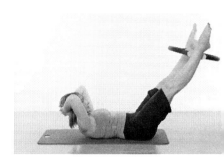

Action

Inhale - to prepare.

Exhale - to engage the core abdominals and extend the legs away from the body as straight as possible and simultaneously curl the head and shoulders off the floor.

Inhale - to bend the knees back to 90 degrees and return the torso back to the floor. The closer/lower the legs are to the floor, the more challenging the exercise.

Target Muscles

Core Abdominals, hip flexors, adductors, gluteals, rectus abdominis

Watchpoints

- Ensure the neck stays long and the shoulders are away from the ears
- Keep abdominals hollowed and only move the legs as far as a neutral pelvis can be maintained
- For tight hamstrings or to make the exercise easier, the knees may stay as bent as is necessary
- Slide the shoulder blades down and apart so that the shoulders stay away from the ears
- Keep the elbows in front of the ears (i.e. within peripheral vision) and the fingers interlaced so that the hands act like a "hammock" cradling the head. This way, the hands take the weight of the head rather than the neck muscles taking the weight and so this avoids neck strain.

Contra-Indications

A curled up position may not be suitable for certain disc-related back problems or osteoporosis

DOUBLE LEG STRETCH – Variation Two – Classic Version

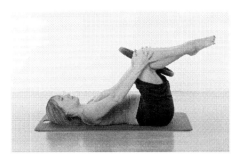

Aim
To work the deep and superficial abdominals, maintain scapula and pelvic stability and challenge co-ordination

Starting Position
Lie supine in the relaxation position with the knees bent. Inhale to prepare. Exhale, engage the core abdominals and lift one leg up at a time until the legs are bent at 90 degrees above the hips. Place the ring in between the knees and place the hands on the outside of the knees. The legs are turned out in the hip socket with the knees apart and feet together. The toes are touching each other and are softly pointed.

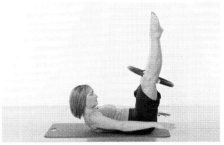

Action
Exhale - to engage the core abdominals

Inhale - and extend the legs up towards the ceiling as straight as possible in a turned out position at an angle of between 70-90 degrees from the body and simultaneously curl the head and shoulders off the floor, whilst straightening the arms so that they are parallel to the floor just above hip height. The toes are softly pointed.

Exhale - to raise arms up to the ceiling whilst dorsi flexing the feet.

Inhale - and continue circling the arms back and out to the side and back to the parallel position just above the hips whilst plantar flexing the foot.

Exhale - to return back to the starting position. The closer the legs are to the floor, the harder the exercise.

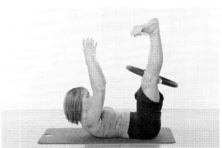

Target Muscles
Core Abdominals, hip flexors, adductors, gluteals, rectus abdominis, scapula stabilisers

Watchpoints
- As the arms circle backwards, the weight of the arms can pull the torso back down towards the floor. Use the abdominals to lift the torso higher as the arms circle backwards to prevent losing height in the torso

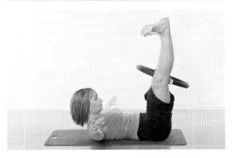

- Ensure the neck stays long with the eyes focused down towards the pelvis
- Ensure the shoulders are away from the ears, particularly as the arms circle behind the head
- Maintain a soft elbow joint
- Ensure the dorsi-flexion and plantar flexion come from the ankle joint so that the toes do not over curl

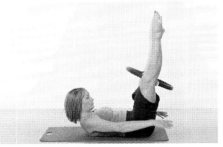

- Keep the abdominals hollowed and only move the legs as far as a neutral pelvis can be maintained
- For tight hamstrings or to make the exercise easier, the knees may stay as bent as is necessary

Variation One (Adaptation) – This exercise may be performed in a parallel position with the legs rather than turned out.

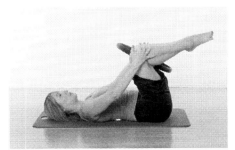

Contra-Indications
The half-curl position may not be suitable for certain disc-related back problems or osteoporosis

DOUBLE LEG STRETCH – Variation Three

Aim

To work the core abdominals whilst maintaining scapula and pelvic stability.

Starting Position

Lie supine in the relaxation position with the knees bent. Inhale to prepare. Exhale, engage the core abdominals and lift one leg up at a time until the legs are bent at 90 degrees above the hips. Inhale to raise the head and shoulders off the floor in a half curl position and hold the ring in the hands, placing the ring so that it is resting on the knees

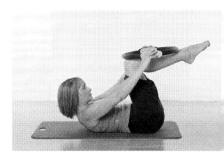

Action

Exhale - keeping the core abdominals engaged and extend the legs as straight as possible away from the body at an angle of between 50-90 degrees and simultaneously straighten the arms behind the head in the opposite direction.

Inhale – to return the legs and arms back to the starting position

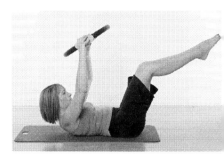

Target Muscles

Core Abdominals, hip flexors, adductors, gluteals, rectus abdominis, scapula stabilisers

Watchpoints

- Ensure the neck stays long with the eyes focused down towards the pelvis
- Ensure the shoulders are away from the ears, particularly as the arms reach backwards
- Try not to let the arms go behind the ears to avoid excessive neck strain
- The further back the arms reach, the more likely the ribs are to flare so maintain good ribcage closure
- Keep the abdominals hollowed and only move the legs as far as a neutral pelvis can be maintained
- For tight hamstrings or to make the exercise easier, the knees may stay as bent as is necessary

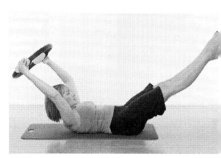

Variation One

This version can be done with the ring either in the hands or between the ankles

Contra-Indications

The half-curl up position may not be suitable for certain disc-related back problems or osteoporosis

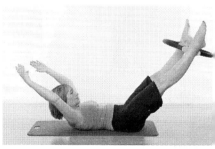

Variation One

CRISS-CROSS

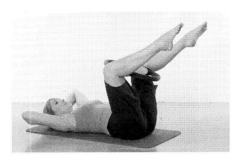

Aim
To work the deep and superficial abdominals and oblique abdominals whilst maintaining a neutral pelvis

Starting Position
Lie supine in the relaxation position with the knees bent. Inhale to prepare. Exhale, engage the core abdominals and lift one leg up at a time until the legs are bent at 90 degrees above the hips. The arms are clasped behind the head and the ring is placed either between the knees or ankles

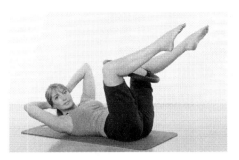

Action
Inhale - to prepare.

Exhale - to engage the core abdominals, tuck in the chin, oblique twist to the right as you lift the head and torso off the floor. The left shoulder blade will be higher than the right shoulder blade. Squeeze the ring as you curl up.

Inhale - to return to the starting position. Repeat to the opposite side.

Target Muscles
Rectus abdominis, transverses abdominis, oblique abdominals, adductors

Watchpoints
- Keep the chin tucked in as if holding a small apple between the chin and the chest
- Ensure the shoulders stay away from the ear
- Ensure the lift comes from the "steering wheel" (i.e. the ribcage) and not from twisting the head or shoulders
- Try not to over twist or one side of the pelvis will lift off the floor (i.e. will tilt from east to west or vice versa depending upon which way the body is twisting)

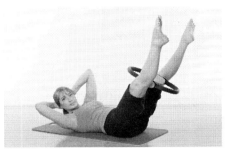

Variation One

Variation One (Progression)
Keep the head off the floor throughout. Straighten the legs at around 45 degrees as you twist.

Contra-Indications
The half-curl position may not be suitable for certain disc-related back problems or osteoporosis. Rotation of the spine may be unsuitable for some back problems.

DOUBLE LEG CIRCLES

Aim

To work the core and oblique abdominals whilst trying to maintain pelvic and scapula stability

Starting Position

Lie supine in the relaxation position with the knees bent. Inhale to prepare. Exhale, engage the core abdominals and lift one leg up at a time until the legs are bent at 90 degrees above the hips. Place the ring between the ankles. Straighten the legs until the knees are directly above the hips. For tight hamstrings, the knees may be bent slightly. The arms are down by the sides of the body.

Action

Inhale - to prepare.

Exhale - to engage the core abdominals and push the legs over to the right and then away from the body towards the floor as far as a neutral pelvis can be maintained.

Inhale - to circle the legs across to the left and then return to the starting position. Repeat to the opposite direction.

Target Muscles

Core abdominals, obliques, hip flexors, adductors

Watchpoints

- Only extend the legs out to the side as far as a neutral pelvis can be maintained to avoid the tendency for the pelvis to lift off the floor (i.e. will tilt from east to west or vice versa depending upon which way the legs are twisting)
- Keep the back of the neck long and the shoulders away from the ears
- As the legs go out to the side, one leg may appear longer than the other

Variation One (Adaptation)

Single leg circles with one straight leg in the air and one leg bent on the floor. The ring is held in the hands with the arms outstretched above the shoulders.

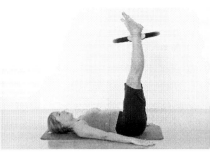
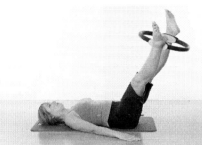
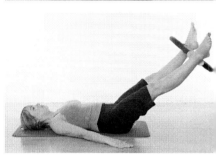
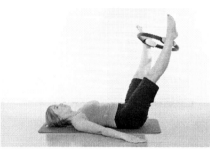
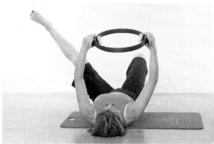

Variation One

HIP CIRCLES

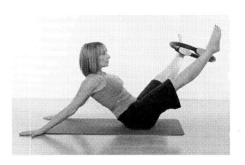

Aim
This is a challenging exercise for the core abdominals to maintain pelvic stability

Starting Position
Sit upright, balancing just back of the sit bones and raise two straight legs in the air (as for Open Leg Rocker). Place the ring in between the ankles or knees. Lean back with straight arms supporting the body and hands on the floor.

Action
Inhale - to prepare.

Exhale - circle the legs to the right in a clockwise direction until a full circle is completed and then return to the starting position.

Inhale - to prepare

Exhale - repeat in the opposite direction.

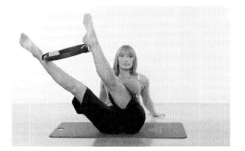

Target muscles
Core abdominals, hip flexors, adductors, scapula stabilisers

Watchpoints

- This is an advanced abdominal exercise where the pelvis can easily be pulled out of neutral. Limit the range of movement to maintain a neutral pelvis and spine throughout.
- Avoid collapsing the shoulders as you circle. Keep the ears away from the shoulders
- For tight hamstrings, the knees may bend a little
- As you circle out to the side, one leg may appear a touch longer than the other leg

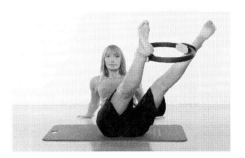

Variation One (Adaptation)
For wrist problems, this exercise may be performed resting on the elbows

Contra-Indications
This may be unsuitable for those with wrist problems (choose variation one instead)

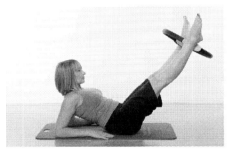

Variation One

CORKSCREW

Aim

To work the core and oblique abdominals; stretch and sequentially move the spine and practise co-ordination

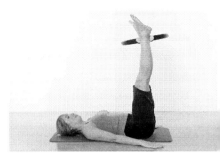

Starting Position

This exercise is a combination of The Plough and Double Leg Circles. Lie supine in the relaxation position with the knees bent. Inhale to prepare. Exhale, engage the core abdominals and lift one leg up at a time until the legs are bent at 90 degrees above the hips. Place the ring in between the ankles. Straighten the legs as much as possible ensuring that the knees stay directly above the hips. The arms are down by the sides of the body with the hands pressing down into the floor lightly.

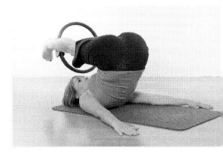

Action

Inhale - to engage the core abdominals and tilt the pelvis, lifting the tailbone, sacrum and lumbar spine off the floor. The aim is to twist to the right as you continue peeling the spine off the floor. Try to get the legs behind the right hand side of the head with the feet on the floor. Then twist the legs to the left hand side of the head.

Exhale - and slowly reverse the movement to return the spine back to the floor, vertebrae by vertebra until the knees are directly above the hips. Use the hands to act as a brake by lightly pressing the palms into the floor. Once the knees are directly above the hips, continue exhaling to push the legs away from the body in a diagonal line towards the right ensuring the lower back does not arch. Then circle the legs over to the left

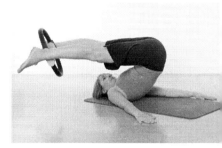

Inhale – to return back to the starting position. The legs make a "figure 8" shape.

Target Muscles

Core abdominals, spinal flexors, neck flexors, hip flexors, hamstrings

Watchpoints

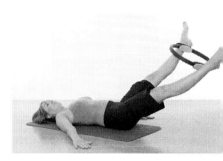

- As you come back to the starting position on the returning phase of the movement, ensure that the head stays on the floor
- Try to keep the shoulders away from the ears
- Try to move sequentially, one vertebra at a time throughout the movement
- Keep the core engaged, particularly on the returning phase
- If the hamstrings or lower back muscles are tight, then bend the legs as required
- The feet may not touch the floor, depending upon flexibility
- On the returning phase of the movement, the closer the legs are to the body, the more challenging the abdominal workload

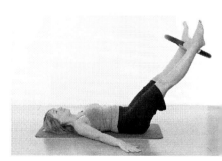

Contra-Indications

This exercise may be unsuitable for neck problems due to increased pressure on the cervical vertebrae. This is unsuitable for osteoporosis.

TEASER– Version One

Aim

To work the abdominals and move sequentially through the spine with control

Starting Position

Lie supine in the relaxation position with the knees bent. Inhale to prepare. As you exhale, engage the core abdominals and lift one leg up at a time until the legs are bent at 90 degrees above the hips. Place the ring in between the ankles. Straighten the legs until they are around 45 degrees from the body (or as near to 45 degrees as possible so that a neutral pelvis can be maintained). Whatever angle the legs start at, they should remain there throughout the exercise. For tight hamstrings, the knees may be bent. The arms are down by the side of the body.

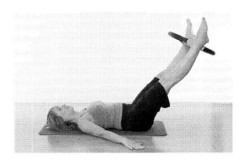

Action

Inhale - to prepare.

Exhale - engage the core abdominals, tuck in the chin and lift the head and torso off the floor and come to a fully sitting position, balancing just back of the sit bones. The body will be in a "V"- shaped position with the arms being outstretched straight at shoulder height.

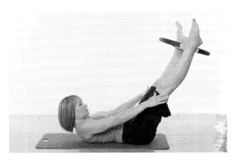

Inhale - to prepare

Exhale - to return the torso back down to the floor, one vertebra at a time, maintaining lumbar flexion in the spine and keeping the legs at 45 degrees.

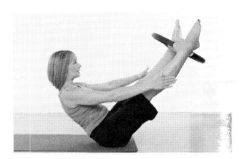

Target Muscles

Core abdominals, hip flexors, rectus abdominis

Watchpoints

- As the head lifts off the floor, ensure the core is fully engaged to prevent the lumbar spine going into extension
- Try to ensure segmental control of the spine when lifting and lowering the torso, vertebra by vertebra
- Try to keep the legs close to the chest when in the fully sitting upright position since the lower the legs, the greater the potential to pull the lumbar spine into extension (to avoid this, the knees may be bent for those with tight hamstrings)
- Ensure the body stays long and tall with the shoulders away from the ears

Contra-Indications

A full cur-up may not be suitable for certain disc-related back problems or osteoporosis.

TEASER – Version Two

Aim

To work the abdominals and move sequentially through the spine with control

Starting Position

Lie supine with straight legs adducted together on the floor and the arms outstretched straight behind the head. Place the ring in between the hands.

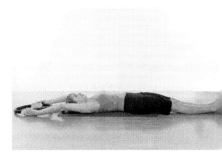

Action

Inhale - to prepare.

Exhale - engage the core abdominals, tuck in the chin and raise the arms off the floor. When the fingertips are pointing directly up to the ceiling, lift the head off the floor. As the shoulder blades start to come off the floor, simultaneously lift the two straight legs until the entire body is in an upright position, balancing just back of the sit bones. The arms will be outstretched straight at shoulder height.

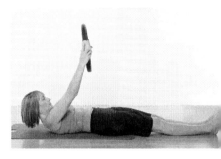

Inhale - to hold the upright sitting position

Exhale - to return the body back down to the floor, vertebra by vertebra, trying to maintain flexion in the lumbar spine throughout.

Target Muscles

Core abdominals, hip flexors, adductors, rectus abdominis

Watchpoints

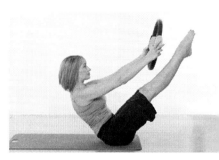

- As the legs lift off the floor, ensure the core is fully engaged to prevent the lumbar spine going into extension

- Try to ensure segmental control of the spine when lifting and lowering the torso, vertebra by vertebra

- Try to keep the legs close to the chest when in the fully sitting upright position since the lower the legs, the greater the potential to pull the lumbar spine into extension (to avoid this, the knees may be bent for those with tight hamstrings)

- Ensure the body stays long and tall with the shoulders away from the ears

Variation One (Adaptation)

On the returning phase of the movement, the knees may bend so that the feet are placed on the floor and then roll back through the spine. The helps to prevent the lumbar spine from going into extension

BACK EXERCISES

THE SWAN

Aim

This exercise aims to increase the flexibility of the spine in thoracic extension. Also the mid back muscles are strengthened which assists in good posture.

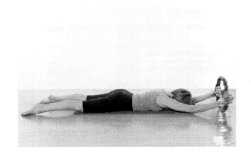

Starting Position

Lie prone with the arms and legs in a star shape. The arms are outstretched above the head with the ring held in between the hands.

Action

Inhale - to prepare.

Exhale - engage the core abdominals, draw down the scapula and raise the head, arms and part of the chest off the floor thereby positioning the spine into thoracic extension.

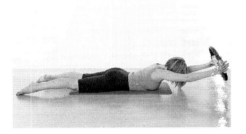

Inhale - to return to the starting position

Target Muscles

Back extensors, trapezius, neck extensors, posterior deltoid, scapula stabilisers

Watchpoints

- Ensure the scapula stabilising muscles are working hard to ensure that the shoulders stay away from the ears

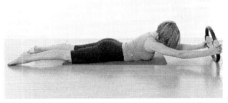

Variation One

- Keep eyes looking at the floor and chin tucked in to maintain length at the back of the neck

- Do not lift too high; it is a thoracic (not lumbar) extension therefore the 12th rib must remain in contact with the floor

- Keep the core abdominals hollowed and try to avoid gripping in the gluteals

Variation One (Adaptation)

The ring stays in contact with the floor and does not lift

Contra-Indications

Certain back problems may feel discomfort upon extension and therefore this exercise may be unsuitable

SEE-SAW

Aim

This exercise aims to increase the flexibility of the spine in thoracic extension. Also the mid back muscles and buttocks are strengthened.

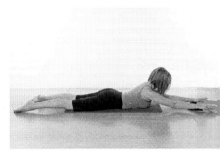

Starting Position

Lie prone with the arms and legs apart. The arms are outstretched above head with the ring in between the hands

Action

Inhale - to prepare.

Exhale - engage the core abdominals, draw down the scapula and raise the head, arms and part of the chest off the floor thereby positioning the spine into thoracic extension.

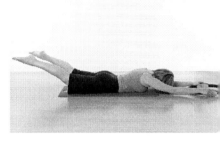

Inhale - to lower the torso back to the floor whilst simultaneously lifting the two straight legs up in the air.

Exhale - to lift the torso whilst lowering the legs.

Keep repeating the above actions and aim for an even speed and a smooth movement (like that of a see saw). Alternate lifting the arms and legs so that when the torso is up, the legs are down and when the legs are up, the torso is down.

Target Muscles

Back extensors, trapezius, neck extensors, posterior deltoid, gluteals, hamstrings, scapula stabilisers

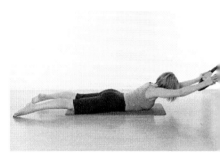

Watchpoints

- Ensure the scapula stabilising muscles are working hard to ensure that the shoulders stay away from the ears
- Keep the eyes looking at the floor and the chin tucked in to maintain length at the back of the neck
- Do not lift too high; it is a thoracic (not lumbar) extension therefore the 12th rib must remain in contact with the floor
- Keep the core abdominals hollowed and try to avoid gripping in the gluteals

Variation One (Adaptation)

To make an easier version of this exercise, there will be no seesaw action (i.e. there will only ever be one half of the body in the air at any one time). Therefore the upper body lifts then lowers completely before the legs raise and vice versa.

Contra-Indications

There is increased pressure in the lumbar spine when both the arms and legs are in the air at the same time. Certain back problems may feel discomfort, therefore this exercise may be unsuitable for them.

SWAN DIVE

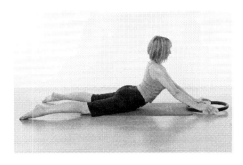

Aim

This exercise aims to increase the flexibility and strength of the spine.

Starting Position

Lie prone with arms and legs in a star shape. The arms are at a "ten to two" position, outstretched above head with the ring in between hands. Raise the torso up into a lumbar extension as far as the back allows (cobra position) and prop the body up with the two straight arms. The hands are placed under the shoulders (or slightly forward of the shoulders)

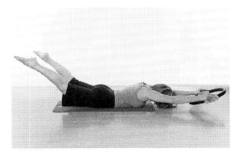

Action

Inhale - to prepare

Exhale - engage the core abdominals.

Inhale - and push the two outstretched arms forwards in front of the body as the body dives down towards the floor, simultaneously lifting up the two straight legs.

Exhale - drop the legs back down to the floor and simultaneously raise the head, chest and arms up above the head towards the ceiling.

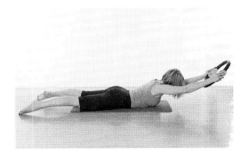

Keep repeating the above actions and aim for an even speed and a smooth movement (like that of the previous See saw exercise). Alternate lifting arms and legs so that when the torso is up, the legs are down and when the legs are up, the torso is down. This exercise is the same as See Saw but with added speed and momentum. This is an advanced exercise that may place extra strain on the lumbar spine. A smooth, rocking motion and even cadence is to be aimed for in this exercise

Target Muscles

Back extensors, trapezius, neck extensors, posterior deltoid, gluteals, hamstrings, scapula stabilisers

Watchpoints

- Ensure the scapula stabilising muscles are working hard to ensure that the shoulders stay away from the ears
- Maintain length at the back of the neck
- Keep core abdominals hollowed
- Try not to "fling" the body up – aim for a smooth movement with an even spinal extension throughout

Contra-Indications

This exercise places great strain on the lumbar spine and may not be suitable for certain back problems

UPPER BODY EXERCISES

FULL PUSH UP

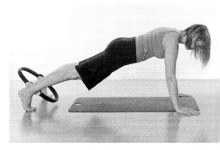

Aim

To work the upper body muscles and use the core abdominals to maintain a neutral spine

Starting Position

From an all four's position, extend each leg back off the floor, one at a time, to come to a full plank position. The ring is placed in between the ankles

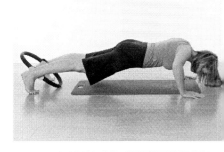

Action

Inhale - to prepare.

Exhale – to engage the powerhouse.

Inhale - to bend the elbows and lower the body downwards towards the floor, squeezing the ring lightly.

Exhale - to straighten the elbows and push the body back up to the starting position.

Target Muscles

Pectorals, anterior deltoid, triceps, core abdominals, gluteals, serratus anterior, adductors

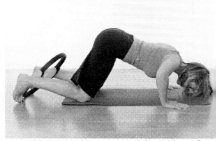

Variation One

Watchpoints

- Ensure the core abdominals are engaged throughout to prevent the back from dipping
- Maintain the length between the ears and shoulders
- Only bend the elbows as far as a neutral spine can be maintained
- Try to avoid collapsing in between the shoulder blades. Engage serratus anterior to maintain the distance in between the shoulder blades

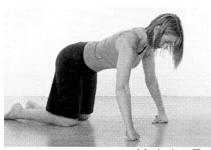

Variation Two

Variation One (Adaptation)

Keep the knees on the floor (box press-up) to make it easier

Variation Two (Adaptation)

To reduce pressure in the wrist joint, this exercise may be attempted on the knuckles of the hand, which will place the wrist in a more neutral position.

Variation Three

The elbows may bend out to the side (working pectorals, anterior deltoid and triceps) or alternatively, the elbows may bend facing backwards to emphasise the triceps

Contra-Indications

This exercise places extra stress on the wrist and knee joints. Take extra care when attempting this exercise for certain clients with problems in these joints, as it may prove unsuitable for them.

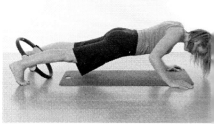

Variation Three

STANDING CHEST PRESS

Aim

To strengthen the muscles of the chest

Starting Position

Stand upright with the arms outstretched at shoulder level and the elbows slightly bent, holding the ring in between the hands

Action

Inhale - to prepare and lengthen the body.

Exhale - engage the core abdominals and squeeze the ring.

Inhale - to return to the start position, keeping the abdominals hollowed.

Target Muscles

Pectorals, anterior deltoid, core abdominals, scapula stabilisers

Watchpoints

- Note that the straighter the arms and therefore the further away the ring is from the body, the harder it will be to squeeze the ring. To make it easier, bend the elbows and bring the ring closer to the body.
- Ensure the elbows are not locked. Keep the elbow joint soft.
- Keep the shoulders away from the ears.
- Pay attention to wrist alignment – a neutral position is desirable

Variation One

As before but with the arms above the head

Variation Two

As before but with the arms below shoulder height

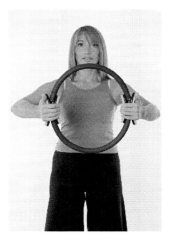

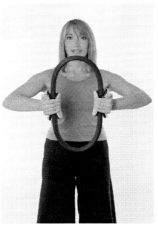

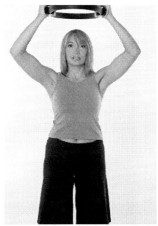

Variation One

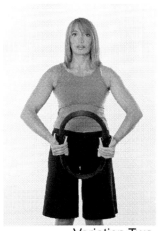

Variation Two

CHEST PRESS SUPINE

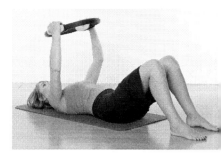

Aim

To strengthen the chest muscles

Starting Position

Lie in the relaxation position with the knees bent and the feet on the floor and with the knees hip width apart. Place the ring in between both hands with the arms outstretched above the chest. The elbows are soft.

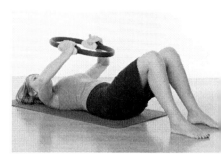

Action

Inhale - to prepare.

Exhale - and engage core abdominals and squeeze the ring, bringing the hands and arms closer together.

Inhale - to return to the starting position

Target Muscles

Pectorals, anterior deltoid, scapula stabilisers

Watchpoints

- Ensure the spine stays in a neutral position
- The back of the neck remains long
- Maintain length between ear and shoulders
- Keep the angle at the elbows constant throughout (i.e. do not bend or straighten the elbows further as the ring is squeezed)
- Maintain a neutral wrist alignment

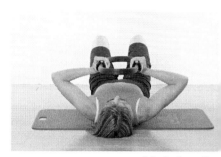

Variation One (Adaptation)

Keep the ring close to the chest with bent elbows (beginners version)

Variation One

STANDING TRICEP PRESS

Aim

To strengthen the triceps

Starting Position

Stand upright, clasping the ring in between the hands with the arms behind the back.

Action

Inhale - to prepare and lengthen the body.

Exhale - engage the core abdominals and squeeze the ring.

Inhale - to return to starting position.

Target Muscles

Triceps, scapula stabilisers, core abdominals

Watchpoints

- Keep the elbows soft and avoid locking the joint
- Ensure the shoulders stay down and away from ears
- Pay attention to the wrist alignment – a neutral position is desirable
- Keep the core engaged to prevent the ribs from flaring, thereby arching the back

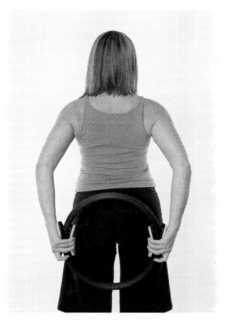

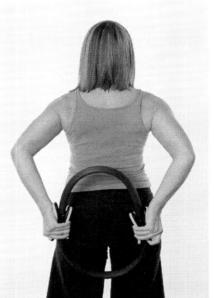

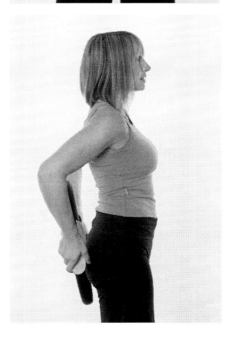

BICEP CURL STANDING

Aim

To strengthen the biceps

Starting Position

Stand upright with the ring resting on the right upper trapezius muscle (between the neck and shoulder). The right hand presses down lightly on the top of the ring to hold it in place.

Action

Inhale - to prepare and lengthen the body.

Exhale - to engage the core abdominals and press down on the ring as far as possible thereby bending the elbow further.

Inhale - to return to the starting position.

Target Muscles

Biceps

Watchpoints

- Ensure the shoulder does not hike up to the ear when pressing down
- Keep the core engaged throughout to ensure a neutral position of the spine
- Maintain an equal length on both sides of the waist

Variation One

Still working the biceps but lying supine in relaxation position. Place the ring so that it stands upright behind the head. Reach both arms behind the head and place both hands on top of the ring and press down as far as possible.

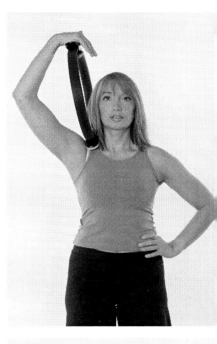

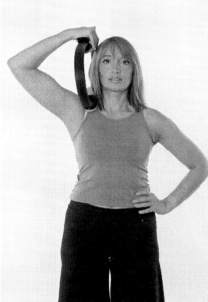

LAT PRESS SEATED

Aim
To work the latissimus dorsi whilst maintaining an upright posture

Starting Position
Sit upright, cross-legged with the ring at the right hand side of the body. The ring is standing upright on the floor and the right arm is outstretched with the right hand resting on the top of the ring.

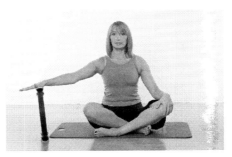

Action
Inhale - to prepare.

Exhale - engage the core abdominals and draw down the latissimus dorsi muscle on the right and depress the ring with the right hand.

Inhale - to return to the starting position. Repeat to the opposite side.

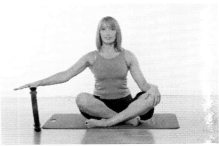

Target Muscles
Latissimus dorsi, core abdominals, scapula stabilisers

Watchpoints
- Keep the waist long and even on both sides to ensure that one side does not shorten as the ring is depressed
- Maintain a neutral spine throughout to ensure spine does not flex as ring is depressed
- Try to keep elbow straight to ensure movement comes from the lats and not from bending the elbow

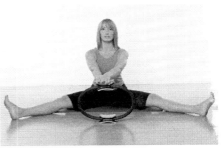

Variation One
Sit with the legs wide apart and the ring on floor in front in between the legs. Place one hand on top of the other and press down.

Variation One

LAT PRESS STANDING

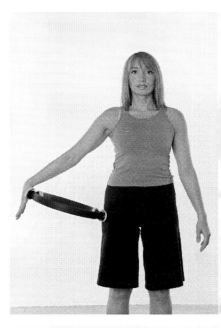

Aim

To strengthen the latissimus dorsi whilst maintaining an upright posture

Starting position

Stand upright with the ring resting sideways against the right hip and hold in place with the right hand pressing it in towards the hip.

Action

Inhale - to prepare and lengthen the body.

Exhale - engage the core abdominals and depress the ring with the right hand so that the ring squeezes further towards the hip.

Inhale - to release to starting position.

Target Muscles

Latissimus Dorsi, core abdominals, scapula stabilisers

Watchpoints

- Ensure the elbow stays soft and not locked.
- Ensure shoulder stays away from the ear to avoid any hiking of the shoulder
- Keep abdominals engaged throughout to ensure a neutral spine
- Maintain an equal length on both sides of the waist

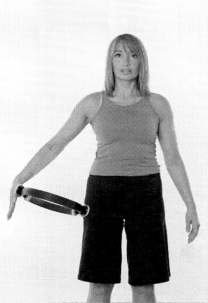

Variation One

Sit cross-legged with the ring at one side of the body and press down as far as possible

Variation Two

Sit upright with the legs wide apart. Place the ring upright on the floor in front, in between the legs. Rest one hand on top of the other on top of the ring and press down.

INDEX

THE STRETCHES

LEG WORK

ABDOMINAL EXERCISES

BACK EXERCISES

UPPER BODY EXERCISES

COMMUNITY WORK SKILLS MANUAL

1999

ASSOCIATION OF COMMUNITY WORKERS

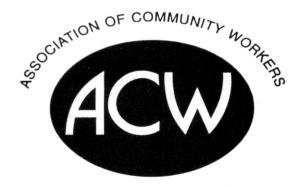

This manual has been published by:

THE ASSOCIATION OF COMMUNITY WORKERS

ACW an association for community workers in the United Kingdom. It is run by community workers for Community workers. It is open to all people who are community workers, whether paid or unpaid, activists or trainers or who have an interest in community work.

ACW is a membership organisation which is independent and is able to contribute to the development of community work theory and practice in a challenging and supportive way.

To order more copies of this publication please contact our office, Stephenson Building, Elswick Road, Newcastle, NE4 6SQ; tel 091 272 4341.

Community Work Skills Manual. © ACW 1994.
Reprinted 1999

ISBN 0 - 907413-22-6

Whitaker/CIP Book Information. British Library Cataloguing in Publication Data. A catalogue record for this book is available from the British Library.

CONTENTS

SECTION 22.
Evaluation

SECTION 23.
Management Committees

SECTION 24.
Local Government

SECTION 25.

Bibiography

Organisations

SECTION 1

INTRODUCTION

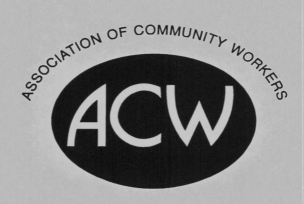

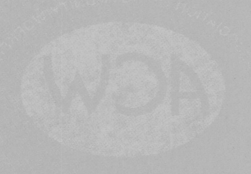

SECTION:	**INTRODUCTION**
TITLE:	**Background**
AUTHOR:	Val Harris

Welcome to this edition of the Association of Community Workers Skills Manual – written by community workers for people who are active in their communities. The manual is a collection of ideas and techniques which will help individuals and groups with their community activities. The first skills manual was published in 1978, the result of 3 community workers undertaking a year in "further study" at NISW (Adrian Lanning, Rita Heeran and Jim Rowan) who decided to put together a reference book which would help them in their work. The original skills manual was reprinted and sold out in the late 1980s.

ACW council decided that the manual should be substantially re-written to reflect the changes in community work over the past decade or so. This manual concentrates on the values behind community work and techniques to improve our day-to-day practice.

We are actively seeking articles for this publication and for the next reprint of this manual which we hope will be in a couple of years time.

SECTION:	**INTRODUCTION**
TITLE:	**How to use this Manual**
AUTHOR:	Val Harris

The manual is divided into twenty four sections, each of which are composed of several short articles, ideas and suggestions for improving our practice on that topic. The full list of section headings and their components can be found on the content pages which is before this introduction. Each contribution is divided into three parts, the narrow column on the left of the first page is the introduction, the wide column details the suggestions or techniques and the final narrow column includes points to note, other useful material and suggestions for other relevant sections to use. At the end of the manual you will find a detailed list of other manuals and useful material, a list of useful national organisations, and full details of the titles and organisations mentioned by contributors. Each article is designed to stand alone – it can be copied and used by groups of people about to undertake a task, or by individuals who wish to raise a particular issue with their group.

This manual is not designed to be read from cover to cover, it is to be dipped in to as the need arises. Some of the suggestions will apply to some groups and not to others so be selective about which ones you choose; many of the techniques can be adapted to suit a particular group.

This manual has been compiled from material written by our members and by other organisations working in the field of community work. Although we have tried to cover most of the main areas of interest it is by no means a comprehensive publication of everything you need to know. We have updated and adapted material from the last manual which we felt was still relevant to today and added in several other sections that were not included in the original manual. We have tried to ensure that as many different perspectives were included as possible and that people were given an opportunity to contribute.

It is important to note that the section of empowerment and participation appears very limited. This is because we believe that all the techniques and ideas suggested by contributors will help people to gain more control and to be able to participate more effectively both within their group and when they come into contact with other organisations. More theoretical works on participation are referred to in the bibliography at the end of the manual.

We hope you find it a useful manual and welcome any feedback you would like to give us, and any contributions for the next one!

Val Harris
Editor

SECTION 2

GLOSSARY

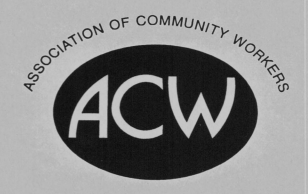

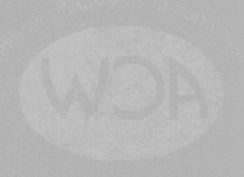

SECTION:	**GLOSSARY**
TITLE:	
AUTHOR:	Compiled by Ann Hindley

The word community has been used to describe so many things that it is in danger of meaning nothing and everything. There are several words and expressions that occur repeatedly with community work writings (and the manual is no exception). We have therefore decided to start with ACW's understanding of the key words and phrases.

Some have been written by our members, others have been culled and adapted from other writings.

ACTIVE CITIZEN

- used by central government to encourage people to provide services themselves rather than expecting the state to provide; it has an emphasis on people's responsibilities rather than their rights – encouraging people to become charitable.

ACTIVIST

- a volunteer/a person who is actively engaged in community activities but without being paid for it.

- a person who gets involved in campaigns to influence policies/services that affect them.

ADVOCACY

- Ideas around the concept of advocacy were borrowed in this country largely from Netherlands and the USA and began as ways in which people with learning difficulties might benefit from representing themselves. The ideas have now spread into work with people with emotional problems and physical difficulties and **SELF, CITIZEN** and **PATIENT OR LEGAL ADVOCACY** are all ways in which power relationships can be shared and rigid systems challenged.

CITIZEN ADVOCACY

- is about working with, and helping, people with often considerable personal physical and intellectual difficulties to better represent themselves. The skill here is to create confidence with people who are often unpractised and unknowing about how complex systems work; of being prepared to explain, deliberately slow down routines and work at your own pace in order to clearly understand what is happening.

- Both self and citizen advocacy are about consciously transferring and devolving power in a sharp, intelligent way in order that everyone can function more effectively.

COLLECTIVE ACTION

- working together with others to achieve a common aim.

COMMUNITY

- that web of personal relationships, group networks, traditions and patterns of behaviour that develops amongst those who share the same physical neighbourhood and its socio-economic situation, or common understandings and goals around a shared interest.

SECTION:	**GLOSSARY**
TITLE:	
AUTHOR:	Compiled by Ann Hindley

COMMUNITY ACTION

- community based campaigns and networks concentrating on issues of concern to that community. Methods can range from the presentation of a petition to a local councillor to non violent protests such as those held by some of the Community Development Projects of the 1970's and the public demonstrations against deportations, or in support of the miners, and the camps set up in 1993 to save the pits.

COMMUNITY DEVELOPMENT

- aims to enrich the web described in "Community" above and makes its threads stronger, to develop self confidence and skills, so that the community (the people) can begin to make significant improvements to their neighbourhood (the place and it's material environment) or it's cause. (adapted from McClellan and Flecknor)

- This leads to community development being a method of working which:

    - Focuses on collective action rather than on individual change,

    - Actively works to counter discrimination and prejudice,

    - Makes working with disadvantaged and oppressed groups a priority,

    - Recognises the importance of formal and informal support and networks in bringing about change,

    - Is about opening up access to resources, services and information to assist people in making informed decisions.

(taken from the paper: Community Participation for Health for All).

COMMUNITY GROUP

- a group acting on behalf of the community or a particular section of the community. A group of people acting collectively for the benefit of the community and possibly with the aim of bringing about some change. (Twelvetrees?)

COMMUNITY ORGANISING

- an American term used to describe the way groups organise to defend/promote the interests of their neighbourhood.

COMMUNITY SOCIAL WORK

- An approach to working which:

    - embraces the functions of a whole social work agency. It is based on collaboration between team members and between social workers and their formal and informal carers.

    - involves taking account of parents, relatives, neighbours, other informal carers and staff in other agencies when planning priorities and other methods of working..

    - is concerned with helping those who are disadvantaged by their social networks to achieve new, more advantageous relationships.

- makes services more accessible and appropriate through involving users in decision making and delivery of services.

- emphasises the strengths and abilities of people to engage in their own problem solving. (Adapted from introductory chapter of Partners in Empowerment).

COMMUNITY WORK

- a process whereby oppressed people gain the skills, knowledge and the confidence to tackle the sources of their problems and to bring about desired changes. (A fuller definition can be found in the next section.)

COMMUNITY WORKER

- a paid or unpaid worker who works as a partner with others in a co-operative venture. A community worker must be skilled in acting as an enabler, a facilitator, a catalyst for action, an energiser. S/he must be able to bring information, support and advice to people so that they make choices about what they want to do. (McClellan and Flecknor)

CONSULTATION

- partial participation: a process in which a more powerful party shares information with a less powerful party and may to some extent allow themselves to be influenced but the power of deciding how much influence is to be allowed and the final decision rests with the more powerful party.

CONTRACT

- A contract is a legally enforceable agreement between two or more parties e.g. a local authority (service purchaser) and a community organisation (service provider). There is a contractual agreement in which the "service provider" promises to fulfil the contract. This type of contractual funding whilst still relatively new is increasingly more common in line with the government's policies and the introduction of the "contract culture".

- Service purchasers tend to closely monitor contracts to ensure the service provider is providing a good service, what is called "value for money".

- Under this arrangement the community organisation has to cost the service they are to provide, for example, staffing, running costs, premises, transport etc., before they agree to take on the contract. Monitoring the service they provide once it's started is important as it can provide evidence to demonstrate to the service purchaser that the contract should be renewed, perhaps with changes, given the experience so far.

EMPOWERMENT

- ways in which knowledge, skills, resources and power can be transferred to people previously on the margin of organisations.

- ways of increasing people's ability to influence decisions.

ENABLER

- one who helps others to realise their potential.

SECTION:	**GLOSSARY**
TITLE:	
AUTHOR:	Compiled by Ann Hindley

ENABLING

- used by some councils to describe themselves as enabling authorities – helping/encouraging community activities to happen, a recognition that they may not be able to directly provide all services themselves.

EVALUATION

- is more than monitoring: it makes judgements about the success or failure of a project/organisation in an informed way: it attempts to assess whether the objectives have been achieved. It involves quality as well as quantity issues.

GRANT FUNDING

- A grant is a sum of money given to a community organisation by a local authority, usually for a period of one year, to fund, for example, a full-time or a part-time worker, the running cost of a community group, or to establish a project. The community organisation puts forward its proposal in the form of an application.

- The granting, monitoring and renewal of a grant varies considerably between local authorities as does the amount of grant given. This is often a political decision taken by the local authority.

- Most local authorities have details available on how to apply for a grant. Check with your local town hall or council offices.

MONITORING

- the systematic collection and recording of information to help an organisation know how it is doing: it helps to account for the work of the organisation.

NEIGHBOURHOOD WORK

- using a community development approach to work with neighbourhood organisations or groups of local people who meet together as peers to try to solve their own problems or those of the locality (particularly those of a social, environmental or economic character) (Twelvetrees)

NETWORK

- a loose semi informal collection of individuals or groups who are in direct or an indirect communication with each other. They operate as horizontal channels of communication within communities (A. Gilchrist)

NOT FOR PROFIT ORGANISATIONS

- an organisation that is either run by a voluntary management committee employing workers or as a co-operative or collective to provide a service and whose excess funds are ploughed back into the provision of services.

PARTICIPATION

- the process by which users become partners in contributing to and sharing in the decisions that affect the lives of the users' groups they represent. There is a distinction between user and community participation. **USER PARTICIPATION** involves working with individuals to enable them to make their own decisions. **COMMUNITY PARTICIPATION** involves groups of people representing the community having a voice in the decision making processes that affects them.

SECTION:	**GLOSSARY**
TITLE:	
AUTHOR:	Compiled by Ann Hindley

PATIENT ADVOCACY

- some times known as LEGAL ADVOCACY means focusing on welfare rights, legal and other advice on one's status in relation to the 1983 Mental Health Act and other pieces of legislation. The aim is to offer independent support and advocacy to any user on any issue relating to his or her experience of the mental health system.

PLURALIST/PLURALITY

- usually used to refer to a variety of welfare services being provided by the public, voluntary and private sectors.

SELF ADVOCACY

- means learning how, for oneself, to take on organisations which resent and prevent everyone's right to participate. Local and central government bureaucracies are often good examples of structures which have become too introspective. (Although, similar problems are emerging as some voluntary organisations become larger). It's about learning how to be prepared and confident when your in someone else's territory; learning the rules which are too often made by others and turned to your advantage. It's also about making it clear to the people who seem to be holding the resources that good practice and equality are legitimate tools that we should all be using. That it's important to insist on knowing WHAT people with authority in organisations ARE doing, as well as how and when.

SERVICE AGREEMENT

- Service agreements have been in existence for some years. They are somewhere in between contracts and grants. For example a local authority will set out in detail the service it requires and a voluntary sector community organisation/project will agree to provide this service.

- The local authority will usually provide a "service specification" for the level and quality of the service to be provided and how the agreement will be monitored to ensure "value for money".

- The funding agency (the service purchaser) and the community organisation (the service provider) will usually exchange letters which formalises the agreement.

- The agreements are usually reviewed annually and tend to last for a period of three years which gives the community organisation a sufficient period of time to recruit staff and give them job security, develop the service and to monitor its effectiveness.

STAKEHOLDER

- a person or organisation who has some influence over another group – this may include funders, or key individuals for example.

STATUTORY SECTOR

- the group of agencies which includes government departments, local authorities and QUANGOs that are set up by statute to provide a particular service but without making a profit.

VALUE BASE

- the principles/ethics that inform community work and its practice.

SECTION:	**GLOSSARY**
TITLE:	
AUTHOR:	Compiled by Ann Hindley

VOLUNTARY SECTOR

- a massive group of agencies ranging from the smallest tenants' association to the National Council for Voluntary Organisations. None of these agencies are set up by Act of Parliament, nor do they pursue commercial profit and they frequently benefit from their supporter's unpaid labour.

SECTION 3

DEFINITIONS OF COMMUNITY WORK

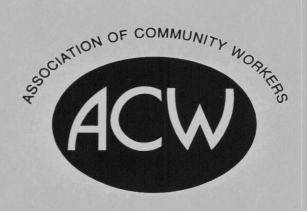

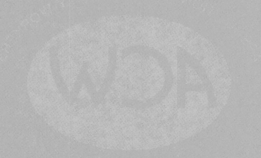

SECTION:	DEFINITIONS OF COMMUNITY WORK
TITLE:	BELIEFS, AIMS AND OBJECTIVES AND WORKING PRACTICES
AUTHOR:	A.C.W.

BELIEFS

1. The organisation and structure of society cause problems of powerlessness, alienation and inequality. To achieve greater equality and social justice, resources and power must be redistributed.

2. Collective action is a proper and effective method of working for social, political and economic change. Community work is a process which promotes such collective action.

3. It is necessary to confront all forms of oppression both within ourselves and within society.

AIMS AND OBJECTIVES

To change power structures by:

*   promoting equality of resources

*   seeking to influence statutory, voluntary and private organisations and make them more responsive to, and open to the needs and demands of community groups

*   assisting groups with multiple disadvantages to gain access to equal opportunities

To spread knowledge by:

*   developing awareness and understanding of issues through social and political education

*   enabling people to develop the expertise and skills necessary to further their own objectives

*   facilitating access to information

To encourage self-determination by:

*   helping community groups to define their own objectives

*   supporting community groups to run mutual aid projects

To promote co-operation by:

*   the developing of community groups to work on issues of common concern

*   seeking to create unity between groups within a locality around issues of common concern, on a basis of mutual respect

*   encouraging the development of alliances in order to achieve common goals and influence decision-makers within society

WORKING PRACTICE

Community workers should work in ways which:

- honestly confront issues of belief and ideology

- start at the point where people themselves identify issues and problems and help them create change in the context of the beliefs above

- always assist people to develop their own leadership and ability to speak for themselves

- respect the contribution made by all people with whom they work, and oppose power relationships

Community workers should not:

- attempt to impose their own or their employing agencies' concealed ideologies or methods of work

- seek to become spokespersons or leaders of the community or community groups, but they do have the same right and duty as anyone else to accept these roles in situations where that appears to be necessary and appropriate.

A WORKING STATEMENT ON COMMUNITY DEVELOPMENT

This is adopted as a move towards our understanding of Community Development.

Community development is crucially concerned with the issues of powerlessness and disadvantage: as such it should involve all members of society, and offers a practice that is part of a process of social change.

Community Development is about the active involvement of people in the issues which affect their lives. It is a process based on the sharing of power, skills, knowledge, and experience.

Community Development takes place both in neighbourhoods and within communities of interest, as people identify what is relevant to them.

The Community Development process is collective, but the experience of the process enhances the integrity, skills, knowledge and experience, as well as the equality of power, for each individual who is involved.

Community Development seeks to enable individuals and communities to grow and change according to their own needs and priorities, and at their own pace, provided this does not oppress other groups and communities, or damage the environment.

Where Community Development takes place, there are certain principles central to it. The first priority of the Community Development process is the empowering and enabling of those who are traditionally deprived of power and control over their common affairs. It claims as important the ability of people to act together to influence the social, economic, political and environmental issues which affect them. Community Development aims to encourage sharing, and to create structures which give genuine participation and involvement.

Community Development is about developing the power, skills, knowledge and experience of people as individuals and in groups, thus enabling them to undertake initiatives of there own to combat social, economic, political and environmental problems, and enabling them to fully participate in a truly democratic process.

Community Development must take a lead in confronting the attitudes of individuals and the practices of institutions and society as a whole which discriminate unfairly against black people, women, disabled people and people of different abilities, religious groups, elderly people, lesbians and gay men, and other groups who are disadvantaged by society. It also must take a lead in countering the destruction of the natural environment on which we all depend. Community Development is well placed to involve people equally on these issues which affect all of us.

Community Development should seek to develop structures which enable the active involvement of people from disadvantaged groups, and in particular people from ethnic minorities and black groups.

SECTION:	**DEFINITIONS OF COMMUNITY WORK**
TITLE:	
AUTHOR:	England Interim Board for Community Work Training and Qualifications

Community Work is about the active involvement of people in the issues which affect their lives and focuses on the relation between individuals and groups and the institutions which shape their everyday experience.

It is a developmental process which is both a collective and individual experience. It is based on a commitment to equal partnership between all those involved to enable a sharing of skills, awareness, knowledge and experience in order to bring about change.

It takes place in both neighbourhoods and communities of interest, whenever people come together to identify what is relevant to them and act on issues of common concern.

The key purpose or is to work with communities experiencing disadvantage, to enable them collectively to identify needs and rights, clarify objectives and take action to meet these within a democratic framework which respects the needs and rights of others.

Community Work recognises the need to celebrate diversity and differences and actively confront oppression however it is manifested.

Community Work is based upon a set of principles and values which underpin practice (see appendix).

Aims And Objectives

Community Work aims to:

1. **Promote co-operation and encourage the process of participatory democracy by:**

- supporting new and existing community groups to work on issues of common interest and concern.

- enabling links and liaisons between groups and individuals to take place, around issues of common concern on a basis of mutual respect, whilst recognising diversity and differences.

- acknowledging the specific experience and contribution of all individuals in communities, to enable them to play a greater role in shaping and determining the society of which they are part.

- promoting models of partnership and organisational structure which empower local communities.

- assisting people to reflect and act together to achieve common goals and to influence decision makers where appropriate.

- assisting groups to use a variety of methods to achieve their objectives e.g. through self help groups, pressure groups, community action, alliances and partnerships.

2. **Encourage self-determination by:**

- helping individuals and community groups to define their own objectives.

- supporting individuals and groups to run autonomous and collectively managed projects.

- developing appropriate organisational forms to ensure self determination.

3.   **Ensure the sharing and development of knowledge by:**

- developing awareness and understanding of issues and perspectives through working towards social, economic and political change.

- enabling people to develop the expertise and skills necessary to further their own objectives.

- enabling people to recognise the values which influence the ways in which they work.

4.   **Change the balance of power and power structures in ways which will facilitate local democracy, challenge inequalities and promote social justice by:**

- recognising that the unequal distribution of power is both a personal and political issue, and that Community Work has a responsibility for linking the personal learning which empowers individuals, through to the collective learning and action for change which empowers communities.

- recognising oppression within society and the necessity to confront all forms of oppression, both within ourselves and within society.

- taking the lead in confronting the attitudes and behaviour of individuals, groups and institutions which discriminate against and disempower people, whether as individuals or groups.

- pursuing the above through the adoption and promotion of explicit anti-discriminatory policies and practices.

July 1996

SECTION:	DEFINITIONS OF COMMUNITY WORK
TITLE:	
AUTHOR:	England Interim Board for Community Work Training and Qualifications

Appendix

Principles and Values

Community Work is based upon the following principles and values:

- That human rights must be respected.

- That society can become a participatory democracy where people contribute as equals.

- That collaboration and collective working within our democracy is not always equal – and that inequalities within communities are severely damaging.

- That people are able to work positively together to change inequalities.

- That community work involves a process of action and reflection moving towards clear goals, set collectively, and regularly evaluated.

- That the community work process must enable the empowerment of those with the least power so that they can participate as equals.

- That groups should become self-determining with those experiencing the problem in control of the outcomes.

- That individuals can take responsibility, for themselves and their own actions and recognise the influence that their values have on other people.

- That individuals groups and communities may need support in orber to deal with conflict and challenge inequality and injustice for themselves.

- Appreciation of each other and the reality of each others' experience – and confirming and validating this is part of a process for real change within society.

- Community Work has been and continues to be influenced by women and Black people and is now also informed by the voices of disabled people.

- Community Work is a dynamic process which is constantly shaped by the experiences of the people actively involved in their struggles against oppression.

July 1996

SECTION 4

COMMUNITY WORKERS
- ROLES, SKILLS AND RESPONSIBILITIES

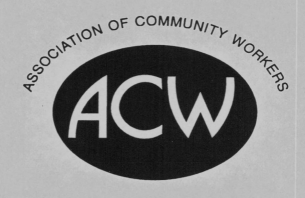

ASSOCIATION OF COMMUNITY WORKERS

ACW

SECTION:	COMMUNITY WORKER – ROLES, SKILLS & RESPONSIBILITIES
TITLE:	SKILLS OF A COMMUNITY WORKER
AUTHOR:	Val Harris

The range of skills that an experienced community worker may be expected to hold has been summarised under ten broad headings. Most community workers will also have specialised knowledge and skills which are relevant to their particular setting or employer.

This section aims to highlight the key core skills needed by someone undertaking community (development) work and as such may be used when drawing up community work job specifications or as the basis of appraisal/reviews of community workers - whether self or employer based.

1. RESEARCH AND INFORMATION GATHERING SKILLS

One of the most important skills involves gathering information from a variety of sources, analysing it, and presenting the results to diverse audiences. The worker may gather information on a particular geographical area, (a community profile,) which will summarise local people's and worker's perspectives on that neighbourhood and detail the existing level of services and facilities available. The highlighted shortfall between the perceived needs of an area and the services available is used to inform community based groups, voluntary organisations and statutory agencies of the value of their current activities and what could be developed in the future. Examining existing material, (such as census small area statistics, changes to the economic base of an area, and the forward plans of different agencies) allows the worker to indicate future potential problems that need to be addressed. Through talking to people in the area an analysis of different communities strengths and needs can be developed, which may give a different picture to that traditionally held by outsiders and policy makers; for instance the needs of black communities, and their resources for meeting them, may vary widely and have substantial implications for service providers; sometimes there may be pockets of poverty within apparently prosperous rural areas. The detailed knowledge of an area that a worker acquires is frequently in demand by agencies and local people who use the worker to find out what is happening or who is the best person to contact about a particular issue. Workers with a specific specialism such as health, housing, or play for examples will gather information around that topic – finding out who is providing what and to whom, and on what basis, and then establishing what gaps are left and how people perceive them as being filled. Sometimes, a service should be provided by statutory authorities adapting their existing provision, another time a self-help group may be the answer. One of the crucial uses of the information gathered is the pulling out of issues and analysing their causes, are they specifically local issues or are they part of a wider, national or international problem or trend. The sharing of this analysis with local people and agencies is equally important as the next section shows.

2. INFORMATION SHARING AND LIAISON SKILLS

In order to plan and deliver services effectively departments and organisations need to have a continuous supply of updated information. Community workers pass on the information they gather to the appropriate people. They frequently pass information between staff of different agencies, and between the local state and community based groups and residents. Community workers act as a catalyst within the community by bringing together people with similar concerns or problems, the basis for collective action. These skills in networking can lead to new groups developing to tackle new problems, and to people from different groups coming together on an issue to prevent duplication of effort.

Organisations can be encouraged to work together to put in joint bids for resources which would not be available to the individual constituent groups, whilst groups can be kept in contact with changes taking place which directly affect them or their environment. Community workers are skilled in meeting new people and of gaining information about their interests and providing relevant information to them.

3.   COMMUNICATIONS SKILLS

Community workers are in contact with a wide range of people and groups, including local residents, professional workers, and councillors. They communicate with all of these people in a relevant and effective manner; both verbally and through writing. They are able to present their ideas to a variety of groups and conferences as well as writing reports and preparing grant applications. Other aspects of communication involve the publicity and marketing of community projects and their work, to attract new members, ensure services are fully utilised and that funders are aware of the benefits of any community based activity.

4.   GROUP WORK SKILLS

The basis of community work is the concept of collective action; of people coming together over shared interests or concerns, either to campaign for services or against threats to their environment, or to provide a service. The skills needed by a worker includes group building, group maintenance, enabling a group towards independence, and the ability to negotiate within and between groups and their members. This requires the ability to work within teams and groups that are loose-knit as well as closely linked, and who are composed of different people with a variety of skills and knowledge, all taking on different roles. The worker will need to understand group dynamics and help others to recognise them and to work towards effective group functioning.

There are a variety of roles that a community worker takes within groups, which depends on the groups age, its activities, and position within its life cycle. Their roles can include acting as a facilitator, a trainer, an organiser, a supporter, an information gatherer or a crèche worker. There is a skill in knowing which role to take with each group and in handling changes over time as the group grows and changes; the overriding aim is always to enable the people involved to empower themselves and to determine their own futures.

5. DEVELOPMENT OF STRATEGIES AND TACTICS

Community workers advise community groups on the options open to them and help them work out the pros and cons of each one. They may advise departments and voluntary organisations on how to approach the local communities, or on ways of beginning to develop community based approaches to their service delivery. They can assist with the prioritising of a group's work, the thinking through of what is possible in the short and longer terms.

Understanding the process of change and the time required to plan, implement and achieve changes is one of the crucial elements that community workers bring to those who are intending to involve "the community" for the first time. Similarly community workers will emphasise the importance of involving people from the very beginning when developing any partnership or participative arrangements between the community and statutory sectors, and will be able to advise on how this might happen. Community workers contribute to the process as well as content of development plans for rural or urban areas, or for user, or potential user, involvement in service design, and for positive action programmes. The need to review and to evaluate the progress and outcomes of such plans is now accepted, and again community workers can contribute suggestions for the techniques and processes that can be used in these tasks. In developing strategies and tactics community workers frequently take on a pro-active role, encouraging people and organisations to decide what they want to do rather than waiting for events to overtake them. This will often involve community workers in assisting groups to plan campaigns and thus they will need a thorough understanding of the different ways that campaigns can be mounted and the pros and cons of each approach. As the world changes so community workers need to be able to respond, and they should be constantly looking for new ways to work within communities which reflect the changes in our society.

6. MEETING SKILLS

For groups to be able to function effectively, and for partnerships to develop people must be able to meet together effectively. Putting people in the same room does not tend to guarantee that anything is achieved; and hence there are a variety of skills that community workers bring to making meetings effective. These range from the way to lay out a room, to how to set agendas so everyone is involved, and ensuring that people are briefed effectively, that they can contribute their expertise appropriately, that any agreed actions are recorded and followed through, and that the aims and purpose of the meetings are regularly reviewed.

Community workers can both model good practice and help groups to devise guidelines for their own procedures.

7. RESOURCE GATHERING

Resources will be needed by both community groups and statutory agencies if they are to make their existing services more effectively or if they are to develop new services or campaigns. The level of resource will range from those who need small amounts to publicise their activities to attract more members or users, to those who need substantial capital to build a new centre or the revenue for the staff to expand a successful pilot project. Community workers can gather information on new and existing sources of funding, some of which may not be available to local government but only to charities, or which requires matching funding, or is only available to a certain areas. The workers will present their findings to the groups who can then decide who to approach for what. As resources become harder to attract so the skill in targeting potential funders and in writing applications to their requirements becomes more specialised and community workers will need to link to the specialised help that is becoming available.

Once resources have been obtained they need to be managed and so the community worker may be assisting groups to establish the necessary systems to ensure that they are used effectively and carefully monitored.

8. TRAINING AND EDUCATION

The aim of community work is to facilitate the empowerment of people: this requires community workers to be adept at passing on their skills to others, particularly members of community based groups, so that their expertise becomes held within the community rather than by an outsider. Through working with groups and key individuals on particular tasks community workers will be helping people develop skills in presenting their case, of making themselves heard, of ways of organising their group or their activity more effectively. They may be asked to run a more formal training programme, on a particular issue that a group wants to gain more knowledge of, or in a skill area that the group want to acquire. Community workers may also be asked by other professional workers to run workshops for example, on working with groups, or how to organise public meetings. The importance of the process in community work, as well as its outcomes, is frequently seen in the growth in skills and confidence of people who become active within their own communities.

9. SELF MOTIVATING

Community workers, by the nature of their work, have to be able to take initiatives, to be willing and capable of taking risks, and adept at changing course and following new issues and opportunities. They have to be self starting, able to work on their own, and to develop their own support networks which will enable them to cope with multitude of crisis and conflicts that will arise, within the communities and between the community and local government. The employment patterns of community workers frequently leaves them isolated and without adequate levels of support or supervision; they are often the only people within their team/area with any detailed knowledge of community work.

10. ADVOCACY

At times the community worker will need to act as an advocate on behalf of communities or groups within them, and to perform this task within the principles of self-determination, the promotion of independence and empowerment; not an easy task! The skill lies in knowing when it is acceptable (or even beneficial) to take on this role and when to maintain a low profile, leaving it to others to speak for themselves.

11. MANAGEMENT OF PEOPLE.

People are the key to all community activity, whether they are volunteers, students on placements, trainees on various training schemes, or paid workers, and it is often the community worker who is given the task of supervising many of these people.

Whenever people work together on issues and projects there is the potential for conflict and it is often the community worker who takes on the role of mediator, of trying to help people to work through their differences in a constructive manner which allows the group, and the individuals, to develop and be able to use conflict constructively rather than letting it split the group and leave people feeling angry and hurt.

SECTION:	**COMMUNITY WORKER – ROLES, SKILLS & RESPONSIBILITIES**
TITLE:	
AUTHOR:	

SECTION:	COMMUNITY WORKER – ROLES, SKILLS & RESPONSIBILITIES
TITLE:	PROCESS OF COMMUNITY WORK
AUTHOR:	Val Harris

The skills needed by a community worker will vary over time and with the different stages of the community work process that they are engaged with. Regardless of the subject/issues involved there is a similar process involved in any piece of development work that is undertaken. Workers may be involved in the whole cycle but will frequently find themselves taking over from someone else's work – for example a student on placement may have gathered background information on an issue which has highlighted the need for a particular group which you are expected to follow up; your post may be the result of an application to attract new resources an area or a centre, or you may be replacing an established community worker and need to review the role of the worker with these existing groups.

Points to note

The completion of any stage may lead to the cycle starting again – for instance a group may decide that there is a particular issue that needs tackling but it is inappropriate for them to do it – so the workers may be asked to gather information and bring together another group to tackle the "new" problem.

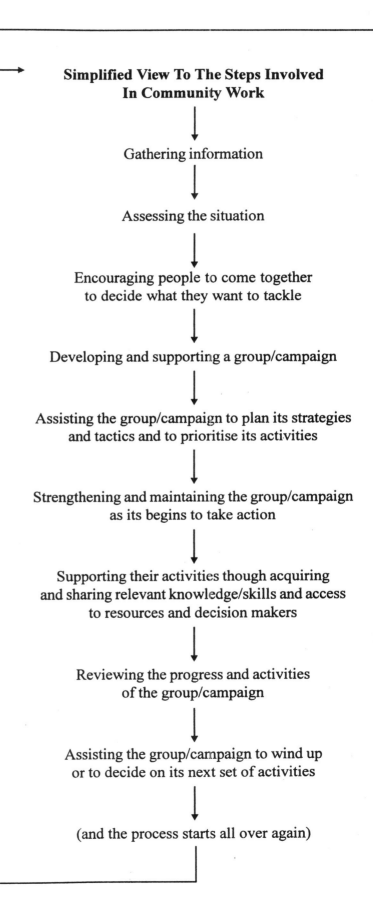

**Simplified View To The Steps Involved
In Community Work**

↓

Gathering information

↓

Assessing the situation

↓

Encouraging people to come together
to decide what they want to tackle

↓

Developing and supporting a group/campaign

↓

Assisting the group/campaign to plan its strategies
and tactics and to prioritise its activities

↓

Strengthening and maintaining the group/campaign
as its begins to take action

↓

Supporting their activities though acquiring
and sharing relevant knowledge/skills and access
to resources and decision makers

↓

Reviewing the progress and activities
of the group/campaign

↓

Assisting the group/campaign to wind up
or to decide on its next set of activities

↓

(and the process starts all over again)

SECTION:	COMMUNITY WORKER – ROLES, SKILLS & RESPONSIBILITIES
TITLE:	ROLES OF A COMMUNITY WORKER
AUTHOR:	Alison Gilchrist

A role might be defined as a work function which encapsulates a particular approach or set of tasks which others can reasonably expect the worker to perform. The community worker has a variety of roles, which can be broadly categorised into five main functions: organiser, advocate, challenger, developer and supporter. These can be arranged on a continuum from directive intervention to an active, but non-directive approach. The role which the worker plays on any occasion depends on a range of factors in the situation, but most importantly on how she can help other people to get things done.

ORGANISER

In the initial stages of helping a group to set up, the community worker might adopt the rather directive role of organiser, taking on responsibility for getting things started by arranging meetings, sending out publicity, organising positive action measures, such as childcare and interpreting arrangements.

Often community workers will do much of the "behind the scenes" organisation for a group, following up contacts, undertaking administrative tasks, such as book-keeping, servicing meetings, producing a newsletter or generally ensuring that the group members maintain contact with one another.

ADVOCATE

This should be a rare role for community workers, whose aim is usually to enable people to speak for themselves and develop a collective voice in negotiating situations. Sometimes, however, there are constraints or pressures which justify the worker speaking on behalf of others to argue for a position based on a degree of consultation and consensus. Circumstances which might support this option might be lack of time in the decision-making process before the people affected by a decision have had time to gain the confidence and skills to articulate their own views in what might be an intimidating forum. Or there might be access issues, which cannot be overcome with the time and resources currently available. This may particularly affect work with disabled people or people whose first language is not English.

The worker should be careful in the role of advocate that they do not go beyond their mandate to represent the views of others.

CHALLENGER

One of the chief purposes of community work is to change things, particularly to question and combat current inequalities in the distribution of power and resources. The worker therefore sometimes has a role to play in challenging prejudices, practices or policies which have the affect of discriminating against some sections of society.

People often hold attitudes and assumptions about themselves and others which perpetuate disadvantage and oppression. These might be expressed through language which is offensive or through hostile or patronising behaviour. The community worker should challenge these (and enable others to do so for themselves) in a variety of ways, including humour, private discussion, open debate, policy proposals and modelling anti-oppressive practices. In adopting this role, the worker must also be prepared to deal with any conflicts, resentment or feelings of disempowerment that result and to recognise that the role of challenger can be both uncomfortable and controversial.

DEVELOPER

However, the community worker should usually be trying to move their professional relationship with users to be more that of developer. The key aspect to this role is that the worker is enabling the people she is working with to acquire new capabilities and to enhance their existing skills, knowledge and understanding.

This process might be through encouraging people to share these with others in the group, learning through role play or observation or through more formal training opportunities. Often this involves working closely alongside individual members of a group on a particular task, giving practical advice, support and feedback so that they eventually feel confident to perform the task on their own.

Informal discussions or workshops also provide opportunities for people to share and develop their knowledge by reflecting on their own experience and gaining information on specific areas on public life (such as the workings of local government).

SUPPORTER

This role involves more interpersonal methods of working, such as counselling, advising, building self-esteem and generally encouraging people to work through difficult situations. It might include talking through an idea or a problem with an individual or group, listening to someone's grievances, staying in touch with a member of a group who is experiencing difficulties in their life and not able to attend regularly, being a friendly and accessible point of contact between people in the community and your employing organisation or simply ensuring that people can make use of facilities and resources that they need in their work (such as use of a telephone, photocopier or meeting space.)

When in the role of supporter, contact between the worker and community users will normally be on the initiative and terms of the user. As such the worker will not have specific goals other than to provide emotional and practical support for the user in their chosen course of action.

The role selected may depend on a number of factors, including the policies of the employing agency, the preferred style of the worker, the wishes of the users and the actual circumstances prevailing (e.g. time and resources available, the experience and personalities of other people involved, including levels of motivation, skills, and range of attitudes).

The choice of roles is negotiable between those concerned and will probably change as a strategy unfolds.

SECTION:	COMMUNITY WORKER – ROLES, SKILLS & RESPONSIBILITIES
TITLE:	THE ROLE OF A COMMUNITY WORKER IN A SMALL ORGANISATION
AUTHOR:	Alison Gilchrist

Small organisations in the community sector usually begin as a concern expressed by people about certain issues that affect their own lives or which are of general public concern. Through voluntary effort, often over several years, small groups gain a degree of credibility and responsibility within their field which can no longer be sustained solely through the willing, but unpaid work of those directly involved in the group. At this stage, funding might be sought to employ a worker to undertake some of the administrative tasks of the organisation or to develop a more professional approach to particular aspects of the work.

Community workers are often appointed with rather vague job descriptions (usually focused around "community development") and encompassing unrealistically high expectations of what can be achieved in the time available, with minimal budgets and frequently short term contracts. The term community development is itself rather a mystical concept, whose particular tasks and processes will depend to a great extent on the circumstances of the setting and the wishes of users and potential users. A worker newly employed in a small organisation, and managed by a hard-pressed band of volunteers and users, may find themselves trying to juggle a number of competing demands and expectations. It is therefore important to be clear from the outset how the role is to be defined and what sort of things the worker can reasonably be expected to do in their hours of employment.

Community Development is about helping people to work together to do things that they would like to do, or to solve problems that they have identified in their lives or the local community.

Ideally, it is not about doing things for people, but about enabling them to do it for themselves.

This might involve helping people to organise an event, a self-help group or a service for others to use. Or it might be helping people make changes in a situation, which they or others find difficult or unsatisfactory. This might involve help with:

- organising meetings,
- publicity,
- campaigns,
- fundraising,
- setting up a committee,
- administrating a project,
- employing workers or
- linking up with others who are involved in similar work.

Each of these could include providing guidance and assistance with applying for grants, recruiting and supporting staff, organising events such as festivals and fundraising initiatives, training for management committees, a newsletter, posters and leaflets, setting up accounts systems and managing budgets, putting people in touch with one another in a support group, supervision and support of sessional staff and volunteers, helping group members to deal with internal conflicts and disagreements and numerous administrative tasks behind the scenes.

Community Development involves working with people (individually and in groups) in ways which encourage, enable and empower them to do things for themselves. This process might entail people learning new skills, building self-esteem and confidence, having a sense of their own rights in a difficult situation, knowing who to contact for useful information and resources, and developing a different understanding of how things work in organisations and society as a whole.

Community development is also about promoting Equal Opportunities in relation to:

- participation in decision making

- access to employment, services and resources, and

- fair treatment by others

It is important that community development is carried out in such a way as to combat inequalities within organisations and to help members to take part equally in whatever is going on. Often this means recognising that previous ways of doing things might have discriminated against some sections of the community, so that they felt left out, that their needs were not being recognised or generally disadvantaged in other ways. Usually these are the results of discrimination within the wider society or prejudices, based on fear or lack of knowledge. Unless community development adopts an anti-discriminatory approach to the work, then it is likely to fail in its commitment to challenging inequalities.

The community development worker actively supports people (usually those working on a voluntary basis from their own communities) to carry out their own ideas, set up services which meet their needs and solve problems which they come across. The processes by which this happens should ensure that the people involved gain confidence, skills, knowledge, awareness and a sense of being an equal member of the wider community. The emphasis is not on the final product (an event, newsletter, group activity, welfare service or whatever) but rather on how that goal has been achieved, and how the people involved have gained as a result. Community development is not primarily concerned to organise or run things for other people, but to support them in learning how to work with others to do it for themselves, so that eventually they make all the decisions and take all the responsibility without being dependent on the worker for their time, skills or motivation. The worker can then move on to develop other initiatives.

Working in a small organisation poses specific problems to do with isolation, self-servicing for administrative tasks, poor quality or infrequent supervision, and burn-out. It is vital that community workers in these situations set up support systems for themselves, perhaps using models of peer consultancy or non-managerial supervision or with a colleague in a similar agency. They must also be clear to their employers about professional boundaries, time management and work programme priorities.

Obviously this accountability will be maintained through consultation with users and managers. Open discussion and regular work reports should ensure that all members of the organisation understand the role of the worker and know what they can expect from them in ways which are mutually supportive and constructive.

SECTION:	COMMUNITY WORKER – ROLES, SKILLS & RESPONSIBILITIES
TITLE:	ANALYSING YOUR ROLE WITH A GROUP
AUTHOR:	Adapted from the original Skills Manual by Val Harris

The roles that community workers can undertake within groups are many. The actual role you take on will be determined by the state of the group's development as well as by the ones that are deemed acceptable by your employer.

The role that you fulfil will change over time; for instance when a group is first starting it will need more help with the basics of how to organise itself, while later on it may turn to you to provide updated knowledge on legislation and funding sources for a service they want to develop.

ANALYSING A COMMUNITY WORKER'S OWN ROLE IN A GROUP

Using the examples below as a guide, you can clarify and analyse your role(s) with a group.

For each group you work with complete a separate sheet.

Name of Group .... Date ....

Roles you could take	Purpose of this role	The action you take	Comment on your actions	Changes you want to make to your role

Overleaf, List 1 will give some of the roles involved in helping a group decide where it is going, and List 2 gives some of the roles involved in building and maintaining a group.

Comments

1.   This list of roles is not exhaustive
2.   The roles, purposes, and action taken can all be re-written to harmonise with particular objectives, assumptions and views of community work held by individual workers. These lists are not definitive.
3.   The technique should not be read as implying that the listed roles should all be incorporated in a worker's relation to a group.
4.   Actual roles taken in particular situations may depend on the workers' capability, orientations and objectives as well as the nature and needs of the group.
5.   The lists (or other similar sorts of lists) can be used to analyse all group members' roles, not just that of the community worker.

SECTION:	COMMUNITY WORKER – ROLES, SKILLS & RESPONSIBILITIES
TITLE:	ANALYSING YOUR ROLE WITH A GROUP
AUTHOR:	Adapted from the original Skills Manual by Val Harris

List 1: Helping a group achieve its goals

Role	Purpose	Action taken
Initiator	to establish an order to the meeting; to give direction and purpose to the group.	proposing tasks, goals, defining problems, suggesting procedures and solutions.
Information seeker	to find out whether the group knows certain facts; to encourage the group to seek facts.	request relevant facts.
Information giver	to enable the group to be better informed; to help the group avoid reliance on opinion.	offer relevant facts.
Opinion seeker	to find out individual opinions.	ask for opinions.
Opinion giver	to provide a basis for a group to start to come to a decision.	evaluate and elaborate group members' suggestions; simply state own opinions.
Clarifier	to reduce confusion.	define terms, interpret ideas, spot ambiguities, define issues, suggest options, give examples, explain.
Summariser	to draw ideas together.	repeat and relate certain statements, link themes, show contradictions, offer conclusions.

List 2: Helping to build and maintain a group as a working unit

Role	Purpose	Action taken
Encourager	to enable others to feel recognised and that they have a contribution; to facilitate communication.	be responsive and friendly to others; draw out a silent member, suggest procedures for discussion.
Commentator	to call group's attention to the existence of certain reactions, ideas or suggestions.	express own feelings, restate others.
Harmoniser	to relieve tensions and/or encourage group cohesion.	injecting humour, suggesting compromises.
Create yardsticks	to make group aware of direction and progress.	express group concern, suggest directions and targets, analyse progress towards goals.
Interpreter	to explain, interpret what someone has already said.	paraphrase initial speaker.
Listener	provide stimulating interested audience for others.	accept ideas of group, go along with the group.

Accountability is a key concept in community work and applies in different ways to all the actors in a community work setting.

Accountability is about taking responsibility for your actions and ensuring that others know just what you're doing and why and how, and being prepared to act on others' criticisms or recommendations

The settings where accountability applies include:

- community workers to their employers,

- community workers to the groups with whom they're working,

- community groups to the wider community,

- groups receiving funding to their funding agency.

Without accountability, power can easily be concentrated in a few hands without challenge. Accountability allows for challenges of power. Two important tenets of community work are those of empowering the community and ensuring the dissemination of information. Accountability involves both of these.

MECHANISMS BY WHICH ACCOUNTABILITY CAN BE ENSURED AND MAINTAINED

- Community workers can make regular reports to their employers. Workers need to ensure that those who are employing them know what they're doing and why and how and receive some feedback. The employers themselves need to be accountable to an electorate or a funding body.

- Where a community worker is working alongside a community group, it is important that she keeps them fully informed about her work in connection with that group so that they retain ownership of that work. Firm guidelines need to be laid down about the limitations on the responsibilities of the worker in this context. Negotiating these early in the relationship is a good idea.

- Community groups which purport to be speaking or acting on behalf of the wider community, whether geographical or a community of interest, need to make provisions in their constitution for ways in which it will be answerable. These could take the form of a newsletter or regular open meetings. Meetings need to be open so that members or the open public are able to ask questions and receive full and informed answers.

- Groups receiving funding from public bodies need to make plans for the monitoring of the work that is being paid for and ensure that either all the members of the group are fully aware of the progress or that a small sub committee is appointed to do so. Accountability, with respect to money, means knowing where and how the money has been spent and proving it. This is why that clause in the constitution stating that: "The Treasurer shall keep proper accounts" is so important.

- Accounting to the funder for money spent both in terms of a set of audited accounts and a report is important for several reasons. Public money is collectively owned and it is therefore right that the public know how this money has been spent. It is also important for your own survival if you want money from that source again.

SECTION:	**COMMUNITY WORKER – ROLES, SKILLS & RESPONSIBILITIES**
TITLE:	
AUTHOR:	

SECTION:	**COMMUNITY WORKER – ROLES, SKILLS & RESPONSIBILITIES**
TITLE:	**POLITICS AND THE COMMUNITY WORKER**
AUTHOR:	Roger Green

Working in a community is very often about taking sides. About fighting discrimination, oppression and inequality, about supporting people improve their lives and their communities by helping them to organise and take action. This may mean that at times you upset and come into conflict with perhaps your own employer or groups that hold some power in the community, for example, the local council, the police or maybe a government department which is involved in a new road scheme.

To be active and to survive within your community and indeed your job, you need to be politically astute and skilful. Not all community workers will be employed by local councils or community projects which are sympathetic to their employee (the community worker) being involved in taking action which may cause conflict and which is seen as being of a "political" nature. What strategies can you adopt to support you in continuing to fight for one of the key principles of community work, a more just society?

STRATEGIES FOR GETTING SUPPORT

1. Getting the support of fellow workers in your workplace

This could be done by:

- keeping them informed of what's happening
- asking for their support
- talking it through with them
- listening to their views and feelings
- not being afraid to admit you might be wrong and revising your plans.

2. Joining a Trade Union

Membership of a trade union:

- will give you support outside of the workplace
- it should give you legal representation if you should ever need it
- attendance at local branch meetings will bring you into contact with other activists
- it could help you build alliances

3. Building a support network for yourself within the community

This could be sympathetic local councillors, community groups you are working with, chairpersons and secretaries of tenants associations and activists and key individuals in the community e.g. a local head teacher, a religious leader, or a journalist on the local newspaper as well as other workers from different departments/ councils

4. Membership of a professional association such as the Association of Community Workers will:

- give you a professional network to access
- give you knowledge of how other community workers are working in different parts of the country
- encourage you to attend conferences and meetings and meet other community workers
- give you confidence and support
- help you to evaluate your own community work practice

SECTION:	**COMMUNITY WORKER – ROLES, SKILLS & RESPONSIBILITIES**
TITLE:	
AUTHOR:	

SECTION:	COMMUNITY WORKER – ROLES, SKILLS & RESPONSIBILITIES
TITLE:	THE COMMUNITY WORKER AS AN AGENT OF CHANGE
AUTHOR:	Alison Gilchrist

Community work is about social development through change. This will involve change at a number of levels, including changing people, changing organisations, changing communities, and ultimately working towards changing the social distribution of power and resources. Broadly speaking these changes can be categorised as psychological developments, new practical arrangements and negotiated political settlements.

PSYCHOLOGICAL DEVELOPMENTS

These refer to changes which take place in the minds of individuals or which relate to adjustments in the dynamics of a group. The former might include learning new skills and knowledge or the development of insights or deeper understanding into aspects of the person's life. It might include consciousness raising or developing empathy and awareness of the situation of others. This could involve challenging prejudices and internalised oppression, and helping people to develop a more critical approach to the media and the sometimes oppressive nature of language. Community workers are also concerned to support individuals in their personal growth and development, encouraging them to talk through problems, try out new roles and skills, become generally more assertive and more confident in tackling difficult situations.

At a group level, the worker aims to develop collective problem-solving methods, in which group members can communicate and interact on an equal basis. This will ensure that a group is able to discuss issues of common concern, make decisions based on strong participation, and then carry these out effectively and in ways which value the contributions of everyone involved. The worker's role as change agent might involve helping the group to form in the first place, helping it to develop ways of managing itself (roles, procedures and guidelines for meetings, negotiating skills, dealing with internal conflicts, etc.) and undertake tasks which move the group towards its agreed goals.

The worker might also help the group with its relationships with the "outside world", liaising with the relevant authorities and networking with similar or umbrella organisations. Finally, the worker must also consider ways of assisting groups through different phases, including periods of turmoil, demoralisation and eventually, sometimes, its dissolution. The process of a group finishing are as important for the individuals involved, and this role for the community worker is often overlooked or underestimated. It may include dealing with unresolved conflicts, a sense of failure in the part of some or all members, tying up loose administrative ends and generally making sure that the affairs of the group are either closed or in good enough order for other people to pick up at a later stage.

PRACTICAL ARRANGEMENTS

The community worker often finds themselves concerned with changes of a very practical nature, usually involving the acquisition, allocation and management of resources. A key issue is one of equal access; both to the methods of democratic processes (meetings, decisions, information, consultation exercises), and to services and facilities. In this respect the worker will ensure that new and existing resources are made available to members of the community and develop a range of positive action strategies to facilitate the effective participation of anyone who is interested. For example, practical changes might involve childcare arrangements which enable people to attend meetings, the provision of interpreters at events, transport and the use of accessible venues, information being presented in translation and other forms, and a range of refreshments available which encourage people from different cultures to feel welcome and valued. Usually these practical developments will require additional funding or adjustments to an existing budget. The community worker is likely to be involved in either of these aspects by applying for grants and donations or managing changes in the financial priorities of the organisation.

The community worker is also concerned that people feel that they have a right to make use of public facilities, such as community buildings and the resources they hold. Positive images and statements around anti-discriminatory practice can enhance this, but also a friendly approach to the use of the office telephone, photocopier, computer and other facilities can improve a group or individual's effectiveness in very practical ways.

POLITICAL PROCESSES

Community work is fundamentally concerned with political processes, recognising that many of the problems experienced by people result from political decisions about financial priorities and power imbalances. Empowerment might be defined as increasing someone's ability (individually or collectively) to influence decisions which affect their lives. Politics is concerned with the distribution of power and resources across a defined population, such as a city, county, nation or community. On a formal basis politics operates through parties and policies, but informal and hidden power dynamics are equally important, especially when considering the different dimensions of oppressions and disadvantage.

For the community worker to tackle these, they must be prepared to deal with potential conflicts and resistance to change. It helps if the worker is able to assist those affected to develop an analysis of the power distribution in a particular situation. This will enable the group to identify where decisions are being made and how they might organise themselves to influence these. Political power is complex. To some extent it is vested in authority and democratic roles, but it is also hidden in traditions, culture and "common sense" notions about status, rights, values and the position of individuals in society.

Decisions can be presented as clear policy or legislation, which can be amended or replaced. This also applies to codes of practice or guidelines. Many decisions are, however, shrouded in the assumptions and prejudices of the policy makers, and manifest themselves as institutionalised discrimination. These need challenging through raising awareness, equality training and campaigning. The people in power must be re-educated to understand and respect the experience and perspectives of people who are oppressed. They must be compelled to take these views into account in the decision-making process. Or they must be replaced by those who can.

Clearly, none of the changes outlined at each of these three levels (psychological, practical and political) can occur in isolation from the others. The community work approach is to develop strategies which enable people who feel themselves to be relatively powerless to work with others to make those changes in their lives which they identify as important and desirable. Sometimes the focus will be on the personal growth of an individual, sometimes it will be about challenging local or central government policies. Whatever the aims, the community worker should ensure that the processes by which these are achieved are determined by the people involved and are developmental in themselves.

Community development aims to identify and nurture leadership qualities within people who are rooted within neighbourhoods or communities of interest. Leadership might be defined as "the use of authority or influence within a group or community to help it achieve its aims", and equally refers to the role played by a single individual (paid or unpaid) or where responsibilities are shared collectively and more or less equally by members of a group.

Leadership is an important concept in community work in helping to understand the power dynamics that are operating in a particular situation, and to intervene in ways which help a group to function more effectively and democratically.

Positive leadership of a group has two aspects – managing internal and external relationships.

It helps people to focus their thinking on a particular issue, to share ideas and information creatively, and to deal with internal conflicts and disagreements constructively.

Leadership facilitates communication of the group's identity with the outside world. This might involve representing collective opinion to authority in order to influence decision-making in the interests of the group, or simply acting as an information channel between members of the group and other agencies.

In many communities "leaders" emerge either through a process of self-selection or they are appointed as unofficial spokespeople by media journalists, anxious to find a "personality" who may be both controversial and readily available.

Sometimes individuals may find themselves in a leadership role, by virtue of their professional or religious status (e.g. the Imam at the local mosque, the head teacher, community worker, etc.) or, more rarely, they may be democratically elected to a position in the community (such as councillor, chair of the tenants' association) with the expectations that they will represent the whole community on a wide range of issues and concerns.

Although community workers may find themselves in certain circumstances in positions of leadership, their role is rather:

- to identify and nurture potential or embryonic leaders,

- to support existing leaders who are using that role constructively or democratically, or

- to challenge examples of authoritarian or unaccountable leadership.

A fundamental principle of community work is a more egalitarian distribution of power within and between groups. This can often involve the process of empowerment of people who experience discrimination, whilst challenging those styles of leadership which perpetuate oppression and disadvantage.

This redistribution of power can be achieved in a variety of ways.

Positive measures such as:

- encouragement, confidence-building, skills training, (e.g. in assertiveness or chairing),

- making space for people to explore options,

- giving constructive feedback after meetings and other forms of informal support can all contribute to enabling someone to take on and sustain a leadership role.

It is equally important for a community worker to be able to "help" an individual either to:

- withdraw from a leadership position which is having damaging consequences for themselves or others in the community,

- or to adapt to a less oppressive style.

The methods used might include acknowledging that someone is "burnt out" or generally over-burdened with commitments, thus giving them "permission" to resign, or questioning how they feel about their role as leader.

Critical feedback should always be constructive, and wherever possible support and training offered so that the person has an opportunity to change their approach.

Leadership is a set of functions, rather than a role.

It is about facilitating participation in decision making processes, and it is about the development of positive and co-operative working relations within the group and with the outside world.

There needs to be a balance between the needs of the group, the needs of individual members and the achievement of agreed collective goals.

Good leadership will manage these competing demands on time and resources, and may require skills in listening, negotiation, organising, group work, communication, advocacy, and facilitation.

QUALITIES OF LEADERS

Charisma, knowledge and wisdom, experience of achieving change, confidence, good communication skills, "in touch", strong commitment and motivation, ability to inspire respect, trust and loyalty, sense of fairness objectivity, strategic thinking, etc., etc.

These qualities may not reside in just one individual and the notion of collective or shared leadership has several advantages.

It allows for skills, ideas, information and knowledge to be shared within a group.

It distributes the tasks more evenly, so that the workload does not fall on just one person or core group.

It recognises that a group may go through phases during which different capabilities may be more relevant or the group may set itself other priorities.

A collective sense of leadership will tend to accommodate these changes more flexibly and allow for differences of opinion to be more openly expressed in decision making.

Some points that should be considered in relationship to leadership include:

IDENTIFYING "NATURAL LEADERS - WHO DEFINES WHO AND WHEN?

Evidence:

responses and references by others in the group or community; a person's own behaviour, articulateness, body language and willingness to take on responsibilities. Beware the power seeking individual, but value those who are prepared to accept leadership roles.

OPPORTUNITIES AND PROBLEMS ARISING WITH COMMUNITY LEADERS.

Positive:

source of knowledge and opinion, endorsement of new proposals and change, respected influence (opinion-former).

Negative:

leaders can often reflect oppressions in society, isolation/detachment of leaders from the "led", loss of leaders due to "burn out", removal, discrediting or a coup.

SECTION:	COMMUNITY WORKER – ROLES, SKILLS & RESPONSIBILITIES
TITLE:	AGREEMENT BETWEEN WORKER AND GROUP
AUTHOR:	Tseggai Johannes – former Head of Community Development Team Refugee Council

It is becoming increasingly common and seen as good practice to prepare a written agreement between community workers and community groups. The aim is to be clear about what is expected of each other and to make the most of the available time, energy and skills of the paid worker.

The agreement encourages a shared commitment, responsibility and accountability and mutual respect between the community worker and the group.

The Refugee Council has a Community Development Team which works in all 32 London Boroughs. They work with community organisations, networks, umbrella groups and the voluntary sector in general.

In recognition of the logistical problems presented by their aim to be available and accessible to new communities they have devised a series of check lists to elicit the particular services required by a particular group, and on the basis of these a formal agreement is prepared.

In this section we reproduce some of these formats which have been amended to make them applicable to most community work settings. They can obviously be adapted and re-written to suit any particular situation.

STEP 1

Tick the service you feel you need; there is a separate sheet for the work and the roles you expect for your meetings.

LIST OF SERVICES

Constitution ☐

Charity Status ☐

Funding & Fundraising

Funding Strategy ☐

Writing Effective Applications ☐

Filing/Supporting Application Forms ☐

Fundraising Information ☐

Lobbying Funders ☐

Ethnic Minority Grants ☐

Management Skills

Support & Supervision of Staff & Volunteers ☐

Interviewing Skills ☐

Recruitment & Selection of Personnel ☐

Creating Work Programmes ☐

Evaluation ☐

Managing Projects ☐

Communication Skills

Chairing Meetings ☐

Minutes Taking Skills ☐

Presentation Skills ☐

Preparing your Annual Report ☐

Networking ☐

SECTION:	COMMUNITY WORKER – ROLES, SKILLS & RESPONSIBILITIES
TITLE:	AGREEMENT BETWEEN WORKER AND GROUP
AUTHOR:	Tseggai Johannes – former Head of Community Development Team Refugee Council

Trustees & Management Committees

Duties & Responsibilities of MC as Trustees ☐

Managing a Voluntary Organisation: MC in Action ☐

Responsibility as an Employer ☐

Equal Opportunities Policies ☐

Finance

Financial Planning – Budget & Cashflow Forecast ☐

Basic Book Keeping ☐

Bank Statement & reconciliation ☐

Financial Management & Control ☐

PAYE & NI ☐

End of Year Accounts ☐

Training

Equal Opportunities Policies/Code of Practice ☐

Recruitment & Selection of Personnel ☐

Duties and Responsibilities of MC ☐

Fundraising ☐

Finance ☐

Cultural Awareness ☐

Others: (please specify)

MEETINGS

Conferences ☐ ☐ ☐

Seminar ☐ ☐ ☐

Workshop ☐ ☐ ☐

Annual General Meeting ☐ ☐ ☐

Extra Ordinary Meeting ☐ ☐ ☐

Other (please specify) ....

THEME ....

VENUE ....

DATE ....

ORGANISED BY ....

TIME ....

ROLE:

Facilitator ☐ ☐ ☐

Notes Taker ☐ ☐ ☐

Resource Person ☐ ☐ ☐

Panellist ☐ ☐ ☐

Organiser ☐ ☐ ☐

Other (specify) ....

Attended by ....

Any written material for our records ....

....

STEP 2

SAMPLE OF AGREEMENT

1. **AGREEMENT BETWEEN COMMUNITY DEVELOPMENT TEAM**

Community Development Worker ....

and

.... (NAME OF ORGANISATION)

Contact Person ....

2. Community development team aims to empower organisations by helping them develop confidence, knowledge and skills to take action on issues that affect them.

3. Community Development Worker will:

   a. facilitate the development of the organisation by providing information, guidance and support to committee members and staff of the organisation in the following areas:

      i)
      ii)
      iii)
      iv)
      v)
      vi)

   b. Carry out this function by any of the following methods:

      i) Discussion and advice session.
      ii) Attend meetings of the organisation.
      iii) Accompany committee members and/or staff to meetings with other agencies.
      iv Training workshops, seminars, conferences, etc.
      vi) (others ...)

   c. Maintain confidentiality and security of all information provided by the organisations.

4. The organisation will:

   a. Provide all relevant information requested by the worker.

   b. Be clear about what it wants to achieve.

To make the most of this system you need to work out ways of recording the work you have undertaken jointly with the community worker, which can then be used as the basis for monitoring and reviewing the value and effectiveness of the worker's input and involvement with you.

The CDT of The Refugee Council can be contacted at:

3 Bondway, London SW8 1SJ

Fax: 0171 582 0929

Tel: 0171 582 6922

c.   Ensure adequate attendance and participation in any workshop/seminar etc., especially if this was requested and arrange specially for the organisation.

5.   The period of time agreed is a minimum of   hours/ meetings. However this may be reviewed at any time after the first 3 months.

6.   Meetings will take place at any of the following venues:

a)   Organisation premises.

b)   CDT office.

c)   Other venues arranged by either party.

7.   Nothing in this agreement will exclude the organisation asking for additional support and advice when appropriate.

8.   The CDT worker and the organisation will endeavour to resolve any misunderstanding/disagreement that may arise. However if this cannot be resolved the matter may be raised with CDT leader.

9.   Both parties will give at least 24 hours notice of cancellation of pre-booked appointments and every effort made to find alternative dates.

SIGNED BY .... Date ....

On behalf of COMMUNITY DEVELOPMENT TEAM

SIGNED BY .... Date ....

On behalf of .... (organisation)

SECTION:	**COMMUNITY WORKER – ROLES, SKILLS & RESPONSIBILITIES**
TITLE:	**AGREEMENT BETWEEN WORKER AND GROUP**
AUTHOR:	Tseggai Johannes – former Head of Community Development Team Refugee Council

SECTION 5

TACKILING INEQUALITIES

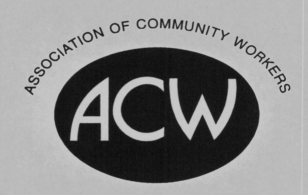

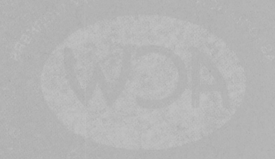

SECTION:	**TACKLING INEQUALITIES**
TITLE:	**WRITING AN EQUAL OPPORTUNITIES STATEMENT AND POLICY**
AUTHOR:	Adapted from Equal Opportunites in Recruitment and Selection

This section looks at the importance of writing and publicising a statement on equal opportunities, then goes on to show how you develop an equal opportunities policy that is practical and effective.

These steps are clearly inter-related. It is no good writing a statement and then not developing the detailed policies or codes of practice that implement it. Equal opportunities policies must lead to action through specific aims and objectives based on systematic examination of the organisations policies and practices in employment and service delivery.

There is also no point in writing a statement and then not publicising it – members of the community need to know and believe that the organisation is taking these issues seriously before they will consider becoming involved.

The Statement

Writing a statement is the first step of work on equal opportunities. It is a public declaration of intent to let people know where you stand on equal opportunities. It is generally very short and intended to be publicised in a similar way to the aims of the organisation.

Equal Opportunites in Recruitment and Selection – This booklet was produced for Nottingham Task Force by Gill Taylor. It is available from Nottingham CVS, tel (0115) 947 6714, who have given their permission for these extracts to be printed here.

THE STATEMENT

The first step for an organisation is to become informed of the facts of discrimination, nationally and locally, and how widely it happens, even when people don't mean it.

For example if you only employ people who are already known to your staff or management committee you will find it hard to change the balance of your staff team.

If you recruit people only from a very small local area you may be indirectly discriminating by not opening job opportunities up to people in areas with a different mix of ethnic residents.

The next step is to examine your organisation and to ask questions about the priorities you set, how you employ people and who you consult about the work:

• Does the membership of the management committee reflect the local population including black and ethnic minority people, women, disabled people, lesbians, bisexuals and gay men?

• Do the people who use your services reflect the local community?

• Do workers reflect the local community?

If you cannot answer yes to these questions, it is important to realise that it is your organisation that has to change, not the community around it.

What to put in your statement

Your statement needs to be an unequivocal commitment to non discrimination on certain grounds and must state how the organisation intends to achieve genuine equality.

The statement should be unique to your organisation and should be properly thought out. It is no good just copying someone else's statement.

The statement should apply to employees and users. Each group should be specifically discussed and notes made of what action needs to be taken under the detailed equal opportunities policy. It is important not to promise what you are not going to deliver!

SECTION:	**TACKLING INEQUALITIES**
TITLE:	**WRITING AN EQUAL OPPORTUNITIES STATEMENT AND POLICY**
AUTHOR:	Adapted from Equal Opportunites in Recruitment and Selection

The statement should say:

• Why you are opposed to discrimination in general.

• What forms of discrimination you intend to tackle.

• How you intend to tackle discrimination in employment and in which areas of your work.

• How you intend to promote opportunities for all groups in the community.

A SAMPLE STATEMENT

1. This statement describes the action NEWVOL community group is committed to taking to make equal opportunities a reality in employment/recruitment/membership/service delivery

2. NEWVOL is taking these steps because it recognises that discrimination has operated to the disadvantage of many people and NEWVOL wishes to challenge the organisational arrangements and personal behaviours that perpetuate discrimination.

3. NEWVOL aims to ensure that no potential or actual employee or user of NEWVOL's services receives less favourable treatment on the grounds of:

    • race

    • ethnic or national origins

    • sex

    • being married

    • sexual orientation

    • disability

    • etc

PUBLICISING THE STATEMENT

Once you have written the statement you need to tell people about it. The main aim of a statement is to show that you mean to change, and the people in your community who use your services need to know this.

The statement should be publicised as part of your annual report, produced as a separate sheet or leaflet and distributed locally. It should become a part of your general publicity leaflet when this is reprinted.

The statement should be circulated widely in the local community among people who are likely to be interested. Consider having a public meeting to launch it.

THE POLICY

A policy is a more concrete step towards developing equal opportunities in action.

You need to write down the steps you decide to take on equal opportunities in a policy because:

- It makes you accountable.

- It is more efficient.

- It allows workers to work with something specific.

- It prevents misinterpretation and misunderstandings.

- It prevents new staff or management committee having to go over old ground.

- It makes implementation plans easier.

- It helps you to clarify your aims and decide what needs to be done.

- It is essential for monitoring and evaluation.

Consultation at the development stage is vital. Use the expertise of workers as regards any gaps they feel there is in the service. Consult with the users you have about any problems they think there are and ways you could improve. Use this information in developing the policy.

The policy can be developed over a period of time according to the priority you place on different areas of work. You need to write a more detailed section on each area you said you would tackle in the statement.

Under each statement you need to include:

- Specific action to be taken.

- Clear rules and procedures.

- Detailed instructions to staff or management.

- Any targets you have decided to set.

SECTION:	**TACKLING INEQUALITIES**
TITLE:	**WRITING AN EQUAL OPPORTUNITIES STATEMENT AND POLICY**
AUTHOR:	Adapted from Equal Opportunites in Recruitment and Selection

EXAMPLES OF STATEMENTS

"The council is an equal opportunities employer. The aim of its policy is to ensure that no job applicant or employee receives less favourable treatment on the grounds of sex, race, colour, nationality, ethnic or racial origin, being married, disability, sexual orientation, age, trade union activity, political or religious belief.

Selection criteria and procedures will be kept under to ensure that individuals are selected, promoted and treated on the basis of their relevant merits and abilities. All employees will be given equal opportunities and where relevant, special training to progress within the organisation.

The council is committed to a programme of action to make this policy fully effective" *(Greater London Council. 1985)*

"............ is committed to actively oppose racism, sexism and all forms of discrimination faced by minority ethnic people, by woman, by people because of their sexual orientation or by disabled people.

"............ declares, therefore that it will introduce measures that will combat all direct or indirect discrimination in its employment practices and in its provision of services and will campaign with groups in the borough fighting to achieve these ends.

"....... intends to ensure that equal opportunity employment becomes a reality in practice and not simply a paper commitment.

"..... will seek to implement a programme of positive action to make this policy fully effective by ensuring that no job applicant receives less favourable treatment on the grounds of race, colour, nationality, ethnic or national origins, sex, being married, sexual orientation, disability or age.

Selection criteria and procedures will be monitored and regularly reviewed to ensure that individuals are selected, promoted and treated on the basis of their relevant merits and abilities. All employees will be given equal opportunity and, where appropriate special training to progress within the organisation."

(Model used in equal opportunities: Some Steps Towards Race Equality In Employment, Southwark Council for Voluntary Service. 1984)

SECTION:	**TACKLING INEQUALITIES**
TITLE:	**WORKING WITHIN ASIAN COMMUNITIES**
AUTHOR:	Shahida Akhtar

To be able to successfully work within Asian communities requires community workers to consider particular issues and develop skills and knowledge which may not be needed when working in white communities. On this page Shahida Akhtar highlights some assumptions that need to be removed from our thinking in order that we can address particular issues before we even begin to make contact with people. Shahida then produces a checklist of good practice that we should be aiming to achieve.

MISTAKEN ASSUMPTIONS

- that Asian workers will sort out all the problems of Asian families and communities.

- that any Asian worker can work within all the Asian communities without appreciating the differences in language, culture, organisations.

- that all Asian families are the same, that they all have the same needs; group stereotyping without appreciating the differences between families based on background, class, history etc.

ISSUES

- of sexism operating to block the work of Asian Women workers; need for separate work and support networks.

- of different groups to meet different needs and the basis of these groupings.

- of organising appropriate support workers: e.g. in mixed groups you may need a Bengali speaking person as well as one fluent in Hindi/Urdu.

- of who to address when visiting a house; talking to the male initially and through him to the women.

- of how you present yourself; how you gain credibility and introduce your agency; how to let your personality come across.

- of not looking at issues in one way only; e.g. it is not just about providing transport to get people to a group but also people's concerns about the views of their neighbours/stigma of being picked up and taken to a group.

- of checking what services already exist; not making assumptions, to prevent duplication.

- being clear about your role and ways of working and checking other people's expectations of roles and work.

- of how to build supportive networks.

- of racism, and claims of racism, and the abuse of both of these, and how to distinguish and deal with them.

- of people not being willing to challenge or contribute within a group but to attack or undermine outside of the group; need to be very clear that it is safe to express their interests/ ideas in the group or else it will be too late once the meeting is over.

- of how to engage people who do not go to centres and will not answer the door; how can you pass on information to them?

CHECKLIST OF GOOD PRACTICE

- black people on panels for interview.

- white people willing to listen to black people.

- check dates of festivals/religious events/Ramadan.

- when home visiting: introduce yourself and your agency; explain purpose of visit; show an interest in children and family.

- smile at people; your personality to redress the power imbalances and to be seen as part of the group.

- when using interpreters or talking to people for whom English is not their first language, speak slowly and break up your speech into short sections.

- do not make promises you may not be able to keep; help people to be realistic about what can be achieved and when.

- invite all family members to meetings.

- give your contact number at the end of every meeting.

- accept hospitality but be clear about what you like and dislike.

- use local venues.

- to achieve quicker results work through existing groups, e.g. ask for 10 minutes at the end of a language class.

- use local gathering places: launderettes, school gates, grocery shops, video shops.

- find sympathetic shopkeepers who will display posters of meetings.

- negotiate with community representatives who see themselves as gatekeepers prior to setting up a new group.

SECTION:	**TACKLING INEQUALITIES**
TITLE:	**WORKING WITHIN ASIAN COMMUNITIES**
AUTHOR:	Shahida Akhtar

Calandars of festivals can be obtained from SHAP, the National Society's RE Centre, 23 Kensington Square, London W8 5HN.

Breaking New Ground, Community Development with Asian Communities, by Jean Ellis. Publisher CPF, 1989. ISBN 0 7199 1238 S.

- develop good relationships with centre co-ordinators and they can give you access to groups using the centre.

- co-work with other workers and projects; invite people to help with specific tasks and volunteer to do things for them which play to your strengths and expertise.

- childcare: consider whether you need a creche; can children be left with relatives? Otherwise hold the creche in the same room as the meeting and ask people to bring favourite toys.

- if you are providing refreshments: keep meat and vegetable dishes separate, don't mix up different flavoured crisps, or biscuits with and without animal fats, label food where necessary. Hindus and Sikhs are primarily vegetarian; Muslims avoid pork, ham and bacon; have fresh juices and water available. Be aware of fast days.

- make the group safe for people to be able to say what is important to them; make it clear you want their ideas during the meetings.

- use the skills and knowledge within the group to plan and organise activities; keep handing back the responsibility for the group to its members.

SECTION:	**TACKLING INEQUALITIES**
TITLE:	
AUTHOR:	

SECTION:	**TACKLING INEQUALITIES**
TITLE:	**WORKING WITH REFUGEE COMMUNITIES**
AUTHOR:	Christine Dixon

Britain is, or it should be, having signed the Human Rights Declaration, providing asylum for refugees. At the same time there is a state encouraged fortress attitude. The majority of refugees are completely disadvantaged by their situation with black and Asian refugees, women, children and the elderly carrying the additional burden of discrimination. Community development is essential as state provision is minimal and individual isolation and powerlessness the norm.

In considering work with refugee communities some or all of the following will have to be confronted:

- Experiences are beyond the experience and, probably, imagination of indigenous workers.

- Cultures are different and beyond knowledge.

- Workers don't know any other language but English.

- Ignorance of situation and country of origin in society generally and in other workers.

- Racism and other factors will block development opportunities and access to resources and funds ... and the help of community workers.

The following is a step by step approach to working with refugee communities:

(1) Find out if there are refugees in your area by contacting:

- your local council

- the Refugee Council

- the Home Office

- local voluntary organisations e.g. CABS

If there aren't any ask why.

(2) Find out where the refugees are from and inform yourself about the country of origin, the situation and history etc.

Sources include:

- The Refugee Council

- The Minority Rights Group

- Newspaper articles and periodicals e.g. Guardian, New Internationalist, Amnesty etc.

- TV documentaries

- Local library

(3) Offer help e.g. meeting place, photocopying, mailing etc.

(4) Provide information on how the system works locally.

(5) Campaign for an interpretation and translation service and for publicity to be produced in appropriate languages.

(6) Raise awareness of issues – e.g. Asylum bill. Experts can be invited from the Asylum Rights Campaign (ARC) and Refugee Organisations.

(7) Include refugee communities in community events and on mailing lists for meetings and conferences.

(8) Find out about national infrastructural support development – e.g. the Refugee Council are in the process of developing regional offices and refugee communities have national organisations – e.g. The Kurdish Cultural Centre and organisations offering specialist help such as The Refugee Support Centre.

(9) Encourage local voluntary and statutory organisations to put refugees on their agendas and develop policies.

(10) Assist and encourage communities in holding cultural/social events.

(11) Develop joint work with host communities, e.g. shared premises, playschemes, youth clubs.

(12) Make a service profile in an area and monitor use by refugees.

(13) Encourage links between different refugee communities.

USEFUL CONTACTS

1. The Refugee Council
   3/9 Bondway
   London, SW8 1SJ
   Tel. 0171-582 6922

2. The Refugee Support Centre
   King Georges House
   Stockwell Road
   London, SW9
   Tel. 0171-733 1482

3. The Kurdish Cultural Centre
   14 Stannary Street
   London, SE11 4AA
   Tel 0171-735 0918

4. Minority Rights Group
   379 Brixton Road
   London, SW9 7DE
   Tel. 0171-978 9498

SECTION:	**TACKLING INEQUALITIES**
TITLE:	**COMBATING RACISM**
AUTHOR:	Keith Popple

Definition:

Racism is a shorthand term for the theory that the world's population is divisible into unequal and hierarchical categories based on physical differences, particularly skin colour. The dominating powerful groups, who are largely white, impose their conceptions on the rest of the humanity.

Tackling Racism:

While we live in an unequal society which uses racism to divide and rule people, the black community will continue to experience mistreatment by institutions and individuals. Community workers with their commitment to a just, humane and more equal society have an important role to play in combatting racism in their work place and in the communities they serve.

In this section we suggest some strategies for tackling racism.

There is no single way of tackling racism. It demands commitment and the concerted use of different strategies by individuals, groups, communities and institutions over a long period in order to make an impact. Progress can appear slow and unrewarding, but the goal of a truly multi-racial, anti-racist society is one that liberates both black and white people.

The following are a number of ways of confronting racism:

1. Does your organisation have an active anti-racist policy that is continually monitored and if necessary revised after consultation? If it not, encourage the creation of one, perhaps using a model policy from an organisation that does have one. Consider the idea of appointing a suitably experienced consultant or trainer to help your organisation devise the policy ensuring that all members participate in its creation.

2. Don't abdicate from dealing with racism in your work. Work with others to think through and act upon racist attitudes and behaviour. Consider how you can both understand the experiences of white people living in the community you serve while working out how best to challenge racism. If you feel inexperienced in this aspect, ask to attend suitable training opportunities and offer to assist in the training of other members in your organisation.

3. Remember that racism is a problem for white society. It can arouse strong feelings among white people which need to be dealt with sensitively and effectively if you are to successfully continue the challenge of combating racism. Nothing is gained by initially condemning white people for being racist. Such an approach to tackling racism stems from the belief that racism resides within the individual rather than recognising that the individual is largely a product of a racist society.

4. Support black groups but be careful not to believe that means you need do less in combating racism in white dominated groups and communities. Similarly support black people in the organisation you work for but don't expect them to be "specialists" in anti-racist work. This is your task.

5. Be wary of multi-cultural approaches that do not recognise that black people experience racism. Multi-cultural approaches usually stop short of tackling racism preferring instead to emphasise the differences between people of different cultural groups, often focusing on the exotic and unusual.

SECTION:	TACKLING INEQUALITIES
TITLE:	COMBATING RACISM
AUTHOR:	Keith Popple

6. Be clear that racism is one powerful form of negatively separating and distinguishing people. Sexism is another way as is disablism and heterosexism. Recognise that theses forms of discrimination are separate but connected and making those connections with people leads to powerful alliances that can assist in changing peoples circumstances.

Institute of Race Relations:

  2 - 6 Leeke Street,
  London WC1X 9HS
  0171-837 0041

has a catalogue of useful books, posters and audio-visual material.

The Commission for Racial Equality:

  Elliott House, 10 - 12 Allington Street, London SW1E 5EH.

SECTION:	**TACKLING INEQUALITIES**
TITLE:	**WORKING WITH LESBIAN AND GAY GROUPS**
AUTHOR:	Val Lunn

Lesbians and gay men are estimated to be 1 in 10 of the population. This means that we are community workers, management committee members, community association members and city councillors. And of course we are a "community". But don't be surprised if your organisation is not working with lesbian and gay groups and doesn't even have a list of lesbian and gay groups in the area. The needs of lesbians and gay men are rarely acknowledged or considered by service providers in either the statutory or voluntary sector.

Lesbians and gay men have learnt that support from local government is unreliable and that the only organisation we can rely on is self organisation. Most lesbians and gay groups exist independently and are self funded. You only have to look as far back as the 1980s to see why. At the beginning of the eighties we saw some councils such as Haringay and Islington, not to mention the GLC, coming out in support of lesbians and gay men. They acknowledged heterosexism, the name given to the oppression of lesbians and gay men, gave funding to lesbian and gay groups, sent their workers on heterosexism awareness training and named lesbians and gay men in their equal opportunities policies. They encouraged lesbians and gay groups to form links with local government and raised expectations and hopes for permanent and radical changes. By the end of the eighties, the Local Government Act 1988 was introduced to prohibit the "promotion" of homosexuality by local authorities and there was an unprecedented backlash against the gay community which was viciously blamed for HIV and AIDS. Confused? Yes so were we.

On the whole lesbian and gay groups are not actively supported by community workers or encouraged to use community centres. Nor do they expect support from or make demands of community workers or community centres. And anyway, why should community workers be working with lesbians or gay men? Surely what people do in bed is their personal choice? Why do they think they're any different to anybody else? And if only they kept quiet about it instead of going on about it all the time nobody need know. Heard any of those? The attitude that being lesbian or gay is only about who you have sex with denies the extent to which heterosexism affects the daily lives of lesbian and gay men. Heterosexism shows itself in a whole range of ways, all of which exist to restrict and penalise lesbians and gay men and to remind us that we have stepped out of line. The reality is that what lesbians and gay men don in bed results in lesbians and gay men being sacked from their jobs, losing custody of their children, being prosecuted for so-called sexual offences for which there are no heterosexual equivalents, made homeless, beaten up and labelled mentally ill. Heterosexism undermines the principles of community work which are opposed to all forms of oppression and seeks to empower individuals, groups to communities so that they can influence change in ways desirable to themselves.

The other comment that I heard from community workers is that there is no visible need. But is there no visible need because you assume that everybody is heterosexual and you don't see lesbians and gay men? If that is your assumption, then the likelihood is that lesbians and gay men will not identify themselves because they will have decided that it probably isn't safe to identify themselves. And so we arrive back were we started ...... there's no visible need. If there are no "out" lesbians or gay men in your project, the likelihood is that it's not a safe project. And why should lesbians and gay men want to identify themselves? Because if they don't, you assume they're heterosexual and although lesbians and gay men have some needs in common with heterosexual members of the community, they also have different needs. It's also important to know that lesbians have needs that are different from the needs of gay men and that lesbians and gay men are also black, white, Jewish, Irish, young, old, parents, non-parents, are disabled, working class, middle class, unemployed and all the other different aspects of our lives and have needs that are not just based on our sexuality. Community workers need to be asking themselves whether they respect the right of an individual to a sexuality that is not heterosexual. Do you value the specific experiences, perspectives and contributions that lesbians and gay men and bisexuals bring with them? Acknowledging, accepting, valuing and respecting difference is at the heart of anti-oppressive practice.

Although the repercussions for being out and visible can be high risk and dangerous, increasing numbers of lesbians and gay men take pride in who we are, refuse to live our lives in the closet and want to participate fully and actively in our local communities.

The following ideas can be used by community workers and management committee members/community association members who want to acknowledge lesbians and gay men in the community and begin to look at ways of providing a service to them.

1. It's worth beginning by checking out basics.

*   Does your organisation acknowledge lesbians and gay men as workers or service users?

*   Is there ever any discussion in your organisation about lesbian and gay men or current issues affecting their lives?

*   Do you know what the current issues are? The Pink Paper, a free national weekly newspaper for lesbians and gay men is available from most radical bookshops or on subscription.

*   Are lesbians and gay men included in your equal opportunities policy (if you have one)?

*   Is the harassment of lesbians and gay men a disciplinary offence?

*   Do you advertise your services to lesbian and gay men?

*   Do you promote and publicise positive images of lesbian and gay men, (an organisation called Pop Against Homophobia has produced a series of positive image posters.)

It is vital that you don't set lesbians and gay men up to fail. If the reality is that your organisation cannot provide a safe environment for lesbians and gay men, then perhaps you should be looking at supporting separate provision for lesbian and gay groups. The Community Support Team in Nottingham, for example, worked with a group of lesbians and gay men to obtain funding for a lesbian and gay community centre.

2.   Whether the answer to all or any of the questions above is yes or no, attempting to work on an intellectual level alone will rarely be enough. Even if your organisation has a progressive or radical understanding of oppression and/or an equal opportunities policy that names lesbian and gay men, this does not necessarily mean that it will want to actively and openly support or work with lesbian and gay groups. Myths and stereotypes about lesbians and gay men, and arguments about why you shouldn't be working with lesbian and gay groups will surface again and again. What you may be taking on is a long process of awareness raising in your team, your management committee/community association, amongst your user groups. Most of the heterosexual community workers I spoke to didn't feel well enough informed themselves to do this. Convincing your employers of the need for heterosexism awareness training, particularly if your employer is a local authority may be tricky but not impossible. Training may also be available from other sources. In response to a training needs questionnaire sent out to community workers in and around Nottingham, Nottingham Community Work Training Group is organising Lesbian, Gay and Bisexual awareness training for local community workers. To check out your Local Community Work Training Group phone the Federation of Community Work Training Groups.

The names of heterosexism awareness/anti-heterosexism/bisexuality awareness trainers may be available from your local Council for Voluntary Services office, Lesbian Line or Gay Switchboard. By the way, be prepared to reassure people who think heterosexism awareness training means that your trying to eradicate heterosexuality.

3.   It's important to think carefully about what is and isn't achievable and to consult lesbians and gay men to make sure that your work is based on need and prioritises individual safety. There's not much point, for example, in setting up a local group for lesbian mothers if when they go home, they get a brick through their window because there's been no awareness raising in the community. One community centre I know began by organising lesbian and gay social events that were advertised city wide. The community centre gained a reputation for being lesbian and gay friendly without risking the safety of local lesbians and gay men.

4.   It's important to be informed about what section 28 of the Local Government Act 1988 says and doesn't say. It applies only to local authorities and states that local authorities should not:

a)   intentionally promote homosexuality or publish material with the intention of promoting homosexuality.

b)   promote the teaching in any maintained school of the acceptability of homosexuality as a pretended family relationship.

Although section 28 has never been tested in law, it has been used extensively by local authorities to justify censorship and discrimination. Until section 28 has been tested in the courts, we must rely on legal opinion as to what "promote" means. Lord Gifford concluded that "promote" means that local authorities are actively trying to persuade individuals to become homosexual or experiment with homosexuality. It is not unlawful for organisations to give advice and assistance to lesbians and gay men, provide and support services to lesbians and gay men and discourage discrimination against lesbians and gay men on the grounds of their sexuality. For more information about section 28 contact the civil rights organisation, Liberty.

5.   One of the ways being lesbian or gay differs from other oppressions is that it's not always obvious who is lesbian or gay. It's important not to make any assumptions about people's sexuality. It is easy to assume that because nobody has chosen to identify themselves as lesbian or gay, that there are no lesbians or gay men already working in or using your project. Asking a woman, for example, if she's got a boyfriend or a husband is a sure tell-tale sign of heterosexism at work. It's also important to recognise that some lesbians and gay men will find it more difficult to be open about their sexuality. Black lesbians and gay men who are constantly confronted by racism may find the discrimination against them compounded if they are open about their sexuality. Lesbian and gay parents may risk losing custody of their children. Lesbians and gay men who choose to be "out" are likely to be abused and harassed unless there is a clear, stated and working commitment to challenging homophobia, the name given to anti-lesbian and gay attitudes and behaviour.

Finally, and perhaps most obviously, consult the local lesbian and gay community. Find out what they want. To get a list of local lesbian and gay groups contact Lesbian Line or Gay Switchboard. Their phone numbers are usually in the local phone directories.

Liberty
0171 403 3888

Federation of Community Work Training Groups
256 Glossop Road, Sheffield
0114 273 9391

The Pink Paper
0171 608 3053

Pop Against Homophobia
0171 323 0180

National Association of Councils for Voluntary Service
3rd Floor, Arundel Court, 177 Arundel Street, Sheffield S1 2NU
0114 278 6636

SECTION:	**TACKLING INEQUALITIES**
TITLE:	**PUTTING BI-SEXUALITY ON THE COMMUNITY WORK MAP**
AUTHOR:	Rick Gray, Jo Eadie, Alix Marina

People who are seen to be attracted to their own sex are assumed to be lesbian or gay. People who are seen to be attracted to the other sex are assumed to be heterosexual. This assumption is made because we have all been brought up to believe that we are only attracted to either men, or women (this is called monosexuality, which means "attracted to one sex"). When someone does have feelings for people of both sexes they are expected to grow out of it and choose one or the other.

This is not the case. Many people experience attraction for both men and women in the course of their lives. Sometimes at the same time, sometimes at different times. This double attraction is called bisexuality (meaning, "attracted to both sexes"). For the most part bisexuality is either ignored, trivialised or confused with homosexuality. It is common for the needs of bisexual people to be seen as the same as lesbians and gay men, so that, for instance, bisexual people are referred to lesbian/gay organisations which may not be sympathetic to them.

Being bisexual does not necessarily mean that someone has relationships with both men and women in the course of their lives, nor does it mean that someone has relationships with men and women simultaneously (although that's quite possible). It just means being attracted to both women and men, and this can translate into many different ways of living and loving.

It is important to recognise that:

1. Bisexuality is a sexuality in its own right.
2. People's sexuality is not fixed, and can change in many ways, including which sex you are attracted to.
3. A person's sexuality is generally reduced to who they sleep with, but their is much more to it. For example, somebody who has relationships with men can find women attractive as well – or may even find women more attractive!

One way of gaining an accurate picture of the complexity of sexuality is to complete the questionnaire which is used in Bisexuality Awareness Training. It can be used by individuals or by groups to raise awareness and challenge limiting beliefs. This has been adapted from a grid designed by Fritz Klein, an American psychologist, in 1980.

An Adaptation of the 'Klein Orientation Grid'

	What has it been? *past*	What is it now? *present*	What would you like it to be? *ideal*
Sexual Attraction: Who do you have sexual feelings for?			
Emotional Involvement: Who do you love and care for?			
Sexual Behaviour: Who do you have sex with?			
Sexual Fantasies: Who do you fantasise about?			
Social Preferences: Who do you share your social time with?			
Aesthetic Appreciation: Who do you find beautiful?			
Closest Person: Who is closest to you?			
Sexual Identity: How do you describe your sexuality?			
Lifestyle: What cultures/communities do you live in?			
Political Identity: Where are your alliances?			

(See Fig. 1 — rows Sexual Attraction through Closest Person; See Fig. 2 — rows Sexual Identity through Political Identity)

Fig. 1

1	2	3	4	5	6	7
other sex only	other sex mostly	other sex some- what more	both sexes equally	same sex some- what more same sex	mostly same sex	only

Fig. 2

1	2	3	4	5	6	7
hetero only	hetero mostly	hetero somewhat more	hetero/ gay/ lesbian equally	gay/ lesbian somewhat more	gay/ lesbian mostly	gay/ lesbian only

SECTION:	TACKLING INEQUALITIES
TITLE:	PUTTING BI-SEXUALITY ON THE COMMUNITY WORK MAP
AUTHOR:	Rick Gray, Jo Eadie, Alix Marina

1.   Points to make about the grid

This questionnaire is designed to raise awareness in people who have up to now only seen themselves, and others, as either heterosexual or lesbian/gay, which is why bisexuality does not appear on the scales.

2.   The questionnaire enables people to address the variance in their own sexuality, as well as seeing the sexuality of others less rigidly. There are no right or wrong answers, and what you score does not prove that you are "really" bisexual, heterosexual, or lesbian/gay. It enables people to accept all the differences within themselves, without having to organise all parts of themselves so as to fit together in a monosexual way. e.g. just because a man only sleeps with other men it doesn't follow that he has to call himself gay – and conversely, just because a man calls himself gay it doesn't mean he only sleeps with other men!

FURTHER READING:

"Bisexual Lives": Off Pink Publishing Collective (Off Pink, UK, 1988). A collection of life stories by bisexual people - eye opening and inspiring.

"Two Lives to Lead - bisexuality in men and women": ed. Fritz Klein and Timothy Wolf (Harrington Park Press, USA, 1985). A collection of psychological and sociological essays, aimed mainly at professionals.

"Bi Any Other Name": ed. Loraine Hutchins and Lani Kaahumanu (Alyson Publications, USA 1991). A very large collection of life stories, political theory, psychology. Very powerful.

"Bisexuality - a reader and source book": ed. Thomas Geller (Times Change Press, USA 1990). A mixture of academic essays, poems, life stories and news reports.

"Closer to Home - bisexuality and feminism": ed. Elizabeth Reba Weise (The Seal Press, USA, 1992). The latest, and most exciting, wave of the bisexual revolution.

Contacts:

Bifrost is a national bisexual magazine/ newsletter, available from:
Bifrost, PO BOX 117,
Norwich NR1 2SU.

The National Bisexuality Phoneline:
7.30 - 9.30 pm

0131 557 3620 Thursday

0181 569 7500 Tuesday and Wednesday

Both organisations have full listings of local and national bisexual support and social groups.

SECTION:	**TACKLING INEQUALITIES**
TITLE:	**PUTTING BI-SEXUALITY ON THE COMMUNITY WORK MAP**
AUTHOR:	Rick Gray, Jo Eadie, Alix Marina

Bisexuality is threatening to clear-cut monosexual beliefs, and hence stereotyping has been used as a way of making bisexuality seem dangerous, unimportant, or invisible. This section outlines the most common prejudices around, along with some possible responses:

COMMON ASSUMPTIONS – AND WAYS OF COUNTERING THEM

BISEXUALS ARE...

- Sitting on the fence, confused, undecided, really gay, really straight, closet gays, going through a phase, just being trendy.

- Promiscuous, unable to have long-term relationships, unfaithful, unreliable, never monogamous, never celibate, always going to leave you for someone else.

- An HIV risk.

RESPONSE

- Bisexuality is a sexuality in its own right.

- None of these are a question of a person's sexuality. Anyone can behave in any of these ways. Bisexual people, like anyone else, can choose to be celibate, monogamous, in a long term relationship – or not!

- The risk of contracting HIV from someone you have sex with depends on how safe your sexual activities are. What that person's sexuality is has nothing to do with it.

Community work is concerned with being responsive to the needs of all different groups. The needs of bisexual people have to be taken seriously. You may not think that in your work you come into contact with bisexual people, but it's almost certain that you do.

RECOGNISING THE NEEDS OF BISEXUALS INVOLVES:

1. Acknowledging the existence and validity of this sexuality, and acknowledging that there is oppression directed towards people who are bisexual.

2. Being aware of individual prejudices – both your own and others – and institutional discrimination, and challenging them.

3. Getting informed on the realities of bisexual lives.

4. Finding out and making available information about bi groups, phonelines, publications, films etc.

5. Encouraging openness and discussion of the issues.

6. Making contact with local and national bisexual organisations.

You may have only seen a part of the lives of co-workers, clients, carers, and friends. Assume nothing.

SECTION:	**TACKLING INEQUALITIES**
TITLE:	**PUTTING BI-SEXUALITY ON THE COMMUNITY WORK MAP**
AUTHOR:	Rick Gray, Jo Eadie, Alix Marina

SECTION:	**TACKLING INEQUALITIES**
TITLE:	**THE LANGUAGE OF DISABILITY**
AUTHOR:	Val Harris

For people who are trying to ensure that good equal opportunity practice takes place it can be difficult to keep up with acceptable terminology, but for people who are often discriminated against it can also be very offensive and/or upsetting to be labelled in a way that they do not feel is acceptable.

The list suggests some of the acceptable and unacceptable terms that exist in our everyday language – at this point in time. Language is always changing as people describe themselves in different ways and no list will remain acceptable and up to date for long, it is important that we keep listening to how people describe themselves and take our cues from them. These suggestions reflect the definition of disability created by disabled peoples organisations:

> "The disadvantage or restriction of activity caused by a contemporary social organisation which takes little or no account of people who have impairments and thus excludes them from participation in the mainstream of social activities."

ACCEPTABLE:

Disabled People, this is preferred by some people because society disables people by the way it is organised and designed.

Physical/Sensory Impairment, this is used to refer to a condition, rather than the above which is about the social context.

Service User, this is a phrase that can be used for any person with a disability who uses a service, rather than a client.

Wheel Chair User, this is more factual than wheel chair bound.

Down's Syndrome, is preferred to Mongolism.

Hearing Impaired, some people, particularly those who are not completely deaf, prefer the phrase. However there isn't total agreement – those who have a high degree of hearing loss may prefer to be called Deaf, as they are proud to be who they are and see no stigma attached to it.

People with learning disabilities or **learning disable people**, replaces terms such as mentally handicapped, educationally subnormal.

UNACCEPTABLE:

The Disabled, this makes people sound like an object, and as if they are all identical.

Handicapped, this term has doubtful origins, but certainly became attached to the stigma of people who can only live off charity (with cap in hand!).

Special Needs, this term is part of the Victim Blaming Mode – people with disabilities have no special needs but society has needs if it is to accommodate them and benefit from their presence, e.g. A building's need for a lift.

Invalid, or In-valid! This term invalidates people.

Mentally Handicapped, this has become attached to the stigma of the institutionalisation and degradation these people have suffered (both historically and in the present).

Wheelchair Bound, how many people do you know who are tied up to their wheelchairs? For many people their wheelchair is their means to freedom rather than their prison.

Disabled Toilet, would you like to sit on a disabled toilet? If the toilet is fully functional call it an accessible toilet!

SECTION:	**TACKLING INEQUALITIES**
TITLE:	
AUTHOR:	

SECTION:	**TACKLING INEQUALITIES**
TITLE:	**WORKING ON DISABILITY ISSUES**
AUTHOR:	Alison Gilchrist

The community work approach to disability issues generally adopts the social model of disability, which argues that people with impaired, different or under-developed bodily and/or mental functions are prevented by society from achieving their individual potential and from participating as equal citizens in many democratic, cultural, recreational, educational and economic activities. This results in inequalities in opportunity and marginalisation for many disabled people, which are determined by the structure of our society, rather than the impairments of individuals.

Work on disability issues is concerned to challenge those policies, procedures, practices and prejudices which discriminate against disabled people. This will involve supporting disabled people to organise and advocate for themselves, and also tackling the obstacles which make this difficult. A parallel strategy will be to encourage and assist the integration of disabled people into mainstream activities.

Key words in this area are that disabled people should be guaranteed rights to choose from the same range of options that are available to non-disabled people, and they should be able to articulate and implement that choice with dignity and as autonomous individuals. As in all areas of work, the core principles of empowerment, participation and access apply so that disabled peoples are involved in all aspects of decision-making and carry out the chosen strategy.

Disable people are increasingly organising their own campaigns, services and support groups, based on principles of self-determination and self-advocacy. Disabled people expect to be consulted on a collective basis about policies and to manage resources that are available for their use. Disabled people seek to challenge the restrictions and stereotyping that many experience resulting in segregation and isolation. Through self-advocacy and the support of non-disabled allies, an approach is promoted which encourages integration, equal participation and the celebration of difference.

In order to achieve these aims, the community worker involved with disabled people must ensure that access issues are fully addressed and properly resourced. Positive action measures which improve access and conditions for disabled people almost invariably makes things easier for non-disabled people as well.

Access doesn't just mean whether or not you can get a wheelchair into a room. It refers to communication and understanding, making sure people have access to the information they need, time and needs to reflect, discuss with others and contribute to debate on own terms. This may mean the provision of hearing induction loops, BSL interpreters, Braille, large print, and using simple language, signs and diagrams, personal assistants and note takers.

Access issues also apply to the personal comfort of participants and the facilitation of informal group processes, making sure that toilets are near and can be used with dignity and privacy, that refreshments include any special dietary requirements, that the facilities are user-friendly and that trained (and paid) personal assistants are available for anyone attending the event or activity. Meetings should include regular breaks, allow sufficient time for interpreting of all items, and should be non-smoking. Distractions and background noise should be kept to a minimum if people need to concentrate.

Transport to and from events should provided either through taxis or accessible minibuses. Expenses should be paid immediately and so expense forms and petty cash must be available at the meeting.

Often, the barriers that prevent or deter disabled people from participating fully in activities or discussions are in the minds of non-disabled people. Patronising or pitying attitudes focus only on the labels of impairment or mental illness and can result in further marginalisation and disempowerment of disabled people. Disability equality training is a means to explore these prejudices and assumptions and ensure that joint activities take place in a spirit of equal partnership and participation. Challenging disablist language is an important aspect of this process of raising awareness amongst non-disabled allies and policy makers.

Disability Equality Training Trainers' Guide:

K. Gillespie-Sells & J. Campbell

Published by CCETSW/The London Boroughs' Disability Resources Team.

1991 ISBN 09044 88 896.

Available from:

CCETSW, Derbyshire House,
St. Chad Street, London WC1 8AD

SECTION:	**TACKLING INEQUALITIES**
TITLE:	**EMPLOYING WOMEN IN VOLUNTARY ORGANISATIONS**
AUTHOR:	adapted from NCVS' Women's Contribution to the Voluntary Sector

The Voluntary Sector benefits from women's contribution, as paid and unpaid workers.

If organisations are to retain, and benefit from, the many skills and amount of energy women bring with them, good working conditions are essential. There are many forms of discrimination that women workers have to face. This section contains a checklist to the key questions that employers should address if they are to meet the needs of their women workers, and particularly the needs of black women, women with dependents, lesbians and disabled women.

Women make up nearly half the workforce of this country - yet they are to found mainly in the lower paid occupations and low grades. Their skills, knowledge and expertise are often not valued or utilised to the full. Women often find themselves trapped into part time and low paid jobs which take account of their caring responsibilities. All the studies show that women still provide the bulk of community care and child care in this country.

Despite all the legislation and a growing awareness of women's contribution to the economy of this country, women still find themselves discriminated against in many ways. They have often been disadvantaged against by the education system which has not allowed them to fulfill their potential, they may have had less encouragement and opportunity to continue with their education after the minimum school leaving age. They may find it hard to return to work after caring for children, to find a job that will utilise their talents and allow them to combine work with caring.

Once in work women can be subjected to sexual harassment, find it difficult to get promoted into senior, managerial or executive posts. They find themselves disadvantaged over wage levels, pension rights and holiday entitlements.

Women's Contribution to the Voluntary Sector by Val Harris is available from Nottingham CVS, tel (0115) 947 6714.

The following questions may help you in examining your current policies and practices.

SELECTION, RECRUITMENT AND PROMOTION

- Do you have any policies and practices that discriminate against women? e.g. do you only appoint men to management or senior positions? Or expect staff to be mobile when in reality they rarely have to travel away?

- Do you have job descriptions and specifications which are non discriminatory?

- Are you only asking for the essential qualifications and experience? Are life experiences seen as valid?

- Does your application form only ask for relevant information? You do not need to know people's ages or marital status for example.

- Do you advertise where women will see the posts? e.g. clinics, libraries, surgeries, community centres.

- Do you have a balanced shortlisting and selection panel? Of black and white people, male and female, and people with differing abilities.

- Do you provide training in equal opportunities for people involved in your selection and recruitment?

- Do you ask all applicants the same questions? Do these relate directly to the job on offer, and not to women's other commitments?

- Do you have a monitoring procedure to check who applies and who gets the jobs?

- Do you have an appeals procedure for people not satisfied with your decision?

WOMEN AND CARING RESPONSIBILITIES

- Do you offer all your posts for job sharing? Most jobs are suitable for job sharing, there are very few that are not.

- Do you recognise and respect your part time workers skills and expertise? Are they treated the same as other members of staff? Do they have decent pay and conditions?

- Do your working hours take into account school/nursery hours, public transport (especially within and to and from rural areas)?

- Do you offer a flexi-time system? Do the core hours allow for caring responsibilities?

- Do you give plenty of notice of changes in working hours, especially if you expect staff to occasionally work weekends and evenings?

- Do you offer career breaks to allow parents to spend time with their young children? The EC recommends up to 3 months during a child's first 2 years.

- Do you allow returners from maternity leave or career breaks to come back to the same job or one with a similar salary and responsibility?

- Do you allow time off for sick dependants? Different organisations have policies on this which vary from 3 – 15 days a year paid, plus other time unpaid.

- If a worker wants to save up their leave to take it in one long period, do you limit the qualifying period for longer leave periods to the same as the annual leave?

- Do you give free choice over when leave can be taken, is there any problem with taking leave during the school holidays?

- Do you know the legal requirements for maternity leave and pay, or where to find out?

- Do you offer improvements to the minimal state maternity leave scheme?

RETURNERS TO WORK

- Do you ever have temporary work which can give some women returners an opportunity to get back to work and gain confidence?

- Do you offer temporary staff the same conditions as other staff?

- Do you provide training opportunities for women to update their knowledge and skills when they return? Will this training be designed to meet their specific needs?

- Do you offer a phased return to work after maternity leave?

- Do you count maternity leave as continuous service for holiday entitlements, pensions and increments?

USEFUL PUBLICATIONS

"Code of Good Practice in the Employment of Disabled People" T.E.E.D., Moorfoot, Sheffield S1 4PQ.

"Equality at Work" E.O.C..

"Equality in Practice - a guide to equal opportunities" (pack of leaflets). Sinnata, Barashad Sheffield Non-Statutory Co-ordinating Group, 1990.

"Equal Opportunities and Childcare" TGWU, 1989.

"Equal Opportunities Employment Policies" North Kensington Law Centre, 74 Golbourne Road, London W10, 1989.

"Equal Opportunities in Voluntary Organisations" Reading List 2, NCVO, 1990.

Equal Pay Act 1970, amended 1983, HMSO.

"Equal Pay for Work of Equal Value - A Guide to the Amended Equal Pay Act" E.O.C..

"Guidelines for Equal Opportunities Employers" E.O.C., 1989.

"How Equal are your Opportunities; a guide for working parents" NALGO, 1989.

"Implementing an Equal Opportunities Policy" CVSNA, 1987.

"Indirect Discrimination" Byre A, E.O.C., 1987.

"Job Evaluation Schemes Free of Sex Bias" E.O.C..

"Job Sharing - Improving the Quality and Availability of Part-time Work" E.O.C., 1981.

"Monitoring an Equal Opportunities Policy – A Guide for Employers" Commission for Racial Equality, 1984.

NALGO Negotiating Guidelines; Job Sharing.

NALGO Negotiating Guidelines; Part-time work.

"Part-time Workers; TUC Factsheet" TUC.

SECTION:	**TACKLING INEQUALITIES**
TITLE:	**EMPLOYING WOMEN IN VOLUNTARY ORGANISATIONS**
AUTHOR:	adapted from NCVS' Women's Contribution to the Voluntary Sector

"Positive Action and Equal Opportunity in Employment" Commission for Racial Equality, 1985.

"Positive Action – Equal Opportunities for Women in Employment – A Guide" The Commission of the European Communities. Directorate – General Employment, Social Affairs and Education. HMSO 9282574008.

"Pregnancy and Maternity" TUC Factsheet, TUC.

"Priority for Equality" Local Government Information Unit, 1991.

Sex Discrimination Act 1975, 1986, HMSO.

"Sex Discrimination Act and Advertising" E.O.C., 1986.

"Sex Discrimination in Redundancy Payments" LACSAB, 41 Belgrave Square, London SW1 8NZ, 1986.

"Sexism, Sexual Stereotyping and Women Volunteers" Advance, 1985.

"Sharing, Caring – Caring, Equal Opportunities and The Voluntary Sector" Thompson C. NCVO, 1985.

"So You Think You've Got it Right?" E.O.C., 1983.

"TUC Charter for Women at Work" TUC, 1990.

"TUC Guide to the Employment of Disabled People" TUC, 1989.

"Trades Unions Working for Equality; a Resource List" TUC, 1989.

Many local authorities have guidelines on sexual harassment and racial harassment; several have prepared reports on violence within the workplace; a detailed list is provided in "Responding with Authority", National Association of Local Government Women's Committees, 1991.

EMPLOYMENT POLICIES AND PRACTICES

- Do you offer the same pay and holidays to men and women?

- Do you have a working and effective equal opportunities policy?

- Does it have a section on sexual harassment, which supports and protects the victims? For example do you accept the woman's account and then investigate it fully, do you suspend the alleged perpetrator rather than the victim while you investigate?

- Does the sexual harassment policy cover lesbians and disabled women, who are often on the receiving end of sexual harassment?

- Do you have policies to deal with racial harassment?

- Do you provide facilities for disabled women? For example is your building accessible? Do you make the most of grants available for adaptations and equipment for staff with disabilities?

- Do you have policies and procedures to protect staff who might face violence or aggression in their work? For example do you provide self-defence training, allow joint visits, have booking out systems that are checked regularly? Do you try and ensure that the access to the building is well lit?

- Do you have good health and safety policies which protect pregnant women, Visual Display Unit (VDU) users, and keyboard users from Repetitive Strain Injury (RSI)?

- Do you provide training and guidance on such potential problems and ways of reducing stress?

- Do you provide access to training opportunities, and offer secondments for qualifying and longer courses?

- Do you provide no smoking areas?

- Does your pension fund discriminate against women, can part-timers join? Does it allow for additional voluntary payments?

- Do you review/appraise your staff and provide them with opportunities for training and personal development?

- Do you ensure that training is geared to the needs of women, caters for part-timers, breaks down traditional job barriers?

- Can you provide workplace creches?

- Do you pay childcare, or other caring expenses, if staff have to work at different times than their usual hours? For example working longer hours, evenings or their days off?

- Do you ensure that part time workers do not lose out on holiday entitlements because they normally do not work on traditional bank holidays?

- Do you expect women to undertake stereotyped roles that are not included in their job descriptions? Preparing food for lunches, making drinks, washing up etc?

USEFUL CONTACTS

National:

Equal Opportunities Commission, Overseas House, Quay Street, Manchester, M3 3HN, 061 833 9244.

HMSO, St. Crispin's, Dukes Street, Norwich, NR3 1PD, 0171 873 0011 / 0121 643 3740.

Labour Research Department, 78 Blackfriars Road, London, SE1 8HF, 0171 928 3649.

Liberty (NCCL), 21 Tabard Street, London, SE1 4LA, 0171 403 3888.

NALGO, 1 Mabledon Place, London, WC1H 9AJ, 0171 388 2366.

New Ways to Work, 309 Upper Street, London, N1 2TY, 0181 226 4026.

NIACE/REPLAN, 47 New Walk, Leicester, LE1 6TE, 0116 255 0798.

TUC Equal Rights Department and TUC Publications, Congress House, Great Russell Street, London, WC1B 3LS. Factsheets are free with a SAE; publication list available, 0171 636 4030.

Transport and General Workers Union, Transport House, Smith Square, London, SW1P 3JB, 0171 828 7788.

WASH (Women Against Sexual Harassment), 242 Pentonville Road, London, N1 9UN, 0171 833 0222.

Working with older people raises two important matters that must be borne in mind. The first is ageism and the second may seem contradictory but concerns the physical factors that often accompany old age.

Ageism is a poorly recognised form of oppression. It is just as insidious and patronising as sexism and racism. We tend to talk about old people behaving in a certain manner or having "funny little ways". We tend to talk about them in the third person plural although it's quite likely that we shall all be there one day. One phrase that is particularly indicative of ageism is "they get like that, don't they?".

The Language of Ageing

A European survey in 1991 * showed that there was no clear consensus from older people on how they should be addresed. Across Europe the majority were split between senior citizens and older people, with a clean rejection of the term "elderly" or anything to do with golden age/years. In the U.K. there some reaction to any connotation of oldness, which was shared by Denmark but not the rest of Europe. Age Concern tends to use the term "older people" and caution that pensioner organisations may well give a different answer. The main point is to listen to how people define themselves.

Age & Attitude – E.C. Survey 1991. Details available from Age Concern England, Astral House, 1268 London Road, London SW16 4ER. Telephone: 0181 679 8000. Fax: 0181 679 6069.

The "over 60s" are not an homogenous group. There will be different generations within that group, different races, cultures, genders, levels of educational attainment, sexual orientations, levels of mobility and physical ability. A liking for bingo and first world war songs doesn't come with the first pension book. It's also worth remembering that old people still make mistakes and making allowances for them can be very patronising.

It needs to be borne in mind that certain physical characteristics are statistically more common in older people and these need catering for if older people are to be made welcome in your organisation.

Think about the accessibility of your premises and your toilet facilities, about induction loops and information provided in large print. There are less car owners in the older age groups and most councils provide bus passes so think about holding meetings, events, etc., on bus routes. Media scares about pensioners being attacked have also caused some people to be nervous about being out after dark so any event planned for an evening may create problems.

Attitudes can also be a problem. Older people may feel excluded if their views are never listened to or they are patronised or always expected to make the tea. In fact, pensioners and those who have already retired are a valuable resource to any voluntary organisation in terms of time, experience and energy. If you have an age limit for volunteers or paid workers in your organisation, maybe you should think about whether it is really relevant.

Ideas for attracting older people include posters in post offices, doctors' surgeries, halls and building where pensioners' groups meet.

Asking to speak at a pensioners' Action Group Meeting or at a pensioners' group. Seeing if the local Age Concern has a local newsletter or mailing that you may be able to put an item in.

Check which of the national pensioners' organisations have newspapers because they may be worth advertising in.

SECTION:	**TACKLING INEQUALITIES**
TITLE:	
AUTHOR:	

SECTION 6

EMPOWERMENT AND PARTICIPATION

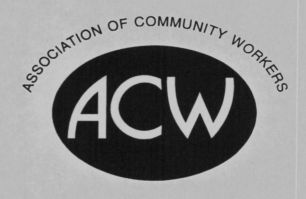

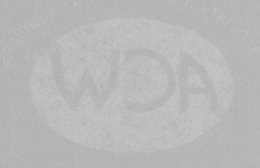

SECTION:	**EMPOWERMENT AND PARTICIPATION**
TITLE:	**EMPOWERMENT**
AUTHOR:	Alison Gilchrist and Peter Durrant

Two contributions discuss the notion of empowerment as it as it applies to community work.

Alison Gilchrist outlines some of the key principles which underline the understanding of empowerment as a concept whilst Pete Durrant warns us against the over use of the word and the suggests some practical ways that community workers can transfer power to those they are supporting.

ADDRESSES

Nottingham Advocacy Groups
9a Forest Road East
Nottingham
NG1 4HT

British Council Of Disabled People
Litchurch Plaza
Litchurch Lane
Derby
DE24 8AA
Tel: (01332) 295551
Fax: (01332) 295580

Empowerment is generally viewed as a fundamental principle in community work, and many related fields of professional work with people which aim to promote growth and responsibility. It is also increasingly mentioned by politicians (especially those on the left) as an important aspect of the processes of political change.

The ideology of empowerment is complex, and the motivations of those promoting it will vary depending on the political outlook of the person or agency. For example, a conservative approach, using a consensus model of society, might promote empowerment of people in order to achieve notions of individual freedom and "self-help" forms of service delivery. Whilst, a radical ideology, based on a conflict model, would see empowerment as a means to mobilize disadvantaged people to make greater demands on the state and a re-distribution in the allocation of resources. In between these lie ideas around pluralist aims of consultation and the active citizen.

The process of empowerment can operate at several different levels

- the individual

- the group

- sections of society or communities of identity

- institutions

In order to understand what level is most appropriate or likely to be most effective, it is important to analyse what factors are currently influencing the decisions which affect people's lives. This will affect the mechanisms of empowerment, which might be psychological, social, economic or political. Some examples may help illustrate these different approaches:

PSYCHOLOGICAL: increasing confidence, skills and knowledge.

SOCIAL: promoting a more diverse and tolerant culture in which prejudices and discriminatory behaviour are challenged.

ECONOMIC: a re-allocation of resources (e.g. increased funding), or the encouraging of withdrawal of labour or money (e.g. rent or labour strikes).

POLITICAL: changes in policy, increased representation or consultation, access to decision-making and information.

Community workers need to think carefully about what is often an over-used term. Can we really "empower" people in the sense that we are prepared, or able, to deliberately transfer all, or some of our own (and others) power and resources? For people employed in local authority, voluntary sector and independent settings it should, nonetheless, always be a central issue. What are the actual ways through which we might demonstrate to people on the receiving ends of often complex services that the transfer of power is possible? Some routes might include:

(a)   Publishing, in as open and direct a way as possible, why, and how your organisation functions. As part of this approach it's important to think out the values on which the, hopefully, helping approach is based. Include descriptions of gaps and problems and ways in which cooperative structures can be explored and consolidated.

(b)   Working on ways through which users should have as much access as they require to YOUR working territory. Empowerment will only come about if we're prepared to develop reciprocal structures. This isn't to say that, sometimes, in the interest of protecting others some confidences do not need to be kept. What it does say is that, in general, written and private opinions about "consumers" are examples of NOT empowering people. Learning how to be straight with ourselves and the people we're working WITH, as opposed to FOR, is how we should all be learning how to be consciously devolve our existing power structures.

(c)   Ensuring that everyone contributes to decision-making and policy information. Some examples of how this can be achieved are through primary and secondary cooperatives; and Cooperative Development Agencies through the country are facilitating this approach. Credit Unions, or community banks, help us all to pool our resources and save, and borrow, money at advantageous rates whilst strengthening neighbourhoods. For people who are recovering from mental ill health, user involvement groups licence people to reinforce their rights to be involved in whatever the helping strategy will be. The Nottingham Advocacy Group is perhaps the best established user participation and involvement group within the field of mental health. Whilst the coalition movement aims to act as a forum for debate, analysis and expression of opinion on all issues relating to physically disabled people.

SECTION:	**EMPOWERMENT AND PARTICIPATION**
TITLE:	**EMPOWERMENT**
AUTHOR:	Alison Gilchrist and Peter Durrant

What these and other groups have in common is that they are committed to sharing and consolidating the principle that everyone should have the right to a more or less equal share in. the administration an development of the organisation. Their obvious advantage over statutory groups is that they have an investment in sharing and equalising power from the beginning.

For community workers and activists the sharing and transfer of power is an essential method of working. This well demonstrated and researched style of work leads to more democratic structures and means that EVERYONE has the option of participating and sharing accountability; that EVERYONE has the option of agreeing, or disagreeing, in the important matters which affect our well-being. If we retain influence and power for ourselves there is no way in which corporate discussion and action can be effectively achieved.

One of the tests of the nineties for community work is to see how well we can translate intellectual acceptance of ideas, which are often more talk than action, into projects that offer an enhanced role for consumers and lead to better services which are more sensitive to all of our needs.

SECTION:	**EMPOWERMENT AND PARTICIPATION**
TITLE:	
AUTHOR:	

SECTION 7

GETTING TO KNOW A COMMUNITY

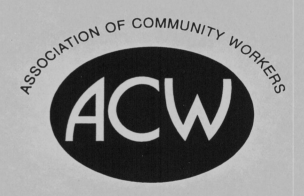

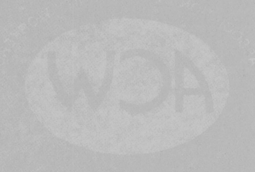

SECTION:	**GETTING TO KNOW A COMMUNITY**
TITLE:	**AIMS AND ISSUES**
AUTHOR:	Alison Gilchrist, Roger Green

Before embarking on any kind of community work strategy it is vital to build up an accurate picture of how a community operates, what internal strengths, resources and problems it contains, how the community sees itself and what external forces are effecting people in that area or with its identity.

Whichever local council department, agency or voluntary sector project the community worker is employed by they will be based in premises somewhere in a community, for example, the setting may be either in a community centre, a neighbourhood project based in a house, shop or other premises, council area offices or even a town hall. Wherever it is the community worker needs to know and understand the community they are working in if they are to be an effective worker in that community.

In order to make an assessment, you need to gather information and views from as wide a range of sources as possible. These might include official surveys and reports, talking to a variety of people with positions in the community, personal observations, newspaper cuttings and casual conversations. All these are valid, but it is important to recognise that some may be more reliable and relevant than others. You need to develop an overview of the communities needs and resources to enable you to make recommendations and to whom; on which issues to take up and to develop feasible strategies, which mobilise resources and enable people to make progress towards their own goals.

AIMS OF THE PROFILE

To enable the community worker to gain the following:

- a "feel" of the community they are working in.
- factual information about the social, political and economic composition of the community.
- an understanding of some of the issues within the community.
- to allow the community worker to "gain entry" into the community.
- to give the community worker a view of what services and resources (and lack of) are available in the community.
- a knowledge of what active community groups there are.

It is essential that at every stage members of the community are themselves involved in gathering and sifting information and opinion, and are fully consulted about priorities and strategies for action.

There are three main methods of community research:

- factual information gathering
- consultation
- participant observation

The data collected in this way can be placed along a continuum from "hard" (statistics, directories, official reports, etc.) to "medium" (newspaper articles, community surveys, posters, leaflets, minutes of meetings, etc.) to "soft" (personal opinion, impressions, chats, eavesdroppings,etc.)

Be aware of how biases and omissions might distort your research. These can creep as easily into official reports as personal conversations. Ensure that you put aside your own prejudices and political agendas when talking to people, make sure that you meet with a representative sample of people in the community, taking into account their age, ethnic background, gender, sexual orientation and any experience of impairment or mental distress. It is also important to talk with "key" people in the community, they can give you useful overview information and it forms part of the process of building up good working relationships and networks for future use or help you understand potential obstacles and blocks.

Value the skills, knowledge and experience of people in the community. Identify the useful organisations for communication, support and material resources. Build on what already exists, but also be prepared to challenge how they might currently be accessed or distributed.

SECTION:	**GETTING TO KNOW A COMMUNITY**
TITLE:	
AUTHOR:	

SECTION:	**GETTING TO KNOW A COMMUNITY**
TITLE:	**WHAT INFORMATION TO GATHER**
AUTHOR:	Alison Gilchrist

You should not spend to much time on this at the initial stage, perhaps a month or so, but remember to keep your mind open and be prepared to update your information as you go along and as circumstances change.

The kinds of questions you might want to ask about a community include:

- how does the community define itself?
- what is the shared identity of members (if any)?
- are there geographical boundaries?
- what is the history?
- what is its size?
- who chooses to belong to the community?
- who chooses not to?
- what is the demographic make up of the community?
- what resources and facilities are available to it?
- what human strengths and resources an are available?
- what problems and issues face people in the community – individually and collectively?
- how is information communicated within the community and the rest of the world?
- what networks and channels of communication exist?
- what political dynamics affect people in the community (economic factors, local policies, government legislation)
- what democratic forces and opportunities exist within the community?
- who are the influential people?
- how is the community viewed in the outside world?
- what conflicts and differences operate within the community?

As a community worker, you might be interested in exploring these issues in relation to employment, health, housing, pay, environment, different forms of oppression and any other social welfare issue.

Try to get a feel for what it might be like to be a member of the community, but bear in mind that your experience will nevertheless be different depending on your age, class, ethnic background, gender, sexuality, relative disability or other factors which influence how you are able to get around the community and interact with other people. It is also important to be around at different times of the day, as this can influence the impression you build up of the community.

SECTION:	**GETTING TO KNOW A COMMUNITY**
TITLE:	
AUTHOR:	

Gathering information about an area or in preparation for starting a new group / project or as part of a campaign often involves interviewing key people.

The purpose of this technique is to provide a basic framework for an individual preparing for and conducting such interviews either with one person or several people. The basic purpose of the interview is to obtain information.

PREPARATIONS:

a) Planning for an interview

- Consider what you want to find out, what you already know and what you want to achieve.

- Identify the appropriate person or persons you should, or need to, interview. Have you met her/him/them before? Do you know or merely think that they have the information you want or are they in a position to obtain the information for you? Is an interview necessary?

- Consider what the person you are seeking to interview may want from you. Are you prepared to trade?

- Will you need more than one interview? If so consider what you want to achieve in the first interview.

- Anticipate likely friendly and hostile responses and consider how you can capitalise on and overcome such responses.

- Who are you representing – yourself or an organisation? How are you going to explain your interest if you need to ?

- Should you have anyone with you? If so, who, and which of you does what?

- How are you going to make the appointment / arrange the interview? Should you use an intermediary? When and where do you want the interview to take place? How long is the interview likely to last?

- Would it be helpful to roleplay the interview beforehand?

- Will a denial or no comment be as informative as a confirmation of a piece information?

- Check in advance that it is okay to tape the interview if that is what you want to do.

b) During the interview

- Introduce yourself and anyone with you. Explain your interest.

- Listen and watch both the verbal and non-verbal communication.

- Check you have gathered the desired information / responses.

- Where necessary clarify and check the meaning of any ambiguous statements.

SECTION:	**GETTING TO KNOW A COMMUNITY**
TITLE:	**INTERVIEWING PEOPLE**
AUTHOR:	Adapted from the Original Skills Manual by Val Harris

- When the interview is ending you should:

  i)   summarise / check the information obtained

  ii)   lay foundations for any further contacts if wanted.

c)   After the interview

- Write up any notes and record the interview.

- Transcribe the tapes in writing if you have agreed to or you wish to ensure any agreed action is recorded.

- Confirm any points

Comment:

While the checklist is not of universal application several of the points raised are relevant to many interpersonal interactions; however the points raised here should be supplemented by further reading if you are engaging in negotiations, recruitment interviewing or conducting a meeting.

SECTION:	**GETTING TO KNOW A COMMUNITY**
TITLE:	**GATHERING INFORMATION - A CHECKLIST**
AUTHOR:	Alison Gilchrist, Roger Green

1. **INFORMATION BASED IN YOUR OWN AGENCY OR PROJECT**

    *   Start from where you're at – your workplace

    *   Can you get any information from discussion with other workers e.g. their impressions, factual details and experiences.

    *   Do an analysis of what services/resources your agency/project currently offers to the community.

    *   Talk and listen to existing users of your agency/projects services. Get their view of the community.

2. **"WALKABOUT" – GETTING YOUR OWN VIEW OF THE COMMUNITY.**

    *   The aim is to get a "feel" of the community, an impression.

    *   Get out and walk around the community you're working in and/or drive or cycle around it if the area is too large e.g. a city or a group of villages.

    *   Visit the local shops or shopping centre, pubs, launderettes, libraries, parks etc.

    *   Buy a map of the local area.

    *   Talk to and listen to local people.

    *   More structured interviews with key people and officials.

    *   Look at the local papers, listen to the local radio station if there is one.

    *   This method may give you a biased view of the community and also a fragmented one based on who you have talked to and where you have visited. However it does give you a view, an image of a community which you can build on.

3. **FACTUAL INFORMATION ABOUT THE COMMUNITY**

    *   This method can give you hard information on the community. It can be obtained from local libraries, council offices, locally based government departments.

    *   **Politics:**
        *   What political party controls the local council?
        *   Who is the local Member of Parliament?
        *   What political parties and organisations are active in the community?

- **Housing:**

  - What types of housing are there and where are they located? e.g. council housing, estates, owner occupier, housing cooperatives and housing associations, private rented, empty properties, multi-occupied properties.

  - Are there people squatting? Are there hostels?

- **Employment/Unemployment:**

  - What type of industry exists and where is it located?

  - How many people do they employ?

  - Are there any industrial estates?

  - What is the local unemployment rate? How is this broken down? i.e. male/female, age, race etc.

  - What trade union branches are there?

- **Local Transport:**

  - How is the community served by transport? e.g. British Rail, buses, community transport, taxis and mini cabs.

  - Frequency of service?

- **Leisure and recreational facilities:**

  - What facilities exist locally? e.g. leisure centres, sports and social clubs, church halls, community buildings.

- **Land Use:**

  - How is land used in the community? e.g. shopping areas, residential, industrial, housing, railways, waste land.

- **Population:**

  - What is the population of the community, how is it made up and how is it distributed? e.g. class, age, gender, ethnic groups, religion, culture.

- **Council Departments and other agencies:**

  - What are they, where are they located and what services do they provide? e.g. Housing, Social Services, Education (schools, youth clubs, adult education, colleges), Department of Social Security, Police, Probation, Health.

SECTION:	**GETTING TO KNOW A COMMUNITY**
TITLE:	**GATHERING INFORMATION - A CHECKLIST**
AUTHOR:	Alison Gilchrist, Roger Green

Community Development by Bernadette
Barry and Laurie Bidwell.

SCVO 18/19 Claremont Crescent,
Edinburgh EH7 4QD
Tel: 0131 556 3882

- **Voluntary Sector Agencies and Community Groups:**

  - What voluntary sector agencies and projects, and community groups are there?

  - Where are they located?

  - What is their role in the community? Who do they work with?

  - How active are they?

  - What services and resources do they offer?

  - What informal networks exist?

- **History of the community:**

  - Read up on the history of the community. e.g. how it has developed, its social history etc.

  - Read official reports, community newsletters.

  - Statistical analyses of census data for the community.

  - Visit other organisations that are involved in the community and read through their files or annual reports.

SECTION:	**GETTING TO KNOW A COMMUNITY**
TITLE:	
AUTHOR:	

SECTION:	**GETTING TO KNOW A COMMUNITY**
TITLE:	**USING THE INFORMATION GAINED**
AUTHOR:	Roger Green

Any information which is gathered by the community worker needs to be shared otherwise it is of no benefit to the community. How you share this information may depend on two factors, firstly, the personal politics, values and beliefs held by the community worker and their view of community work practice, for example, whether they see their role as helping community groups to develop and supporting them in taking action over issues which affect their community and secondly, it may also depend on the community workers employing agency or project, for example, your job description and job expectations may vary considerably if you are employed by a local council or a voluntary agency.

There are a number of options to consider:

- The information you have collected is shared, either in a written report or verbally, with local community groups. Such a report could highlight the needs of the community as identified by the community and expose gaps in existing services and resources. This information could help local community groups in taking action to secure improved services, resources and funding for the community.

- A report or selected information is presented to your own agency. This could be helpful in, for example, allowing your agency to improve its networking and its service in the community.

- A report or selected information is presented to a number of locally based agencies. Again this needs to be carefully thought through as it could either, for example, improve the co-ordination of the agencies work in the community or have the reverse effect of cutting services as agencies and projects compete against each other because of their differing aims and philosophies which do not always correspond with the needs of the community.

Whichever way the community worker shares and uses this information, either formally or informally, it is important to keep in mind that "knowledge is power".

A final point: any profile is a "snap shot" of a community at the time you undertake it. It will need to be regularly updated as your knowledge of the community develops and the community itself continually changes.

SECTION:	**GETTING TO KNOW A COMMUNITY**
TITLE:	
AUTHOR:	

After completing the initial stages of a community profile you, in a close consultation with others, will begin to develop a strategy of how the situation might be changed in order to meet some of the needs you have identified. It is more than likely that you will not be able to respond to every single need that has been expressed or assessed.

You must prioritise which issues, problems or goals you are going to tackle. The following factors may affect your judgement:

(1)   What is realistic in the given circumstances

(2)   The local and national climate of opinion and interest

(3)   What kind of funding is available

(4)   What other resources are available (especially people)

(5)   The current policies of the agency that employs you

(6)   Your job description

(7)   What has been tried before

(8)   Strength of local pressure, motivation and opinion

(9)   Your personal interests, values, personality and skills

Some Words of Warning:

*   Be realistic about what can be achieved. Aim to change the world, but take a long-term view of this. Make sure that you also survive as a worker and as a human being.

*   Always consult as much as possible, and be accountable for your decisions. This means being able to explain and justify them to relevant people, including your supervisor or line-manager, and your users.

*   Keep on checking out your assessment. You will be working in a constantly changing situation, and your priorities may have to change due to circumstances beyond your control. Try not to get carried away by your own enthusiasm or political commitment. Your motivation alone will not suffice.

*   Beware prejudices and cultural expectations.

*   Develop a strategy which has long-term aims and objectives, but is also flexible enough to respond to needs as they arise, or can adapt to the arrival of new resources.

*   Understand your own impact on the situation – including other peoples' expectations and requirements of you. Self-awareness will help you to realise "where you are coming from", how others perceive you, and how your personality affects your decision-making, e.g. the desire to be liked by certain people, or the excitement of an active campaign, etc.

- Realise that prioritising will inevitably result in some needs that have been articulated being ignored, neglected or postponed. This may lead to resentment, conflict, lack of co-operation and hostility. Be prepared to deal with these negative reactions sensitively, honestly and constructively.

- Be aware of invisible, stigmatised and "unfashionable" needs. Make sure that you seek these out, and do not just rely on assessing demands that are made on you. This could result in you failing to acknowledge and respond to people in the community who are currently not heard, who feel they have no access to you as a resource, or who simply do not know of your existence.

- An equal opportunities approach requires that you are proactive in finding out about needs and resources, and that your practice in responding to these, challenges and combats forms of practical disadvantage, as well as psychological discrimination.

SECTION 8

WORKING WITH GROUPS

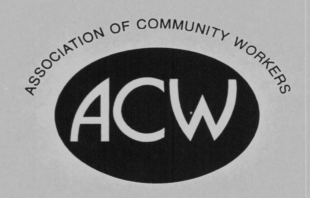

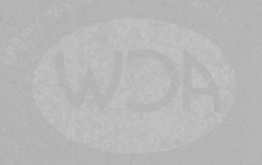

A good deal of the time spent as a community worker is with community groups either helping to bring people together to set up a group, or working with existing groups in the community. With any group there are a number of skills the community worker will use.

This checklist is designed to help you clarify what roles you are taking on with different groups.

SKILLS CHECKLIST

Are you:

- Acting as a facilitator to bring people together as a group. These will be people in the community you are working in who share similar concerns, issues or problems.

- Helping a group to decide its aims and objectives. What do they want to achieve?

- Helping a group(s) to link up (network) with other groups in the community and nationally, if appropriate.

- Supporting individuals within a group e.g. encouraging people to talk, gain confidence to attend, how to chair a meeting, take minutes, set an agenda, how to divide up tasks within the group.

- Helping groups to understand local power structures and how to negotiate with them e.g. local council departments, the police.

- Supporting groups generally e.g. how to advertise meetings, publicity, attracting new members to the group (to avoid a clique forming)

- Being clear what your (the community worker) role is with groups e.g. is it directive or non-directive?, do you want to lead and control the group or do you want to encourage the group to develop at its pace with group members gaining confidence themselves? The latter should be your aim.

- Acting as a resource person/consultant to established groups e.g. on applying for funding and grants, advice giving, equal opportunities policies.

- Helping groups to decide on how to take some form of action, and what type of action, in pursuit of their aims and objectives.

Footnote:

When to withdraw from working with a group is always a difficult decision for any community worker and one that needs careful consideration but a good aim to keep in mind is that you should be preparing to leave a group from your first contact with them otherwise there is a danger the group becomes too dependant on you. A useful general rule to follow is that the skill in working with groups is to "help people to begin to help themselves rather than be helped".

SECTION:	**WORKING WITH GROUPS**
TITLE:	
AUTHOR:	

SECTION:	**WORKING WITH GROUPS**
TITLE:	**SOCIAL ACTION THEORY**
AUTHOR:	Peter Hulse

One way of clarifying the aim of a group and the role of the worker is Social Action Theory (SAT). This was developed during the late 1970s by workers questioning the methods and values contained within existing social work practice based on "welfare" or "justice" models which generally sought to locate problems within individuals, their families or in the community as a whole. These approaches led to the development of programmes designed to either control, modify, correct, appease or punish.

The National Youth Bureau (now the National Youth Agency) provided training sessions on using a different approach to work with young people which was based on the values of community work. The same technique can be applied to other areas of community work.

By using SAT techniques a worker negotiates their relationship with any group they are working with. The group is then encouraged to go through a process which involves exploring:

a)   WHAT are their issues and problems

b)   WHY do the problems exist

c)   HOW can positive change be achieved and then enabling the group to

d)   ACT to implement their plans

e)   REFLECT on and review their plans.

This process is a continuous one and by reflecting on what happens following any action a re-evaluation of the issues is encouraged and further action decided upon and so on, until a solution achieved.

The role of the worker is therefore to provide a process within which those involved can own issues, content and action and become problem solvers themselves.

This method was extremely relevant to community and youth groups aiming to develop and manage projects for the benefit of their neighbourhood.

SECTION:	**WORKING WITH GROUPS**
TITLE:	
AUTHOR:	

A variety of people in a community feel strongly about an issue and they and/or others they know in the community want to come together to pursue their shared interest. This section suggests a way that will enable people in a community to form a community group.

DECIDING WHETHER OR NOT TO SET A GROUP UP

Step 1.

Identify the issue which has some importance within the community. Be clear about its potential in the development of that community.

Step 2.

Gather the names of people in the local community who might be interested. For example, you might go to key people in the community and ask for lists of other people they know who could be approached about the issue. Ask the people who give you lists to also ask the individuals they have listed whether you, the community worker, can pay them a visit. Ask them to explain who you are.

Step 3.

Go and knock on the door of those listed. Spend time discussing the issue and be clear about the interest each person has in it. Notice how they express their feelings about that issue, which aspect they focus on, whether there are other issues they feel strongly about.

Step 4.

Evaluate all that information. Get it written down. Look at it. Go back to the original people who had provided the lists. Discuss with them how a group might come together. Discuss what role you will play and what role they will play.

Step 5.

Go back to your employer. Explain this is the direction you intend to go in and why.

Step 6.

Make a decision to go ahead or not. If you decide not to go ahead then get back to all those people and say why you are not. If you decide to go ahead let people know.

Step 7.

Deciding to go ahead

Go back to all the potential people for the group with a personal visit telling them that you are calling a meeting (date, time, place), say who else is going to be there, what it is going to be about. Make sure you have arranged a room and have refreshments laid on. Be pretty clear that the meeting is going to be productive. Depending on the type of group, you may want to centre it around a speaker or somebody who is going to come in from the outside to take the edge

SECTION:	**WORKING WITH GROUPS**
TITLE:	**ONE WAY TO SET UP A COMMUNITY GROUP**
AUTHOR:	Adapted from the original Skills Manual by Val Harris

off things so that it is not just them trying to talk amongst themselves for the first meeting. It can be valuable to have someone from an established group with similar aims who can demonstrate that it is possible to set up successful groups and who can talk about any potential pitfalls ahead. One or two days before the first meeting put a note through the door, as a reminder.

Hold your meeting.

A community worker may find that a small local group represents a very large area. Or a central group in a neighbourhood may not be representing and articulating issues that affect smaller groups and minorities in that neighbourhood (e.g. a block or a street). Alternatively a central group may be swamped by many local concerns and be unable to make headway on more general issues affecting the neighbourhood. One strategy is to encourage the formation of smaller groupings representing blocks or streets or other natural units in the neighbourhood. The idea is that block or street groups would get on with their own business, taking the load off the central group and also be represented on the central group to take up shared issues. Naturally, local situations vary and the development of 'component parts' can be done to a greater or lesser extent depending on the nature and needs of the situation. There are many ways in which a community worker can encourage people to become involved, and this section outlines a few approaches.

WAYS TO ENCOURAGE MORE PEOPLE TO BECOME INVOLVED.

Finding individuals

The situation may best be met by simply finding individuals who are prepared to act on behalf of a block or a street, without necessarily being elected or formally proposed by their neighbours. Likely people can be found from, for example:

- friends or people who are already active in the neighbourhood

- by developing other activities or events, such as a playscheme and finding 'new' active people in a neighbourhood

- by finding out from 'professional' workers such as teachers, social workers, etc., if there are people they know who might be willing to represent their street or block

- by door knocking etc.

Creating a structure for individuals to work in

The new grouping of individual representatives may become a sub group or sub committee of the existing central group, working on specific issues. For example, on a council estate this might be taking up repair and maintenance problems that affect particular blocks. Alternatively think if the new grouping as additional members of the central group who meet in an extra meeting as an extension of the existing central group meeting.

DEVELOPMENT

- A central committee is elected from a public meeting;

- The members of this committee go around the area with leaflets, doorknocking, loudhailers at a time when most people are in. They do this on several occasions each time focusing on a particular natural area within the estate or neighbourhood.

- The leafletting/doorknocking/loudhailer announces a meeting to be held fairly soon, giving the time and place.

- Hopefully small meetings will take place; someone from the central group or committee makes the purpose of the meeting clear; from this meeting it should be possible to form street or block committees or grouping.

- Block or street committees are asked by the central group if they would like to send someone along to the central group as a representative.

SECTION:	**WORKING WITH GROUPS**
TITLE:	**DEVELOPING NEIGHBOURHOOD GROUPINGS**
AUTHOR:	Adapted from the original skills manual by Val Harris

Setting up block or street meetings

A third option is to spend time finding out who is well liked in a block and who genuinely wants to see a block or street group formed; hold the first meeting in this persons house. Involve at least 2–3 residents in selecting a time and date for this meeting; make the date sufficiently far in advance so that you and any others willing to help organise the meeting can contact all the residents personally; give people you talk to sufficient notice of the meeting; don't worry if not everyone can make it. Put a simple reminder through letter boxes a day or so before the meeting. It might be an idea to give people a number they can call at to say that they cant make it but would be interested in future meetings.

note: where a central grouping already exists in a neighbourhood it is crucial in developing component parts for this central group to agree to this happening and if possible to actively involve themselves in helping it to happen; different approaches reflect different objectives. For example one approach may be more to do with the 'more effective take up of issues using pressure group tactics' while another may be to do with 'developing a sense of community and the maximum use of local resources'.

Thoughts on conducting a meeting

1. The need to develop block or street groupings may be to develop better relations between people in the block or street rather than take up particular 'external' issues. Thus the meetings may have to contain both informal conversations so that people get to know each other and a short business part.

2. People may feel a strong desire to share negative stories and feelings with each other. If this develops the meeting could end up promoting and reinforcing a greater level of depression.

3. The heart of the meeting should be the exchange of good information between neighbours; connecting the needs and concerns of some with the resources and suggestions of others. To build towards this it may be necessary to start of meetings on a positive note; one way is to ask people to introduce themselves and say something good which has happened since the last meeting.

4. Where individuals want to follow up an interest or concern they may want to form a small group of volunteers to work on it before the next meeting; one of the volunteers may act as a convenor.

5. Meetings in the block or street can be held at different peoples houses or flats so that responsibility is shared and people get to know one another better.

Networks are based on informal membership. They assume that all members are equal (though this is not usually the case in practice). They do not have a hierarchical structure and they do not usually have formal policies. Their main purpose is to share information, ideas and support. Participation is optional.

Networks may have officers and regular meetings of the members, but they don't have to. They may act as a consultative body to another authority, and they may elect individuals to represent their perspective to some other body.

Networks may operate on an "ad hoc" basis, coming together to organise a particular event or activity, but this is not seen as its primary purpose, but rather a response to a specific situation or shared need/desire.

Networks may develop a policy position on some issue and advise its members on this, but decisions are not seen as binding.

Usually networks simply provide space to debate and reflect on difficult or new areas of policy or legislation.

Networks do not always have a common identity, nor any resources, except those contributed by members. The individual members may not be aware of each other's existence.

Networks operate as "horizontal" channels of communication within communities. Sometimes they might have a co-ordinating node, which collates and disseminates information, but this is not always the case.

USES OF NETWORKS

Working with people in informal ways and linking them into existing networks or helping them to set up new ones can help people to:

a. develop support and solidarity amongst themselves

b. acquire and promote a positive identity

c. share skills, knowledge and resources

d. develop a common purpose, which may not be represented by a formally agreed goal, but can provide a strategic framework

e. co-ordinate their approach to problem solving or campaigning

f. represent a collective and specific point of view.

HOW MIGHT THE WORKER USE OR CREATE NETWORKS?

The water system model: the worker as a conduit, pump or tap.

Conduit:

The worker is simply a channel or provides channels through which members of a network are kept on contact with each other. This might be through a newsletter or the worker's own brain.

Pump:

The worker organises and encourages people to stay in touch with each other. For example, by organising meetings or deliberately arranging channels of communication, which might not otherwise exist or be constricted. This acknowledges that the flow of information may not be uniform through a network, such to people on the periphery or people whose language or mode of communication might be different.

Tap:

The worker actively feeds in information and ideas to the network, and injects enthusiasm and support from time to time.

Methods and skills of networking:

Mostly these involve informal information gathering and passing on. They include structured conversation, active listening, empathising, understanding, introducing ideas and information, researching, eavesdropping, organising and facilitating.

Networking usually takes place between individuals, or in large, semi-structured groups, where roles are not clearly defined.

Problems and Issues

As a result of the informality and unstructuredness of networks, confusion can arise over the status of collective decisions, especially when these are controversial. The looseness of membership can lead to undemocratic procedures and cliques forming. Inequalities of access to the network, especially when these are determined through casual, occasional and informal contacts, can lead to information not always reaching the parts of the network that might need it most. There are also issues around the confidentiality and general reliability of information.

SECTION:	**WORKING WITH GROUPS**
TITLE:	**IDEAS FOR INTRODUCING PEOPLE**
AUTHOR:	Adapted from the original Skills Manual by Val Harris

It is important that people know who else is in the group or at a meeting. The amount of information that people need to know about each other will vary from simply knowing people's names and possibly their jobs or position, through to sharing personal knowledge of each other, which may be the case in some self-help groups.

This section suggests 3 ways that initial introduction can be made with a group of people who know little about each other or when new people join an existing group.

1. NAMES AND ONE OTHER THING

- People say their name, going round the group

- They also contribute one other thing. This might be, items for the agenda, saying what they came for, saying one talent they think they have, by saying one good thing or new thing that happened during the week, by giving one piece of information about themselves that they wish to share.

N.B. By giving additional information as well as the name there is a greater chance of people remembering it. A list of names and glimpses of faces are soon forgotten.

2. CUMULATIVE NAMES

- The first person says their name

- The second person says their name and the name of the first person

- The third person says all three names

- This is continued round the whole group.

N.B. This name remembering technique is best used in small groups as it can be hard work for those near the end. If the group is larger then one half of the group can introduce themselves followed by the other half.

3. MUTUAL INTRODUCTIONS

- Group members pair up. Preferably with people they don't know.

- Each person introduces themself to the other for about three minutes.

- Someone calls time.

- They change roles for a further three minutes.

- The group re-assembles and each person introduces their partner to the group.

SECTION:	**WORKING WITH GROUPS**
TITLE:	
AUTHOR:	

SECTION:	**WORKING WITH GROUPS**
TITLE:	**CLARIFYING ROLES AND TASKS**
AUTHOR:	Adapted from the original Skills Manual by Val Harris

Every group has a number of tasks that need to be undertaken if it is going to operate effectively. This section suggests two different ways that the group members can identify all of the tasks and decide who will take responsibility for each one.

TECHNIQUE 1: SORTING OUT JOBS

1. Use a large blank sheet of paper to write down all the tasks (major and minor) that group members can think of.

2. The group arranges the tasks in categories (e.g. administrative etc.) Some tasks fall in more than one category.

3. Use the categories and lists of tasks to allocate and clarify roles of group members – some tasks may be undertaken by several people.

TECHNIQUE 2: NEGOTIATING ROLES

1. Each group member simultaneously lists what they would like each other group member to do more of, what the other should do the same amount of, and what the other should do less of.

2. The "role messages" are then exchanged. There may be immediate agreement, or the messages can be use to negotiate roles.

SECTION:	**WORKING WITH GROUPS**
TITLE:	
AUTHOR:	

SECTION:	WORKING WITH GROUPS
TITLE:	SETTING PRIORITIES - DISAGREE GAME
AUTHOR:	Val Harris

Setting a group's priorities

The aim of this exercise is to enable a group to decide on its priorities over a period of time and to establish an action plan. It aims to give everyone the opportunity of contributing their ideas and comments, not just those who are good at talking in groups. It requires some level of literacy but could be adapted to symbol languages without too much difficulty.

You will need several pieces of paper approximately 2"x3" with "I Disagree" printed on one side, an A4 sheet of paper can be ruled out to give 8–10 rectangles and then copied. Everyone in the group will need a pen/pencil and several pieces of paper. Ask each member of the group to write down what they think their group should be doing in the next year (or so many months) – one idea only on the blank side of the pieces of paper. The more pieces of paper people have the longer the exercise will last – so you can say put down 4 main ideas (for example) if you want a quicker exercise.

When everyone has finished writing down their ideas ask them to gather round a table, make sure that everyone is at the same height (i.e. all standing or all sitting). On the table you will have placed the numbers 1,2,3, at intervals along one side: These can represent priorities, or time scales (what we should start with now, what in 3 months, what in 6 months etc.) as long as it is clear what the numbers represent. Everyone puts their pieces of paper in a heap on the table, they are shuffled and everyone takes some (not their own) and decides where they will place them on the table, under what priority/timescale.

It is still an individual choice at this point in the exercise and no one touches the papers laid down by other people. Once all the slips are laid out everyone goes round the table and if they disagree with the priority given to any idea, or they do not understand it then they turn it over so that I DISAGREE shows up. All of the suggestions which are left facing upwards will be transferred on to flip charts and form the basis of an action plan, only those that have been turned over will be debated so it is important to make sure that everyone is happy with the position and content of those left on the table. Pick up all those that have been agreed with in the 1st section and begin to write them up as a list on a flipchart leaving space for an action column. Ask a group member to turn over one that has been disagreed with in that first section and invite bids and comments.

The idea is not to get into long debate but to quickly check out if any one wants clarification about what it means, and then to ask where it should be moved to – the majority view wins! – it may remain where it is, get moved to 2 or 3 or be scrapped. If the issue looks set to lead to a major discussion put it on one side and come back to it later to decide how and when this discussion can be held. The idea is to see where quick consensus or majority decision can be made, so keep the group moving onto the next one, and then the next...

SECTION:	**WORKING WITH GROUPS**
TITLE:	**SETTING PRIORITIES - DISAGREE GAME**
AUTHOR:	Val Harris

As decisions are made so the items are added to the flipcharts for each priority.

Work through each priority in turn and record all the decisions. After a break the group comes back together and works through the flipcharted lists and agrees what actions will be taken, by whom, when and how, e.g. it will be put on the next team meeting agenda, it will be brought to the management committees attention, two or three people will take on the task.

The actual exercise should take 30–40 minutes and then the discussion of action points will depend on the length of the lists but again should be fairly quick – it's about taking decisions rather than holding debates at this stage.

This idea was gathered from a workshop run by Tony Gibson when he was at Nottingham University and working on the "Action For Neighbourhood Change" project.

SECTION:	**WORKING WITH GROUPS**
TITLE:	**GROUP DECISION MAKING**
AUTHOR:	Adapted from the original Skills Manual by Val Harris

The purpose of the technique is to enable a large group to make decisions in a participatory manner and not in a representative or voting manner.

Context: large groups may find it difficult to arrive at decisions. This may be because of their size, the complexity of the issue, the tension in the group etc. Small groups can form from members of the large group to aid decision making. Two general examples of how this can be done are described in this section.

A. USING SMALL GROUPS TO ACHIEVE CONSENSUS

1. The large group breaks into small groups of 6–8 people, to discuss the problem, review possible solutions, develop a proposal for a solution to be presented to the whole group.

2. The large group reconvenes and proposals from the small groups are presented and recorded on a large sheet of paper.

3. The large group looks for common conclusions in the report and sees if a consensus can be reached on these points. Disagreements are identified.

4. Small groups reconvene to work on the contested points and try to develop new proposals.

5. Small groups present new proposals to the large group.

6. The large group tries to find consensus.

Note:

Steps 4 to 6 can be repeated as necessary.

The technique works better when the group sets and abides by the time limits for each step of the process. Forceful facilitators and time keepers may be needed for this to happen. Holding to time limits while trying to solve complex problems may increase the group's feeling of progress.

The technique is not about achieving unanimity but sufficient consensus to take action

B. USING SMALL GROUPS TO DEVELOP A PROGRAMME OR WRITE COLLECTIVELY

1. Having defined what a programme or written document is needed for, the large group brainstorms approaches, issues, possibilities, goals etc.

2. Individuals privately reflect on the brainstormed lists to order priorities, sort out personal reactions and ideas.

3. Results of personal thinking are shared.

4. The large group discusses issues which need to be taken into consideration, might be difficult, need further thought

5. A small group is appointed to develop a proposal or document based on the input from the large group

6. The small group presents the proposal/report

7. The large group evaluates it. This might mean accepting the substance of the proposal, but returning the report to the small group for further minor changes. Alternatively disagreement about substance may require further techniques or a change in the small group personnel.

The small group may need to check comments or small revisions with the larger group informally.

Technique A can be used to follow technique B, i.e. split the large group to consider the report back.

Technique B looks like the formation of a working party. However, the small group works closely to the material from the large group and is accountable to it.

SECTION:	**WORKING WITH GROUPS**
TITLE:	**CONTROLLING DISCUSSIONS**
AUTHOR:	Adapted from the original skills manual by Val Harris.

One of the most common complaints about the way groups work (or don't) is that some individuals dominate discussion and other people say very little. The purpose of these techniques are to limit individuals dominating.

A.   THE CONCH

(A conch is any object that can be held, e.g. match box, tennis ball)

1.   A group adopts the following rule: the only person who can speak is the one holding the conch.

2.   The person who wants to talk takes the conch from the table around which the group is sitting or from the floor if there is no table.

3.   When a person has finished talking they put the conch back where they got it from or pass it to the person who wants to speak next.

note:

1.   if there is a scamble for the conch it can be passed around the group;

2.   the conch may act as the equivalent of the 'loudest voice'; if a person seeks to dominate the discussion this becomes clinging on to the conch. The conch is thus a training tool which the group should be able to do without quite quickly.

B.   MATCHES

(As in boxes of matches, or pieces of card.) The aim is to make people consider the value of what they want to say.

1.   Each person is given the same number of matches/cards; use as many matches/cards per person as the time limit for the total discussion suggests.

2.   Each time someone speaks they give up one of their matches/cards by putting it into the centre of the circle

3.   When a person runs out of matches they cannot speak

note:

if the rule is adopted properly it can reduce the level of interruptions or garbled statements.

SECTION:	**WORKING WITH GROUPS**
TITLE:	
AUTHOR:	

SECTION 9

CONFLICT IN GROUPS

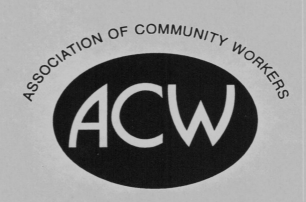

ASSOCIATION OF COMMUNITY WORKERS

ACW

SECTION:	**CONFLICT IN GROUPS**
TITLE:	**CONFLICT AND OPPRESSION – SOME THOUGHTS**
AUTHOR:	Izzy Terry

The understanding and the resolving of conflict needs to be set in the context of power and oppression within our society and within the groups and organisations of which we are part. The more groups and organisations attempt to adopt "equal opportunities" practices, maybe involving and/or employing people from groups under-represented within their organisation, the greater the potential for exploring differences and power imbalances; the greater the potential for conflict.

Too frequently these conflicts are not used creatively; they are either suppressed, the "new" members expected to fit into the existing culture practices and structure of the group/organisation; or if they question or criticise these they are often not listened to and/or individually seen as a "problem" or "trouble maker" within the group/organisation. The potential for change, development and growth is not used or acted on clearly throughout the whole of the organisations'/groups' practices. Too frequently equal opportunities issues are seen solely as interpersonal rather than connected to the structure and practices of the whole organisation.

We need to be aware of:

- Focusing the problem/conflict on the oppressed members of the group rather than the oppressor group members looking at themselves, their identity, values, strategies and actions.

- Forgetting that each individual within the group whatever their composition, e.g. race, class, gender, is also unique with their own values, opinions and experience.

- Over-concentrating on oppression conflicts at the expense of other fundamental problems within the organisation (which may be connected to the former).

- Avoiding addressing issues of power and oppression within groups, organisations and its implications on policy and practice overall ... Whatever the composition of the group members.

- Ranking oppressions, as one e.g. sexism being worse, to be taken more seriously than e.g. racism or classism. To do this doesn't allow for the complexity and interconnectiveness of oppression in any one individual.

- Assuming the notion of "you fight my oppression and I'll fight yours"; we need to be committed to fighting oppression unconditionally.

- How power/oppression issues affect our ability to communicate clearly and directly to each other. e.g. Being patronising, fear and guilt preventing honesty, fear of unfair treatment, defensiveness.

SECTION:	**CONFLICT IN GROUPS**
TITLE:	**CONFLICT AND OPPRESSION – SOME THOUGHTS**
AUTHOR:	Izzy Terry

PROMOTION OF CONSTRUCTIVE CONTROVERSY

As mentioned earlier, such controversy in organisations is healthy and necessary.

It is not possible to address "equal opportunities" or "commitment to the community" if people are unwilling to value and hear everyone's ideas, opinions and contributions.

In order to do this it is necessary in your organisation to create and a climate/culture where controversy is valued and promoted.

Controversies among members should be initiated by highlighting contrasting viewpoints, pointing out disagreements and promoting challenging tasks.

If agreement appears in the group too easily or quickly, time should be taken to reconsider the situation and think about it more, rather than feel relief that an agreement has been reached. All members should be encouraged to be assertive and state their opinions. Don't assume silence of certain members is their agreement.

The more controversy is promoted the more at ease group members will feel at airing their opinions, giving criticism etc.

SECTION:	**CONFLICT IN GROUPS**
TITLE:	**SOME STEPS IN CONFLICT RESOLUTION**
AUTHOR:	Izzy Terry

The characters that make up the word "conflict" in Chinese are "danger and opportunity" (LEAP 1992). Conflict is inevitable in all groups and organisations and we need to discover and develop ways of using the opportunity as well as the dangers of conflict. Conflict becomes destructive and damaging when it is ignored or repressed; or when the only responses to it are to bully, bulldoze or withdraw (LEAP 1992).

Differences in groups and organisations are the basis on which growth and change occur. In effective organisations and groups there is a shared sense of unity – common goals and purpose but also a shared sense of diversity. (S. Adirondack 1989).

Conflict arises when difference can't be satisfactory dealt with; people may be unwilling to accept different values, points of view; or maybe resources are perceived to be unfairly distributed; fear and mistrust may create "outsiders", "enemies", "others"; people may be resistant to change; people may want to hold onto their power and position; or maybe there are unclear or no procedures for exploring differences before they develop into conflict.

USEFUL BOOKS

"Playing with fire" N. Fire and F. Macbeth

LEAP 1992. Training for the creative use of conflict.

"Just about managing" S.M. Adirondack 1989 NCVO; especially chapter 14. Managing differences and conflict.

"Getting to Yes" R. Fisher and William Ury 1989.

The goal of conflict resolution is agreement on special actions, which can be taken by some or all of the parties involved to deal with a particular situation (S. Adirondack 1989). Both parties must choose to take part.

1.   Parties need to be encouraged to meet together at a mutually agreed time and place.

2.   Groundrules/guidelines need to be agreed on e.g. no interrupting, trying to listen to each other, no name calling, being willing to explore a range of solutions.

3.   Giving each party in the conflict opportunity to clarify and define the issues in conflict as they see them; trying to separate facts, opinions and values.

4.   Giving each party the opportunity to clarify why they wish to/need to resolve the conflict e.g. what goals do they share?

5.   Defining what issues/concerns do both parties need to agree about; clarify fact, opinion and values about each issue.

6.   Brainstorm positive ways/suggestions for resolutions of each issue/concern. Try to generate as many ideas as possible, avoiding judgement of their validity.

7.   Agree a specific solution for each issue of concern and the steps to implement it either by consensus or compromise (see glossary). This may take quite a time, beware of rushing this.

8.   Ensure that all parties are willing to implement the solutions even if they don't fully agree with it. Explore what support and assistance they may need.

9.   Agree a procedure for reviewing the situation to be sure that the solution is working out and/or for dealing with those who do not do what they agreed.

N.B. BE AS ASSERTIVE AS POSSIBLE: AND RECOGNISE OTHERS' RIGHT TO BE SO.

SECTION:	**CONFLICT IN GROUPS**
TITLE:	
AUTHOR:	

SECTION:	**CONFLICT IN GROUPS**
TITLE:	**RESPONSES TO CONFLICT**
AUTHOR:	Izzy Terry

To respond to conflict in your organisation, there are essentially three main options:

- Ignoring it
- Imposing a solution
- Members finding their own solution

This section examines each of these.

1. IGNORING IT

This will not solve the conflict and it will often-mean it resurfaces in ways unrelated to the real problem/conflict.

Ignoring conflict previously may have helped create the conflict that exists at present.

This approach is relevant to minor conflicts which do not affect how people work together. Beware of minor conflicts feeling major to some people or minor conflicts actually covering up major conflicts.

2. IMPOSING A SOLUTION

A solution is imposed on the group or team usually from above either in an authoritarian, forceful way or in a sympathetic, caring way. If those involved in the conflict accept this, it's fine but usually they will have less motivation to implement the solution than if they had been involved in the process/decision.

Often this approach does not always get to the root of the conflict, or lasts for a while only for the conflict to resurface at a later date.

3. MEMBERS FINDING THEIR OWN SOLUTION

– With or without a third party. It is usually better for the people involved to come up with their own solutions to their conflict, either by compromise or consensus by problem solving.

Sometimes someone from within the group or from outside may be able to help members to solve the conflict.

Ignoring major conflicts can have a detrimental effect on the effective worth of an organisation and can be the result of one or both parties refusing to resolve the conflict, at that particular time.

Sometimes these parties have tried previously to resolve the conflict but have felt that the other party has not kept their side of the bargain.

Sometimes, it's possible to have a combination of all three steps in an organisation:

Agreed solution to conflict assumed – but then one party fails to keep their side of the deal – Solution is therefore ignored – Imposed solution from above e.g. Management Committee.

SECTION:	CONFLICT IN GROUPS
TITLE:	RESPONSES TO CONFLICT
AUTHOR:	Izzy Terry

GROUPS COMING UP WITH THEIR OWN SOLUTIONS

"Conflict resolution means discussing, negotiating and coming to a joint solution through compromise or consensus." S.M. Adirondack

For this to work, all parties must:

- be willing to listen to each other

- to look at several options not just their own

- to be motivated to finding a solution

- choose a convenient time and place to meet and agree on duration of meeting.

If this does not happen, there may be a need to re-examine why people are in the organisation in the first place – what's their motivation? What are the aims and objectives of the organisation? Is there a common purpose? Is this understood and agreed?

COMPROMISE

Each party gives up part of their goals and persuades the other party to give up part of theirs. They seek a conflict resolution where both sides gain something – the middle ground between the two extreme positions.

Sometimes compromise is the best solution but often parties compromise without really examining all the options because they assume compromise is the only solution.

Sometimes it happens due to lack of time.

CONSENSUS

Both parties view the conflicts as problems to be solved and seek a solution that achieves both their own goals and those of the other party. It can take a long time to draw people out so that consensus solution is possible. One also has to beware of hidden or informal power in the parties which may be used to impose a solution yet give the impression everyone has reached a consensus.

USE OF THIRD PARTY

A third party from within or outside the group may be able to help the people in conflict to move from their fixed positions and work towards an agreed solution. These people must not be directly involved in the conflict and must be given permission to help solve the conflict by both parties. They must be very clear about their role, i.e. to help the parties to resolve their conflict and must not get caught up in the conflict or misuse their authority.

A person in this position should try to be:

- Committed to finding a solution acceptable to all parties.

- Able to recognise and build on points of agreement.

- Be aware of their own values, views and opinions in relation to the conflict and to keep them separate from the process of conflict resolution.

- Committed to equalising the power as much as possible between the two parties.

- Committed to finding out the underlying causes of the conflict with those involved.

- Aware of the affect of people's background and composition in relation to their presentation and perception of the conflict.

- Committed to focusing on the problem/conflict rather than personalities/people concerned.

- Committed to encouraging open communication, honesty and expression of feelings.

(Adapted from the Centre for Conflict Resolution 1978)

SECTION:	**CONFLICT IN GROUPS**
TITLE:	**GLOSSARY**
AUTHOR:	Izzy Terry

Resolution

agreement on how a conflict should be dealt with

Solution

a specific step or series of steps to end the conflict

Reconciliation

building a good relationship within groups who have been in conflict.

Intermediary or third party

a person or group not directly involved in the conflict

Crisis intervention

separating, protecting, or getting help for people in a heated or violent situation

asking people to calm down and talk about what's happening just prior to a heated or violent situation

Facilitator

helps people to listen, to communicate with each other. Can help people out of deadlocked situations.

Mediator

more directly involved in resolving the conflict. Remains impartial.

Advocacy

negotiating on behalf of one party. An advocate supports the party in a conflict e.g. in a situation where that party is less powerful than the other.

Negotiation

discussing each party's needs, demands and interests and agreeing which aspects of each should be incorporated in to a solution.

Arbitration

a legal or quasi-legal process in which the parties in conflict agree beforehand to accept the decision of a third party, if a voluntary agreement cannot be reached

Adjudication/litigation

settlement of a dispute through legal processes

Compromise

each party states their position indicating what they are (or are not) willing to give up. Assumes that all parties have relatively equal power.

Consensus

each party states their position and the goal is to try to find a solution which recognises and values peoples differences. Solution is possibly unexpected by parties. Consensus needs understanding of power within the organisation; beware of a solution being imposed by the most powerful persons while still giving the impression that everyone is participating equally.

Definitions taken from 'Just Managing'
– S.M. Adirondack. N.C.V.O.

ACW SKILLS MANUAL 1994-Reprinted 1999

"Assertiveness is about people becoming clearer about what they want. It's about finding out what we feel in any situation, learning how to express this appropriately and asking for what we need without ignoring the needs of others". (CETU 1990).

Being assertive means:

1. Recognising you have a number of rights which you can use and defend.

2. Valuing your feelings and emotions; they are important.

3. Expressing yourself clearly and directly but still in your own way, i.e. words/accent/style. It means speaking for yourself using the "I" statements.

4. Not putting others down, blaming others, or being bossy. Assertiveness means accepting and respecting other people's rights as being equally important as your own.

5. Challenging situations that exclude or discriminate against you or others from taking part on an equal basis.

6. Separating fact from opinion; there is rarely an absolute truth in any conflict situation. Avoid statements like "the fact of the matter is"; rather say "my opinion/idea is that .....".

7. Encourage others to be assertive; asking others what they want/feel even if it's different from you.

8. Look at and listen to each other. Eye contact is important in helping to see the real person/people in a conflict situation. It is important to listen properly in case the other party gives you new information or a new view on the situation that may make you change your mind.

9. Take one issue at a time. Avoid confusing one issue with another and using examples from the past to illustrate your point.

10. Ensure you understand each other. If you are unclear ask for clarification e.g. "what are you referring to exactly?"

    "So what you are saying is ...., is that right?"

11. Acknowledge and appreciate one another.

    Try and appreciate the others separate from the conflict situation.

    Try and give positive good points especially if you feel the other party has accepted you opinion, say you feel good about it.

12. Being open to change and suggestions from the other party about what change needs to happen.

   It is important that these suggestions are given in a direct not vague/hinting way.

   e.g. "I'd like you to .... to me" rather than keeping quite but looking resentful or saying "maybe you could ....".

SECTION:	**CONFLICT IN GROUPS**
TITLE:	**WORKSHEET FOR INDIVIDUAL WORK**
AUTHOR:	Taken from a Training Day on Conflict - Izzy Terry

Choose a conflict situation we have or have had direct experience of in our work, as the raw material for this case study. This may be a conflict actually in our team at work, or within a group we are or have been working with.

1. Describe the situation, how the conflict arose – what exactly happened?

2. What did we feel when the conflict arose and how did we personally react?

   How did other people involved react?

3. What was at the root of the conflict? Did this emerge clearly at any point? If so, how or by whom was it brought to the surface?

4. What steps were taken to resolve the conflict? Who initiated this process?

5. What happened at the end? Was the conflict resolved? If so, how?

6. Any reflections/conclusions we have drawn from the situation/incident?

SECTION:	**CONFLICT IN GROUPS**
TITLE:	
AUTHOR:	

SECTION 10

MEETINGS

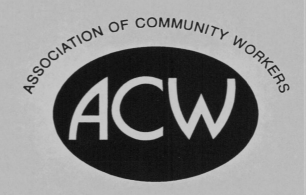

SECTION:	**MEETINGS**
TITLE:	**ARRANGING A MEETING**
AUTHOR:	Adapted from the original Skills Manual by Martin Wyatt

The purpose of the technique is to think in a structured way about the setting for meetings.

CONTEXT: the place in which a meeting is held, the way it is set and the way it is conducted, will convey a lot of messages which people will pick up sometimes without realising it. Meetings can run into problems because not enough thought has gone into the setting they are held in, people's relations to one another, and organisational factors.

THE TECHNIQUE

To help you develop a checklist of items to think about in relation to organising meetings, the list may be used as a prompt.

Who can attend and contribute

location?   creche?

accessible to disabled people?

induction loop/signers for hearing impaired people?

Physical setting

number expected? – amount of space

lighting	acoustics
seating arrangements	no smoking?/ashtrays
refreshments	toilets
writing materials	breaks

People's relations

number expected? – formality/informality

welcome/introductions	collaborative style
guidance to chair	handling outsiders

who is seen to be in control/accountable?

who sets the agenda?

Organisational

notification of meetings	agenda
information	structure of discussion
finance	attendance list
minutes/notes	accountability

For Open meeting/AGM

publicity

relevant papers

purpose

SECTION:	**MEETINGS**
TITLE:	
AUTHOR:	

SECTION:	**MEETINGS**
TITLE:	**FACILITATING EFFECTIVE MEETINGS**
AUTHOR:	Roger Green

Meetings are an everyday part of community work. All community groups and other organisations in the community hold meetings to discuss a variety of topics ranging from applications for grants, organising a public meeting to the groups regular meeting.

If they are poorly organised and managed and without some clear aims of why a meeting is necessary people who attend them will consider them a waste of time and not come back to the next meeting.

The community workers role is often to help organise the meeting and encourage the meeting discuss and cover its business in an open and democratic way as possible. This is achieved by attending meetings, helping the meeting make decisions and supporting individuals both at the meeting and following the meeting.

CHECK LIST FOR FACILITATING A MEETING

- What is the purpose of the meeting? Check out with people.

- What is to be discussed? Help organise an agenda making sure that everyone has the opportunity to add their items.

- Help find a place to meet – which is accessible and acceptable for everybody.

- Will some people need transport to get to and from the meeting?

- Time of meeting – find a time which is convenient to everybody. Remember people's other commitments e.g. care of dependants.

- Will the meeting need a creche? Who will organise and staff it? Or will people need help with caring costs? Where can you get the resources?

- Publicity for the meeting – advertise the meeting and make sure people know the time and place and have any papers or materials needed.

- Organise the tea, coffee and biscuits. (Including non caffeine drinks such as juices and herb teas.)

- Who is to chair the meeting? Will they need support in doing this?

- How will everyone introduce themselves?

- How can latecomers be told what has happened? Will someone tell them as they arrive?

- Try and ensure that everybody has their say. Encourage the quieter people to make their points particularly if the more confident talkative people are taking over the meeting.

- Should individuals agree in advance to present or speak to a particular item? Do they have enough information?

- Will any item provoke conflict? Can this be handled by breaking it into small pieces and taking one part at a time?

- Help the meeting clarify and check out the points discussed.

- Check out the decisions reached by the meeting are clearly understood by everybody and recorded.

- If the agenda is long – what can be held over to the next meeting? What can be dealt with quickly? What needs more time?

- Check out the meeting is clear what tasks have been divided up amongst those present and who is responsible for carrying them out.

- Turn the lights out after the meeting and lock up!

SECTION:	**MEETINGS**
TITLE:	**AGENDA SETTING**
AUTHOR:	Adapted from the original Skills Manual by Val Harris

Purpose of the technique

To encourage group responsibility for the organising, running, and progress of the meeting.

WALL AGENDA

1. Put up a large sheet of paper and write up suggestions from the group for items for discussion.

2. The items suggested can be grouped as they are suggested or after they have all been suggested.

3. Grouping can be done with different coloured pens or by writing items in separate categories or columns.

SECTION:	**MEETINGS**
TITLE:	
AUTHOR:	

SECTION:	**MEETINGS**
TITLE:	**AGENDA FORM**
AUTHOR:	Adapted from the original Skills Manual by Val Harris

The purpose of the technique is to assist participants at a meeting to record essential information during the course of the meeting of a small group or a committee meeting with a task centred agenda.

The technique utilises the form below. Each participant is given, (preferably circulated before the meeting,) a copy of the form with the agenda items filled in and each participant fills in their form as the meeting proceeds.

AGENDA FORM

Meeting of: .... Date: ....,......

Purpose of Meeting: ....

Participants: ....

Agenda	tick as item completed	Action	Person/s responsible	Deadline
1.				
2.				
3.				
4.				
5.				
6. A.O.B.				

Conclusions reached:

Date of next meeting:

Comment:

The form is not appropriate for discussion groups and it is not a replacement for minutes. It is intended as a bridge between the meeting and the circulation of minutes.

SECTION:	**MEETINGS**
TITLE:	
AUTHOR:	

SECTION:	**MEETINGS**
TITLE:	**NOTE TAKING**
AUTHOR:	Adapted from the original Skills Manual by Val Harris

The purpose of the technique is to facilitate taking accurate and informative notes during a meeting and to enable a concise, relevant and accurate report to be written afterwards.

A)

1. Divide your paper in half drawing a line from top to bottom. Use the left hand side of the page only. Leave the right hand side blank.

2. Note the speaker and topic first.

3. Listen and note down key words and phrases. Don't attempt to take down exactly what is said.

4. Learn to follow the meaning of what is being said rather than every word.

5. When notes are completed go back to the beginning as soon as possible and begin reading through. On the right hand side of the page put down the points missed, personal comments, and indications about the emphasis and logic of the argument.

6. Finally write a report from the notes leaving out items which on reflection are not relevant.

N.B. A good report may be more concise than the notes on which is based.

B)

Another way of recording group decisions is using wall minutes.

1. Put up a number of large sheets of paper.

2. Before passing on to the next item the group says what it wishes to record as its view, decision, action taken etc., about the item just discussed. The group should agree on the warding of the wall minutes.

Notes:

1. People may quibble over the warding and content of minutes written by one individual. One individual may not want to be "saddled" with taking minutes. A group minute taking session after discussion on each item can be a response to these situations.

2. Since the wall minutes can be written out after and handed out to the group for the following meeting individuals are reminded about the group decision. It may reduce disagreement about what was decided.

3. A group may want to agree a format for recording items, e.g. decision, action to be taken, who to take action.

SECTION:	**MEETINGS**
TITLE:	
AUTHOR:	

SECTION:	**MEETINGS**
TITLE:	**FOLLOW UP AFTER MEETINGS**
AUTHOR:	Ann Hindley

The committee member likely to have most to do after a meeting is the secretary. It will be their task to write or type the minutes and have them circulated and to ensure that an agenda is drawn up for the next meeting. If the committee is an active one, however, a number of other committee members will have tasks to carry out and these should be recorded in the minutes.

ACTION MINUTES

An effective way of ensuring that everyone knows what they promised to do at a meeting is to prepare action minutes and ensure that they are distributed early. Action minutes involve drawing a column down the right hand side of the page and entering the relevant committee members' initials against each action they have agreed to undertake.

This will act as an easy reminder to committee members of what they agreed to do and provide a way of checking at the next meeting what was agreed and what has and has not been done.

OFFICERS' MEETINGS

Another useful device for both follow up and preparation is that of holding officers' meetings. These will involve the chair, vice chair, secretary and treasurer meeting between committee meetings to chase up matters that need further work and/or discussion. It will also give them an opportunity to prepare for the next meeting by insuring that all information, including financial information, is available, that all tasks not completed are under way and all contacts made. An officers' meeting will also give you chance to delegate chasing the other members who promised to do something.

WORKER'S FOLLOW UP

As a worker working for or servicing a committee, there could be a number of jobs that you personally need to follow up. Or you might want to give support to the other committee members in their work.

The technique of making a list of tasks and prioritising them immediately after the meeting is a start to ensuring follow up happens. It is also best to make appointments before the meeting disperses with those committee members needing help and/or support, before the impetus is lost.

SECTION:	**MEETINGS**
TITLE:	
AUTHOR:	

SECTION:	**MEETINGS**
TITLE:	**GROUNDRULES FOR EFFECTIVE MEETINGS**
AUTHOR:	Val Harris

Groups often find it useful to set their own ground rules which will guide the way they will organise themselves and spell out the behaviour that is expected from each person at the meeting.

There are several ways that ground rules may be set up: one is by a brainstorm – asking everyone to throw in their ideas, and then discuss which ones should be kept or discarded. Another is by producing a list like this one and asking people to add other ones or to change the wording to suit the group.

In meetings everyone should have the right to:

- state their opinions and put forward suggestions.

- have these opinions and suggestions listened to and reacted to.

- understand what is being said.

- disagree with views put forward by others.

- make their contributions without being interrupted by others.

- have minutes (if they are taken) that are an accurate reflection of what is said in the meetings.

- know in advance what the purpose of the meeting is.

- know in advance roughly how long the meeting will last.

- not be personally attacked or put down for their views.

- change their views.

- have an equal right to vote on all decisions unless it has been decided otherwise (e.g. when people have vested interests).

- not be subjected to offensive language.

- not to be excluded by the use of jargon.

- to have their confidence respected.

What ever method is chosen, once a main list is agreed upon, everyone in the group is asked to take on responsibility for keeping to these rules.

SECTION:	MEETINGS
TITLE:	
AUTHOR:	

SECTION 11

GROUP ORGANISATION

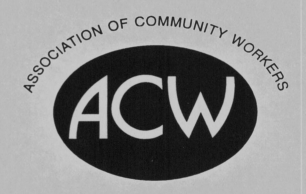

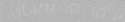
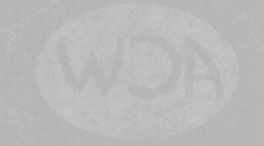

SECTION:	**GROUP ORGANISATION**
TITLE:	**DIFFICULTIES OF BEING ON A COMMITTEE**
AUTHOR:	Ann Hindley

Most community groups and projects are run by a committee of one sort or another. Many people end up on a committee without any information or training in how to be effective as a committee member and so it's not surprising if some committees don't work as well as they could.

If you think your committee is not functioning very effectively it's useful to be able to pinpoint what the nature of the problem might be and then the committee members can do something to improve their situation.

This checklist can be used as the basis for a group discussion on what is going wrong: each one could be put onto a piece of paper/card and people could pick up the ones they feel are most important for them: some blank cards/papers could be included so people can add other suggestions once people have chosen the most relevant cards/pieces of paper. The group can then discuss them one at a time and come up with some suggestions for change.

- jargon and complex language

- intimidating atmosphere

- bad chairing

- clique who know what's happening

- papers and reports arrive late

- meetings difficult to get to

- no expenses or loss of earnings payments

- can't hear

- wrong time for meeting

- don't understand the importance of some items, lack of clarity

- little time to consult other people involved

- lack of independent advice on issues

- being treated as a token or expected to be representative of a diverse group e.g. of all black people

- lack of commitment from other committee members to providing equal opportunities for all

- not knowing what is expected of committee members

SECTION:	**GROUP ORGANISATION**
TITLE:	
AUTHOR:	

SECTION:	**GROUP ORGANISATION**
TITLE:	**GUIDELINES FOR WELL RUN COMMITTEES**
AUTHOR:	Ann Hindley

Committees come in all shapes and sizes which reflect the different kinds of groups and projects they are organising. These are some basic guidelines which will help to ensure that your committee is as effective as possible at carrying out it's aims and objectives.

The following checklist may help you in setting out the ground rules/ guidelines for the way you want to work.

- Do you provide training – induction and ongoing – for committee members

- Do you set standards for when paper and reports should arrive and how they should be written

- Do you make sure reports are written clearly

- Are there summaries of all reports

- Do you organise pre-meeting briefings on major/new subjects

- Do you have a system for getting subjects put on agendas

- Do you have a system on how to get members views on each item

- Do you have the resources to report back to your members

- Do you arrange for feedback to the committee on what happens outside of the meetings

- Do you plan for meetings beforehand

- A good chair makes it easier for committee members

- Are you willing to move venue and times of meetings to suit members

- Can you pay expenses and cover loss of earnings

- Do you have access to use an induction loop in your committee meetings

SECTION:	**GROUP ORGANISATION**
TITLE:	
AUTHOR:	

SECTION:	**GROUP ORGANISATION**
TITLE:	**POLICY MANUAL**
AUTHOR:	Adapted from the original Skills Manual by Val Harris

As groups and projects become established so their membership changes and it becomes difficult for new members to know and understand all the policy decision that previous committees have made.

The purpose of the technique is: to create an up to date reference document of all the policies adopted by an organisation; this can then be given to new members when they join as well as providing a reference for longer serving members.

Conditions for the technique to be of any value:

Technically a policy manual can be established for any organisation providing it makes policy decisions. However unless members of the organisation are prepared to be accountable and implement policy it is not worth the effort. The policy manual is not a prison from which the organisation cannot escape; it presents a starting point. Its purpose is to clarify policy. Nor should the policy manual be used to stifle initiative.

The technique is intended to identify all formal sources (committees etc.) of policy in the organisation.

Collect a complete set of documents (and copy another set as well) which may have policies noted in them e.g. minutes, constitutions, standing orders, contracts of employment, statements of procedures, reports and publications.

Go through all the documents, noting the subject area of any policy, where the decision on the policy was taken, when the decision was taken and briefly note the policy.

Sort your notes into sections so that all references to the same area of policy are together. This constitutes as a policy grouping. Arranging the policy groupings in a logical sequence so that related policy areas are together. Record the sequence – this is your contents list or retrieval system.

Take the other set and go to work with scissors, cutting and gluing onto backing sheets the policies on each subject. This will give a policy statement on each area. There will probably be a few inconsistencies that will need resolving later.

Once you have compiled the policy statements you can use these as a basis for drafting the policy manual. You will need to resolve any contradictions or confusions, and ensure that the document reads well.

Present draft to appropriate policy making body, amend draft and policy as required. DON'T LIMIT DISCUSSION TO INTERPRETING PREVIOUS DECISIONS; IT IS POSSIBLE TO INCLUDE A COMPLETE POLICY REVIEW AT THIS STAGE.

Get copies of the policy manual printed and distributed. Keep a list of all those with a policy manual. When any amendments or additional policy is adopted, ensure that all these on the list receive copies of any new policy statements. Issue clear instructions. With any new statements e.g. "This statement replaces the previous policy on conditions of employment. Please throw out previous conditions!" Or "please find attached additional policy adopted by the general committee on the proposed White Hall Highway, insert after existing policy statement". Updating is made much easier if the manual is in a loose leaf form. UPDATING THE MANUAL IS ESSENTIAL. ALL POLICY STATEMENTS SHOULD BE CLEARLY DATED AND POLICY BODY ADOPTING THE POLICY RECORDED ON THE STATEMENT.

SECTION:	**GROUP ORGANISATION**
TITLE:	
AUTHOR:	

SECTION:	**GROUP ORGANISATION**
TITLE:	**TIME LINE**
AUTHOR:	Adapted from the original Skills Manual by Val Harris

Once a group has decided that it wants to organise an event it is useful to break down all the work that needs to be done and to decide when they need doing.

Thus the purpose of this technique is to establish a sequence of activities which have to take place for a particular event to occur.

The technique:

1.   Draw a vertical line on a sheet of paper.

2.   Divide it into time periods appropriate to the problem.

3.   Mark NOW at the top and the event in question at the bottom.

4.   Write down all the possible tasks or activities which have to occur in connection with the event on a separate piece of paper.

5.   Use the list of tasks or activities and fill in on the time line what has to be done when, by sticking the pieces of paper on with blue tack.

An example:

A team of fieldworkers employed by a local authority wishes to be involved in selecting a replacement for one of their numbers who is about to leave. The kind of participation they can expect to achieve involves the following kinds of activities:

•   drafting an advert

•   working out criteria for selecting a replacement

•   shortlisting applicants

•   interviewing short listed candidates

•   feeding views into a formal interview panel

All the fieldworkers have full diaries and want to work out accurately when they are going to have to make time to become involved. They draw up the time line shown overleaf.

SECTION:	**GROUP ORGANISATION**
TITLE:	**TIME LINE**
AUTHOR:	Adapted from the original Skills Manual by Val Harris

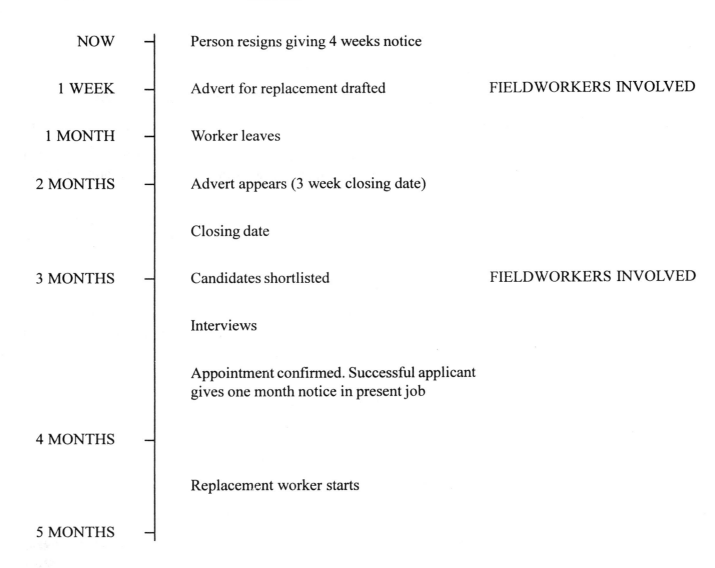

Further points:

In this example the fieldworkers know they will have to keep their diaries clear around the beginning of month 3 if they really want to be involved. They could draw up another time line focusing specifically on the use of time over this two week period, specifying who was going to take on what tasks.

The technique could be used in planning a conference, or a campaign which starts on a certain date, the launching of a publication, the writing of a report or preparations for an Annual General Meeting.

SECTION 12

VOLUNTEERS

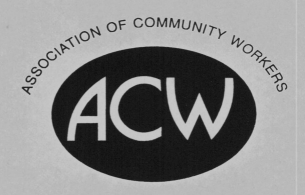

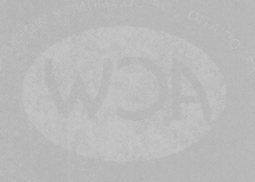

SECTION:	**VOLUNTEERS**
TITLE:	**WORKING WITH VOLUNTEERS: A GOOD PRACTICE CHECK LIST**
AUTHOR:	Roger Green

Volunteering allows people from the community to participate in the life of their community by working for a locally based group or organisation.

Groups and organisations employing volunteers should adopt good practice guidelines which ensure the rights of the volunteers

This is a checklist of points to consider:

Benefits

Taking on volunteers may affect their rights to various benefits and pensions (see DSS/Benefits Agency leaflets).

Equal Partners

Volunteers should be seen and treated as equal members of the group/organisation they are working with, along with paid staff. The relationship between volunteers and paid staff should be complementary and of mutual benefit to each other, the group/ organisation and its users.

Expenses

Volunteers should be paid out of pocket expenses e.g. travel, meals etc. Most voluntary sector groups/organisations pay such expenses.

Influence

Volunteers should have access to and play a part in influencing the work and the decision making of the group/organisation they are working with, for example, this might be representation on the management committee. This would ensure volunteers interests, ideas and experiences are represented.

Every group/organisation should ask themselves: how will the voice of volunteers be heard in their group/organisation?

Insurance

Groups/organisations should have adequate insurance cover for individuals employed as volunteers, for example, Public Liability Insurance.

Job Description

This is sometimes called a "volunteer agreement".

Volunteers need a clear understanding of their role and the duties and responsibilities attached to it. This needs to be in the form of a written job description or person specification.

Managing

Volunteers should have a named person who they are responsible to within the group/organisation for their work. They should be clear as to how they can contact this person and how often they meet with this person to discuss their work. It should ideally be a paid employee of the group/organisation.

SECTION:	**VOLUNTEERS**
TITLE:	**WORKING WITH VOLUNTEERS: A GOOD PRACTICE CHECK LIST**
AUTHOR:	Roger Green

Partners

Volunteers should be recruited on the basis that they are to complement paid employees of the group/organisation, not replace them. They should not be seen as a cheap option.

Police Check

How this is done varies considerably across the country and between groups and organisations.

However it is good practice that all volunteers should have a police check, particularly those volunteers who will work with children and other vulnerable groups

Contact the nearest Social Services office, local volunteer bureaux for advice on this or the local police station.

If in doubt check out!

Recruiting Volunteers

Good practice in recruiting volunteers is ensuring that everybody in the community has the right to apply to become a volunteer.

Staff and volunteers of the group/organisation should reflect the cultural and ethnic composition of the community it is based in and the users of the group/organisation.

Good practice in recruiting volunteers means trying to recruit local people as volunteers where possible to reflect this balance.

Advertising in local newspapers, through local radio, existing networks the group has etc., should all be used. Interviews and the selection of volunteers should be on an equal opportunities basis.

Supervision

Volunteers should receive regular supervision, either one to one or group supervision with a member of the group/organisations staff i.e. paid employee.

Support

Volunteers will need support with their work to help them maintain their motivation, maximise their contribution and involvement to the group/organisations work.

This means identifying their support needs; building support systems for them e.g. regular meetings of volunteers, such as a volunteers forum where they can raise issues and discuss concerns, ideas etc. in a collective setting.

USEFUL ADDRESSES

The Volunteer Centre UK

The Volunteer Centre provides a range of courses, publications, information and a consultancy service on most aspects of working with volunteers.

Address:

29, Lower Kings Road,
Berkhamstead,
Hertfordshire HP4 2AB
Tel: 01442 873311

Resource Unit for Black Volunteering

A national voluntary organisation which aims to promote black volunteering.

Address:

First Floor, 102, Park Village East,
London NW1 3SP
Tel: 0171 388 8542

The National Association of Volunteer Bureaux

NAVB supports a network of over 250 Volunteer Bureaux across the country.

Address:

St. Peter's College,
College Road,
Saltley,
Birmingham B8 3TE
Tel: 0121 327 0265

Trade Union Membership

Volunteers should have the right and be encouraged to join a trade union when employed by a group/organisation. Trade unions, such as, Unison, should be contacted for advice on this.

Training Needs

All volunteers should expect and receive training when working for a group/organisation. Ideally this should take place prior to them working with the group/organisation.

This could take the form of a history of the group/organisation, its aims and objectives and its work with individuals and groups the group/organisation works with.

It should also include training on the skills and knowledge required to work for the group/organisation, for example, group work skills, counselling skills.

Volunteers should also be involved in reviewing and identifying their future training needs.

Valuing Volunteers

Volunteers should be valued for the skills and knowledge they bring with them; who they are as individuals; their experience. Also their local knowledge of the community (which is sometimes better than the group/organisations paid workers and professionals working in the community).

Their commitment, motivation and enthusiasm should also be valued.

SECTION:	**VOLUNTEERS**
TITLE:	
AUTHOR:	

SECTION:	**VOLUNTEERS**
TITLE:	**ASIAN VOLUNTEERS (A CASE STUDY)**
AUTHOR:	Sneh Kashyap

I worked as a Co-ordinator/Trainer for a project called "The Asian Parent Programme" for several years. This project involved working with a team of volunteers who are known as "Asian Community Mothers". In this paper I explain how I recruited Asian people for my project.

In recruiting experienced Asian mothers for training as Community Mothers, the choice is made on the basis of the woman's overall competence and gentleness of approach rather than forcefulness or leadership qualities. There is no doubt that the best way to recruit volunteers for my scheme is through personal recommendation, however there are other ways that I have considered:

- through the local community units

- on local radio

- through the local schools

- by leafletting local houses, shops

but the most rewarding has been by word of mouth.

After recommendation a letter for an open day is sent out to all the people who have responded to discuss and for me to give out the following information:

- what the scheme does, how it is organised and who's who

- a list of things that the volunteers should get involved in

- how training is on offer to them and in any case how they are supported: group support meetings and a one to one support meeting.

As the scheme involves working with small babies and their mothers/families on a home visiting structure the volunteers have to go through screening i.e.

- occupational health checks

- police checks

- declaration of no criminal convictions

- contract on confidentiality

As a good practice I get a form filled which includes: name, address, telephone number etc., and also ask for a reference. This lets the volunteer know that I am being vigilant and responsible in my care for the Asian families we are working with. I try to get the Community Mothers to be realistic when they volunteer their time. This project requires at least 25 hours work a month, and has to be between 9.00 a.m. to 5.00 p.m. so that they are insured and legal.

Sometimes you can over commit yourselves and then find that you have no time left for home life. Therefore I allocate the maximum of 10 families per Community Mother at 2 hours per family per

SECTION:	**VOLUNTEERS**
TITLE:	**ASIAN VOLUNTEERS (A CASE STUDY)**
AUTHOR:	Sneh Kashyap

month and add on group training days and one to one training days which makes a total of approximately 25 hours a month.

Most of these Community Mothers have never been out to work, and may be claiming some sort of income support. In order that they do not lose out on that, we provide a re-imbursement of expenses @ £3.00 per hour.

The introduction of this programme has helped to identify resources within the Asian Community which can provide culturally appropriate support to families in the early years of child rearing.

I can now clearly identify that any service can be delivered effectively by appropriate volunteers provided standards are set to meet the needs. In this case it cannot be right to compel families to conform to those western views of child rearing which are not necessarily appropriate to Asian family life, therefore Asian experienced mothers were the appropriate volunteers to deliver the service and Asian women can do it!

SECTION 13

TRAINING

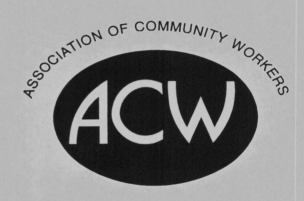

SECTION:	**TRAINING**
TITLE:	**POINTS TO CONSIDER WHEN PLANNING A TRAINING SESSION**
AUTHOR:	Ann Hindley and Gordon Falconer

This article is designed as a check list of some of the things you may need to consider before running a training session. This is in no way an exhaustive list rather it's purpose is to get you thinking.

GENERAL

- Equal opportunities and Equal Access issues are integral to the whole process and everything you do: advertising, recruitment, selection, venue, materials, facilitators, handouts, practical work, refreshments and/or meals, evaluation and follow-up.

- Offer relevant information prior to the session i.e. background reading, list of the participants, map.

- Materials and handouts should be user friendly, relevant and accessible to all.

- Get all the equipment booked well in advance and know how to use it.

- Don't use other peoples material unless you have to. However if you do, and we all do, make sure you've thought about and prepared for it well in advance and credit them.

VENUE

- Get the basics right i.e. comfortable room and surroundings, heating, provide a variety of refreshments e.g. fruit juices, water, tea, coffee, herbal teas, milk and biscuits (non-animal fats), etc., and the group will gladly give their time.

- Does everyone know where the venue is and how to get there? Is it accessible to all? Do you want it to be somewhere local and familiar, on a bus route, impressive and prestigious, accessible? What can you afford?

- Make sure that you look at the premises first. Are they suitable? Is there background noise, is there room for a creche? Is there room to reflect an overhead projector? Are there any convenient power points? Are there tea making facilities? Are the rooms big enough? Are there enough chairs? (Book the venue well in advance.)

PARTICIPANTS

- Be aware of who's coming, how many and where from.

- Do you know if participants have any particular requirements?

- How are participants getting to and from the session?

SECTION:	**TRAINING**
TITLE:	**POINTS TO CONSIDER WHEN PLANNING A TRAINING SESSION**
AUTHOR:	Ann Hindley and Gordon Falconer

FINANCE – HOW MUCH IS IT GOING TO COST?

- Get estimates from local trainers/agencies.

- Price up alternative venues.

- Are you providing a creche? – Carers cost/sitters costs – how much will the room, wages and toy hire cost?

- Are you going to provide refreshments?

- Will you have to hire equipment such as overhead projector or flip chart stand?

- Will the training materials be photocopied by the trainer or will you need to photocopy them? – Allow for Brailling/ signing costs.

- Bookings – set up a system for accepting and acknowledging bookings. Keep a list so that you know when you've got to your maximum. Do you want money with the booking or will you invoice? Remember to say who you want cheques made out to if people are likely to pay by cheque. Give receipts – keep a book.

- When you know the answers, prepare the budget. Have you got this much in your training budget? If not, you need to be looking at charitable sources, Training and Enterprise Council, County Council Economic Development, and ask at your local CVS for other ideas. Are you going to charge and how much per person or organisation? Reflect this in your budget.

PUBLICITY

Make out a list to all the organisations and people who might be interested. Put a press release in the local papers. Prepare a leaflet letter/programme and circulate well in advance. Remember to include details of:

- How to book

- Prices

- Dates

- Venue

- What it's about

- Who the trainer(s) are

- Creche/carers

- Accessibility arrangements.

TRAINERS

Can you do the training? If not, look around for suitable people. Ask your CVS, TEC, Adult Education, WEA. There are a number of directories about. Take up references from other groups who have used them. Make sure that you know how much they charge before you book them and that they have a background in the sort of training that you want. Make your arrangements with them in writing so that there can be no misunderstanding about dates, times, prices etc.

- Facilitator(s) should know what they are expected to do. If co-working have they worked together before?
- Be there to check arrangements and welcome trainers and trainees.

ON THE DAY

- Start on time and be disciplined about your time.
- Don't over plan the session.
- Establish clearly understood guidelines.
- Tell participants there are no right or wrong answers.
- Mix participants up when doing practical work.
- Allow plenty of time for feedback.
- Value and enjoy the practical work. Don't get hung up on the task or the agenda.
- Trust the group – it's their course, so go with them.
- Remember your groupwork.
- Challenge discriminatory practice and views.
- Write things up as you go along.
- Label everything fully.
- Trust your own skills.
- Practice what you preach.

GENERAL

- If you wish to get your course accredited allow lots of time and be prepared for hard work and re-writing.
- Expect the unexpected.
- Have a good time.

TRAINING IS FUN.

SECTION:	**TRAINING**
TITLE:	
AUTHOR:	

SECTION:	TRAINING
TITLE:	NATIONAL VOCATIONAL QUALIFICATIONS
AUTHOR:	Extracts from National Council for Vocational Qualifications publications

"NVQ's" – Another set of initials? – just some more jargon? ... but they appear to be here to stay and community work has developed its own NVQ's. In this article we reproduce some of the main points of the nature of NVQ's and their relevance to people active in the community, whether it be as an activist or a paid worker.

NVQ's provide one route to qualification in community work – one that is based on showing what you can already do and so is very similar to the accreditation process that many people are already familiar with.

NCVQ is committed to the recognition of competence HOWEVER acquired. In the past, awarding bodies have tended to give particular weight to two roles – employment and study – and to pay less attention, for certification purposes, to the family, voluntary work and leisure. In this sense, previous practice has perhaps tended to fall into the trap of equating "work" exclusively with conventional paid employment. Now training organisations – and the lecturers, trainers and tutors who work in them – are being encouraged to recognise competence acquired in all areas of work carried out in the home and family, in the community and in the voluntary sector.

THE VALUE OF UNPAID WORK

Providing credit for competence acquired in unpaid work allows individuals planning their training and career, to take account of the totality of their experiences. It also allows employers to build up a better picture of the possible value of a particular individual to the organisation. This is relevant both to recruitment and, on a more long term basis, to negotiating and planning the individual's progress within the organisation.

Also providing credit for competence gives formal recognition to the value of unpaid work to our society and to our economy. For example, it means that the 1.4 million people who spend more than 20 hours a week caring for sick, disabled or elderly people can now get recognition for their skills.

TOWARDS A WIDER CONCEPT OF WORK

The NVQ Framework is based on a recognition of the dynamic nature of work in our society. At its heart, it represents a system of credit accumulation and transfer designed to help individuals and organisations to see education and training as a continuing career-long process. The system allows workers to update their skills and knowledge as their area of work changes.

CREDIT FOR COMPETENCE

Many features of the NVQ Framework make it easier to provide credit for competence achieved outside conventional paid employment. Amongst these are:

- NVQ's are based on explicit statements of competence. These statements spell out what a candidate is required to be able to do for the award of an NVQ and include criteria by which performance can be assessed. For the purpose of certification, the context in which the candidate achieved competence is not important – work at home is every bit as valid an arena as work on the shop floor.

- All NVQ's are made up of a number of units of competence. Each "unit", representing a discrete area of competence which has value and meaning at the workplace, can be assessed separately and a candidate can receive credit for achieving it. The important point here is that individuals can gain unit credits and then use this as a basis for planning a programme of learning and experience which will lead to the award of a full NVQ.

- The NVQ assessment model relies on evidence of competence which can be collected from a range of sources.

AGREED NATIONAL STANDARDS OF COMPETENCE

Which form the basis for

NVQ STATEMENTS OF COMPETENCE   UNITS OF COMPETENCE   ELEMENTS OF COMPETENCE   WITH PERFORMANCE CRITERIA

These determine

THE NATURE AND AMOUNT OF   EVIDENCE NEEDED FROM A   COMBINATION OF ALTERNATIVE SOURCES

Including

EVIDENCE OF PRIOR LEARNING   AND ACHIEVEMENT   EVIDENCE OF KNOWLEDGE,   UNDERSTANDING AND SKILL   PERFORMANCE AND EVIDENCE

REMOVING BARRIERS TO ACHIEVEMENT AND PUTTING PEOPLE FIRST

- The NVQ system has removed the traditional barriers to qualifications, shifting the emphasis from institutional requirements to individuals needs.

- NVQ's and the NVQ FRAMEWORK provide open access to assessment and clearly stated competence targets and progression routes.

- The National Database makes public and available to all information on qualifications and assessment requirements. It provides users with the facility to map progression routes through the system.

- The National Record gives the individual control of their movement through the system, a means to record their experience and achievement, set targets and timeframes, and continuously asses progress.

- NVQ's have no unnecessary entry requirements such as age, previous qualifications, specified length of experience anyone can put themselves forward for assessment. NVQ's necessitate that informed guidance, counselling, and initial assessment replace arbitrary entry requirements.

CREDIT ACCUMULATION

NVQ unit credit design gives people greater choice in how they get qualified. Credits can be accumulated as and when the individual wishes. Career breaks no longer mean missing out completing qualifications. Unit credits enable those re-entering training to gain early endorsement of their competence.

NVQ units also allow people with learning difficulties or disabilities, for whom gaining a full NVQ may not be a realistic goal, to gain valuable credits within the qualifications system.

THE AWARDING BODIES

NCVQ requires awarding bodies to have an equal opportunities policy, and a means of monitoring its implementation. The policy must be clearly communicated to candidates and organisations involved in the operation of the award. NCVQ's role is to assist awarding bodies in developing policies and practices that promote equal opportunities in NVQ delivery through their centres.

Awarding bodies are encouraged to develop their equal opportunities practices further with regard to:

- the communication and marketing of NVQ's

- access to assessment

- assessment methods

- administration of assessor and verifier selection and training

- providing a recognised appeals procedure

- monitoring and evaluation arrangements

By addressing such issues, awarding bodies are working to remove any remaining barriers that create access problems for both learners and providers. Detailed information is available from the awarding bodies themselves.

SECTION:	TRAINING
TITLE:	ACCREDITATION OF PREVIOUS EXPERIENCE AND LEARNING
AUTHOR:	Toni Baptiste

This article comes out of my experience of completing a pilot study as part of the Work Related Further Education Fund. This study investigated "access to accreditation of previous experience and learning for educationally disadvantaged groups". Like most educational research I feel that just the title of this work is jargonistic and inaccessible so before I go on I want to give some clear definitions of the terms used.

ACCESS

Because of the long history of "free" educational services in Britain and well established Further and Community Education sectors it is easy for people to assume that "we all have access to education, new developments in educational systems and routes to qualifications". Rubbish! Very many studies have shown that access to education is hampered by social class, race gender, disability and so on. For the purpose of my study I was looking at how to enable access to an educational resource for mature returners, women returners, members of black groups (all people of colour). This included people who were also classified as long-term unemployed (it's no surprise that unpaid community workers fall within these categories). These groups are widely recognised as being Educationally Disadvantaged....

EDUCATIONALLY DISADVANTAGED

For my purposes this term is used to indicate and identify people who have not gained access to the system and consequently have few educational qualifications. It does not mean unable to learn, uneducated, unskilled or inexperienced. Everyone has some previous experience and learning but even a well qualified person will not have had all their learning documented and endorsed by qualifications. For example, most people cook, but few people will take a cookery exam, unless they are seeking employment in the catering industry.

ACCREDITATION OF PREVIOUS EXPERIENCE AND LEARNING

This is quite an old piece of jargon in adult education and it basically means taking into account previous knowledge and skills and bringing this into the learning situation. However its meaning has become more sinister with the development of National Vocational Qualifications which is having a profound effect on training and ultimately on all education. Part of the underlying philosophy of this new development is that: *if people have the skills to do jobs, no matter how or where they have learnt, they are entitled to the qualification.* This forms the basis of the very recent focusing in educational services on accreditation of previous experience.

Accreditation of previous experience is an extremely time consuming and costly educational process, which is almost coinciding with the privatisation of further education. Throughout 1991 some Educational Establishments and Training and Enterprise Councils were exploring ways of offering this service to employers and individuals who can afford to pay. At the end of 1991 questions were being asked regarding access to accreditation for other groups and the small pilot study that I was involved in was exploring original ideas of *how to, how best to, and what are the barriers to....*

Here are some practical tips on how individual and groups of community workers can start working towards gaining accreditation, which at its most basic level is working towards recognition and value for what is often highly skilled and unpaid labour:

- Allow yourself the time to sit down and review your life experience, think about your life, skills and any achievements. Any experience you have from voluntary work and previous educational experience.

- Think about what you would really like to achieve. Things that you would really enjoy and would like to develop further. This may be a particular job that you would like to go for in the future or recognition for your experiences of the past.

- Everyone can have different goals; you may be doing voluntary work for the same organisation as your friends but some people may want to credit their administrative experience and some their community work. Think about what **you** really want and need a qualification in. If you are not sure about the options careers advice is available at most colleges and job centres and through discussion with friends and colleagues.

- Once you have decided what you are going for, look up relevant qualifications on the NVQ Database. This is available at some TEC's and colleges. Also look through some college prospectuses. Examine the competencies required.

  ("Competences" are just a list of skills and level of skills that NVQ's are broken down to. A checklist that will list areas of experience and learning such as "able to communicate" "able to manage" "able to type at 30 w.p.m." "design a leaflet" etc.) This can also give you some idea of what level of qualification you are aiming at.

- Look through the notes you have made on your previous life experience and pick out bits that are relevant to your qualification area. For example, if you were going to go for a counselling qualification on the basis of previous experience you would need evidence of previous study of counselling theory, such as attendance of previous courses, and practical counselling experience such as voluntary work you have done in this area and in your private life. It may be that you are

SECTION:	**TRAINING**
TITLE:	**ACCREDITATION OF PREVIOUS EXPERIENCE AND LEARNING**
AUTHOR:	Toni Baptiste

USEFUL ADDRESSES.

THE LEARNING FROM EXPERIENCE
TRUST,
6, Buckingham Gate,
London,
SW1 E6JP.

ACCESS TO ASSESSMENT
SERVICES,
North Lincolnshire College,
Cathedral Street,
Lincs. LN2 SHQ.

THE FEDERATION OF COMMUNITY
WORK TRAINING GROUPS,
356 Glossop Road,
Sheffield
S10 2HW

PUBLICATIONS.

The Assessment of Prior Learning and
Learner Services (1992) F.E.U.

Building your portfolio
A Basic Guide (1990). Anne Woodrow.
F.E.U.

Accreditation of Prior Learning
Report from Telford F.E. College APL
Project (1990) SCOTVEC.

Building Portfolios
A Training Manual designed by and
available from
Swindon Community Work Training
Group
C/O TVSC
1 St. John Street Swindon SN1 1RT

"A Credit To You"
A work related Further Education pilot
study on the accreditation of previous
experience for disadvantaged groups
A. Baptiste. (1992) available from
Clarendon College
Pelham Avenue Nottingham.

only half way there but you will be building on what you have got so far.

- If possible ask people who you have worked for in the past to give you references detailing exactly what your experience was. Dig out old photographs and publicity material. If you have attended any courses find programmes and documentation.

- START DOCUMENTING YOUR EXPERIENCE FROM NOW. Evidence from your past (always difficult if like me you throw bits away!), evidence from now and evidence from the future will all form part of your portfolio (a portfolio is a folder of information including all the relevant bits you have collected).

- Get into the habit of keeping a diary. If you attend any training sessions ask for a certificate of attendance. Keep course programmes. If you do any work where you feel you are demonstrating your skills ask the person who is supervising you for a reference that lays out clearly what you are doing and how competent you are

- Track down a college that is offering courses in subjects that you want to become accredited in and negotiate accreditation of your previous experience. This varies from area to area and it is also clouded by colleges needs to fill courses (bums on the seats) or staff knowledge or lack of knowledge on how to operationalise the policy. Be persistent!

- Finally as a group you might like to think up some ways of supporting each other through the process. Set aside time to do exercises on action planning, skills identification, portfolio building. It may be that as a group you would like to obtain similar qualifications. So you can share information and negotiate with an accrediting agency (e.g. colleges) together.

SECTION:	**TRAINING**
TITLE:	
AUTHOR:	

SECTION:	**TRAINING**
TITLE:	**TRAINING OPPORTUNITIES**
AUTHOR:	Peter Wilde

Community Work Practice is developed and improved by providing opportunities for continued reflection and learning for those involved, whether they be paid workers or unpaid activists. The Federation of Community Work Training Groups was established to bring together groups who are working at a local or regional level to provide such opportunities.

In order for training to achieve its goal it must have the same starting point as community development and be based upon people's experience. It will actively seek to promote models which challenge the power relationships which exist in society (e.g. Black/White, male/female), and for this to be possible 'trainers' will themselves have to be conscious of, and have located themselves in, these issues.

A participatory approach to training is a way of working which most suits the requirements of community development. It is based upon the belief that adults learn most effectively when they are involved in activities which take their own knowledge and experience into account as a basis for reflection and learning.

The member groups of the Federation provide a model for ways in which those involved in community work, at a local level, can collectively both develop their own learning and training skills and deliver a wide range of opportunities for community work learning.

The starting point for many groups has been to develop a short Introductory Course in Community Work (Stage 1). These courses are geared towards those involved in community groups who have not had the opportunity to undertake previous training. Building upon the experience of its membership the Federation has published a training manual to support the further development of such courses. The manual provides a practical guide for a ten x three hour course which includes both a "core" curriculum focusing on the values and processes integral to good community work practice, and a "negotiated" curriculum arising out of the needs and interests of each group of participants. Such courses are increasingly being accredited in some way, often through local Open College Federations.

The development of such introductory courses can provide the "agenda setting" and "jumping off" point for a range of further courses and training events. It can also lead participants onto more individual recognition of skills and experience and development planning through portfolio building.

In partnership with local educational institutions it is possible to develop longer courses (certificate level) such as the Community Work Learning Programme run by the Greater Manchester Training Group through Manchester University, and by West Yorkshire Community Work Training Group with Leeds University. Indeed some local and regional groups are now working to develop the progressive sequence of locally based courses which lead to professional qualification.

The Federation, as part of its work, convened a Forum on Community Work Training and Qualification, which has become part of the developing National Training Organisation and brings together a range of community work organisations who are involved in training and qualification for community work "in its own right", including an accreditation of practice route, already regionally developed through a number of Federation groups.

The proposals developed by the Forum have been widely supported by the community work field and work has led to the establishment of a Community Work Standards Council.

There may well be a local or regional training group near you (see contact list). If not the Federation provides support and advice in setting up training groups. It also publishes a quarterly Community Work Training Bulletin and can offer general advice on developing community work training.

SECTION:	**TRAINING**
TITLE:	**TRAINING OPPORTUNITIES**
AUTHOR:	Peter Wilde

THE PROPOSED RANGE OF ROUTES TO A COMMUNITY WORK AWARD – Nationally recognised

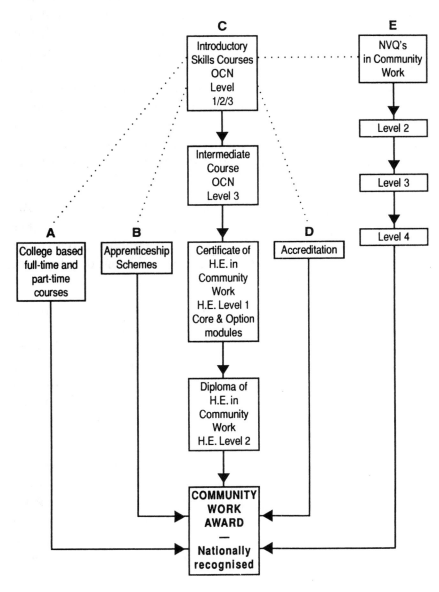

LOCAL AND REGIONAL TRAINING GROUPS CONTACT LIST

Avon Accreditation Unit
c/o Community Development Section
Bristol Central Library
College Green
Bristol BS1 5TL
Tel: 0117 922 2660

Basingstoke CWTG
c/o Hilary Reed
Community Services
Civic Offices
London Road
Basingstoke RG21 4AH
Tel: 01256 45687

Blackburn and Darwen CWTG
c/o Clare Mason
CVS
St. John's Centre
Victoria Street
Blackburn BB1 6DW
Tel: 01254 583957

Cardiff CWTG
c/o Lorna Wallis/Nicola Vale
Voluntary Action Cardiff
Strand House
2 Fitzalan Place
Cardiff CF2 1BD
Tel: 01222 485722

East Anglia CWTG
c/o John Bottomley
CD Team
Latton Bush
Southern Way
Harlow
Essex CM18 7BL
Tel: 01279 446611

Greater Manchester CWTG and Accreditation Unit
c/o Kay Fairhurst
Unit 95
23 New Mount Street
Manchester M4 4DE
Tel: 0161 953 4117

Gwent CWTG
c/o Jim Barnaville
Monmouth Diocesan Team
2 Emlyn Walk
Newport
Gwent NP9 1EW
Tel: 01633 213771

Hull CWTG
c/o Les Braim
29 Anlaby Road
Hull HU1 2PG
Tel: 01482 324474

**Liverpool Community Learning
Network**
c/o Val O'Rourke
Community Rights
Caber House
10-12 Pall Mall
Liverpool L3 6AL
Tel: 0151 255 0588

Mid Glamorgan CWTG
c/o Terry Burns
WEA Office, Room 7
58/60 Commercial Street
Mountain Ash
South Wales CF45 3PW
Tel: 01443 477300

**Northamptonshire Voluntary Sector
Training Group**
c/o Richard Powell
Junction 7
3-7 Hazelwood Road
Northampton NN1 1LG

**North East Region CWTG and
Accreditation Unit**
c/o Margaret Allen
28 Saxondale Road
North Kenton
Newcastle NE3 3RE

Northern Ireland FCWE
c/o Ann Pendleton
3rd Floor, Philip House
123/127 York Street
Belfast BT15 1AB
Tel: 01232 232587

North Lincolnshire CWTG
c/o Stephanie Codd
Tricare Neighbourhood Project
The Lodge, St. Paul's Road
Ashby
Scunthorpe DN12 3DL
Tel: 01724 864786

Nottinghamshire CWTG
c/o Dorothy Holmes
3 Mabel Grove
West Bridgford
Nottingham NG2 5GT
Tel: 0115 981 3469

Portsmouth CWTG
c/o Alana Gooding
Community Leisure Services
Portsmouth City Council
Guildhall
Portsmouth PO1 2AD
Tel: 01705 834809

**Rochdale Black Workers Training/
Support Group**
c/o Ann Ratu
7 Greengate Close
Hurstead
Rochdale OL12 9PX
Tel: 01421 462848

**Sheffield CWTG and S Yorks
Accreditation Project**
356 Glossop Road
Sheffield S10 2HW
Tel: 0114 275 0599

Southampton CWTG
c/o Lucy Collins
TWICS
25 Queens Terrace
Southampton SO14 3BQ
Tel: 01703 333566

South Wales CWTG
c/o Alice Greenlees
WCVA
Llys Ifor
Crescent Road
Caerphilly
South Glamorgan CF8 1XL
Tel: 01222 869224

West Glamorgan CWTG
c/o Jennifer Twelvetrees
West Glamorgan CVS
Pagefield House
Page Street
Swansea SA1 4EZ
Tel: 01792 648888

West of Scotland CWTG
c/o John Starke
246 2nd Avenue
Birkenshaw
Uddingston
Lanarkshire G71 6AY
Tel: 01698 334289

West Yorkshire CWTG
c/o Val Harris
10 Hall Royd
Shipley BD18 3ED
Tel: 01274 582191

SECTION:	**TRAINING**
TITLE:	**TRAINING OPPORTUNITIES**
AUTHOR:	

SECTION 14

SELECTION AND RECRUITMENT

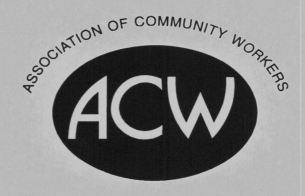

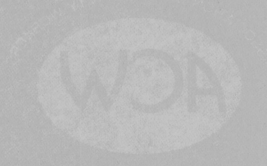

SECTION:	**SELECTION AND RECRUITMENT**
TITLE:	**PRINCIPLES OF RECRUITMENT**
AUTHOR:	Adapted from Equal Opportunities in Recruitment and Selection

Adapted from Nottingham Task Force publication "Equal Opportunities in Recruitment Selection" by Gill Taylor. Available from:

*Nottingham CVS,
33 Mansfield Road,
Nottingham NG1 3FB*

Equal opportunity in employment is about getting the best possible person for a job. It means that you should only select people on their ability to do the work, and no one should be denied a job for reasons that have nothing to do with their competence or capacity.

This section looks at your "recruitment procedure" – all the things you need to do to get the best possible staff for your organisation. Some of this is just a matter of making decisions, but you will find that there are areas which involve time and hard work:

- writing all the different papers you will need at various stages.

- training at least some people in your organisation to interview well.

- actually doing the short listing and interviewing.

The whole lot is your "recruitment procedure", and it should preferably be written down so that everyone involved knows what is supposed to happen.

We start by looking at the principles your recruitment procedure should follow. Then there is a section on advertising, and how to make sure you get good applicants for your job. The next part covers the written information you will send to people thinking of applying for the job, and finally the preparation for an interview and its conduct.

You may start to think that all this effort takes time away from delivering a good service, but it pays off. You will find that an equal opportunities recruitment procedure is actually more efficient, and is time well spent. Your staff are your greatest resource - spend time on them!

The overall aim is to be welcoming, fair and accurate in how·you present the job and the organisation. By creating a good impression you will attract a wider range of people, and by treating them properly you make sure to select the person who really is the best candidate.

The best equal opportunities recruitment follows these principles:

- The whole process is well organised, consistent and efficient.

- You make a special effort so that everyone who might be interested hears about the vacancy.

- Candidates are given informative, accurate information.

- You only look for skills and experience that are relevant to the job.

- There is no direct or indirect discrimination in the shortlisting.

- Interviewing and the final decision are fair and systematic.

- You use a panel of selectors who have had training.

Where to Start?

It might seem daunting to face such a big task, but each change you make for the better will have a positive result. In an ideal world it would be better to review your recruitment procedure without the pressure of a job vacancy. Checking that job descriptions are clear and accurate, drawing up your procedure, and re-writing the written materials are the best way to begin.

However, most often recruitment procedures get pushed aside until a vacancy comes up, and then action is urgent. It is still worth spending time on each section and trying to implement as much as possible.

There is nothing to be gained by rushing. If you get it wrong then you might be stuck with the wrong person for years. Far better to delay for a month or so now, however many immediate problems that brings.

Whom to Consult

One person alone should not have the power to decide on the written information or the adverts. In fact it is so important to get it right that at least some of the management committee must be involved, as well as other staff and any equal opportunities group within your organisation.

SECTION:	**SELECTION AND RECRUITMENT**
TITLE:	**PRINCIPLES OF RECRUITMENT**
AUTHOR:	Adapted from Equal Opportunities in Recruitment and Selection

Reviewing Job Descriptions

Job descriptions need to be reviewed as part of your equal opportunities plan, preferably all at the same time so that changes in one person's job don't clash with someone else's job description. If this is not possible all in one go, then review them for each vacancy or when new posts arise, but if you are only changing part of the organisation, be careful what responsibilities you put on new staff.

SECTION:	**SELECTION AND RECRUITMENT**
TITLE:	**ADVERTISING**
AUTHOR:	Adapted from Equal Opportunities in Recruitment and Selection

Getting the advert right is important, because it must:

- attract people with the relevant skills and qualifications

- be as accurate as possible

- appeal to as large a group of potential applicants as possible.

People can be easily put off applying by the wording of the advert and by the job title. Make the advert friendly and clear, and always put a phone number so that applicants can get hold of you easily for more information Avoid the use of sexist job titles or giving the impression that the job is suitable for only one sex, unless using a "Genuine Occupational Qualification" exemption.

Before you send it off, ask someone who was not closely involved in writing it to check it for these qualities.

The Content of the Advert

Key items for the advert are:

- The organisation's name

- The job title

- Where the job is based

- At least a general idea of the salary (either the amount, or the scale if you use a recognised one), and any allowances

- Your equal opportunities statement (if you have one)

- The closing date

- Where to get further details – include phone number.

You will probably also want to put a general idea of the duties involved and the kind of person you are looking for. You don't want to send out information to a lot of people who then find out they aren't interested or qualified, but you do want to get as many good applications as you can.

You should also include the following if they apply:

* The duration of the post if it's for a limited term

* The hours if it is not full-time

* A statement of any positive action you are taking to fill the post with particular types of people

* A reference to any exemptions you are using under the Race Relations or Sex Discrimination Acts.

Make it clear that all applications will be treated equally and without prejudice. Mention any terms and conditions such as flexible working or carer's leave that would make the post particularly attractive to people who face discrimination in employment. When a post does not require previous experience or where training can be given, then state this. Women especially are more likely to apply if they realise they will be given training.

The Design of the Advert

Advertising is costly. Your money is better used if the advert is well designed. Look through the papers to see what catches your eye and learn from that. Perhaps highlight the organisation's name and logo. Make the advert leap off the page by putting a double lined box around it. Emphasise the equal opportunities statement, job title and salary to attract people to read further.

Placing the Advert

It is important to select the places you advertise in order to reach the people you want without wasting money. Local papers are cheaper than national ones and often have a wide circulation. Always consider using papers that are read predominantly by black and ethnic minority people, women, lesbians and gay men, and disabled people. Many of these are weeklies or even monthlies, so you need to do some research well ahead of time to find out how early you have to book your advert and supply the text. Remember to check if you can get a discount for charities or for payment in advance.

The advert can be placed in Jobcentres throughout your city. It is also well worth preparing a small flyer for local community centres, local radio, employment agencies for disabled people, women's groups, black or ethnic minority groups, lesbian and gay groups. Circulate it to bookshops and centres where people meet too. If you choose the right outlets you can often reach many people who would not see your advert in the paper.

When people respond, always ask where they saw the job advertised, as this information will be useful for decisions on where to advertise in future.

Responding to Enquiries

Just before your advertisement appears you should brief everyone from your organisation who might have to take enquiries over the phone. They should be friendly and encouraging, and should make sure they get the name and address of the caller accurately. If they know about the post they should answer any particular questions, but if they don't they should immediately pass the call on to someone who does. Information should always be sent out promptly after the enquiry has been received.

SECTION:	**SELECTION AND RECRUITMENT**
TITLE:	**THE WRITTEN MATERIALS**
AUTHOR:	Adapted from Equal Opportunities in Recruitment and Selection

The next area you need to think very carefully about is the package of information to be sent out to enquirers. The wording of the different documents needs to show that you have a policy and have thought seriously about equal opportunities. What is not said in the job package can just as easily discourage potential applicants as what is said. The package should contain:

• The job description

• The person specification

• Background on the project or organisation

• An application form

• Your equal opportunities policy

• An equal opportunities monitoring form

• A covering letter

The following paragraphs describe the purpose of each item and what goes into it. In everything you write, avoid using initials or abbreviations without explaining what they mean, as this can be intimidating for people from outside the organisation or the immediate field of expertise.

The Job Description

Job descriptions should state clearly and simply the duties, tasks, responsibilities and lines of accountability of the post holder. The main points to include:

• How the job fits into your organisation, and how it relates to other workers' aims and responsibilities.

• Lines of accountability – who are they responsible to, and for what.

• Lists of duties and targets, specific but realistic. If there are any seasonal or regular tasks, make this plain.

• Details of any induction, supervision, support.

• Details of career opportunities and training available in the job.

• Brief terms and conditions, with any particular perks or factors which will affect people's response.

Some general points on writing job descriptions to encourage people who might otherwise think they were unsuitable:

- Change job titles to remove sex stereotypes.

- Make it clear how much travelling and overnight stays will be involved and whether you pay dependent costs in those circumstances.

- Make it clear how accessible the office is and do not include items which are unnecessary or likely to put off disabled people.

- Tell the reader exactly what skills are needed so that they can assess their ability to do the job.

- Make it clear if the job is open to job sharers, and under what terms and conditions they would be employed. Often disabled people and people with childcare or other responsibilities prefer to work part time or to job share. If you do offer sharing, say who has to find the partner.

Some employers include a catch-all to the effect that "the worker will carry out any duties necessary to implement the equal opportunities policy". This is not adequate. As you introduce equal opportunities to your organisation, you should work out, in as much detail as possible, which particular responsibilities each staff member will have, and put them in the job description.

The Person Specification

Although this will be quite a short statement, it is one of the keys to good recruitment. It should say what skills, experience and abilities are required to do the job. These might include:

- Knowledge and skills

- Education and qualifications

- Experience

- Requirements to travel.

You should be as specific as possible without being intimidating and offputting.

Be sure not to include any skills and qualifications which are not really necessary. The best way to do this is to work through the job description, writing down anything necessary for each task. That way you avoid guesswork if it is a new job, and you don't just look for a carbon copy of the outgoing worker if the job already exists.

Some people like to divide the list into "essential" and "desirable" characteristics. The desirable ones are only used to choose between applicants who are equally good on the essentials.

Background on the Project or Organisation

This should contain general information about the organisation and the specific project where relevant. You may be able to use a copy of your latest annual report instead of writing something new. You need to cover:

- Who the employer is and what the organisation's overall aims are.

- A description of the project: why it was set up? what does it do?

- How the management committee and any other committees work, what the other staff do.

- Where the money comes from and how secure it is.

- Information about the job which is not obvious from the job description, to give a feel for the work.

- A description of disabled access for any building the worker will be using.

The Application Form

The design of the application form is another key area for effective recruitment as it is one of the first contacts an organisation has with a prospective employee. A good application form tells people that your procedures are well thought out and gives them confidence in the organisation; it is easy for them to fill in and helps you to get the information you need for shortlisting.

It needs to be correct in three respects:

1. *ADMINISTRATIVE*

Personal details

The only necessary personal details are name, address and phone number. You do not need to ask a person's age, sex, marital status, health details or number of children on the application form. When applicants see questions like this it can lead to their anxiety about potential discrimination.

After someone has been appointed, the personnel worker can take any personal details that may have to go into the files.

Access needs

You need to ask on the application form whether people have access or other needs in order to attend the interview. This makes it clear that some of your readers might be disabled people rather than all able bodied. A blind person, for example, might prefer to be met at the station if it is their first time in your town.

Past criminal offences

Questions about criminal convictions should not be asked as a matter of course, but included only when necessary. You would need to ask about sex offences or child abuse when recruiting someone with significant unsupervised access to young people, and you might want to check potential finance workers for fraud.

Under the Rehabilitation of Offenders Act convictions eventually become "spent". Provided the time for expiry is met, applicants are not required to disclose them. However, certain jobs are exempt under this Act, including jobs in places required to register under the Registered Homes Act 1984 and those providing young people with accommodation, care, social services or training.

Monitoring where the applicant saw the advert

Monitoring where the applicant saw the job advertised is useful on the application form, but monitoring for equal opportunities should be separate.

2.   *INFORMATIVE*

The main body of the form should have questions relating to the skills, experience and qualities needed for the job. The questions on the application form must be tied in with the person specification. Each point in the person specification should be covered, and it often turns out that there needs to be a specific question relating to each point. This prevents applicants having to add frustrating extra bits of paper in case they haven't said everything the panel should know, and it makes shortlisting easier because all the information is on the right place on the form. Do not include irrelevant questions – for example asking for educational qualifications when expertise gained in other ways is more important.

Try to make the questions friendly and encouraging, so that people put down everything which might be important. You could use wording like:

Please give full details of your skills/experience which you consider relevant to the post, paying close attention to the job description and person specification.

Questions should always be related to the post. On equal opportunities, for instance, if recruiting a personnel worker you might ask:

What experience have you had of following and monitoring equal opportunities in recruitment?

Ask about people's ability to travel, possession of a driving licence, etc., if this is relevant, but do not ask things like whether they could manage to work unsocial hours. This could lead to discrimination against people with dependants and disabled people, and they should be the ones to decide, not you. Such questions can be gone into at a later stage.

3. *DESIGN*

The layout of the form is important. You should leave the correct amount of space for each answer, as this gives applicants a good idea of the importance you attach to each question and how much you want them to write.

Equal Opportunities Policy

You should include your equal opportunity statement and some general information about how it is being put into practice.

Equal Opportunities Monitoring Form

As well as a monitoring form, the package should include an envelope so that applicants can return the form separately from their application. This is important in giving applicants confidence that the information they provide is not going to be used against them in their application. It is vital to explain how you will use the monitoring forms and keep them confidential, and who will have access to them.

Classification

The Commission for Racial Equality recommends the following classification system for ethnic monitoring:

White
Black: Caribbean
Black: African
Black: Other (please specify)
Indian
Pakistani
Bangladeshi
Chinese
Other (please specify)

SECTION:	**SELECTION AND RECRUITMENT**
TITLE:	**THE WRITTEN MATERIALS**
AUTHOR:	Adapted from Equal Opportunities in Recruitment and Selection

A SUMMARY OF ACTION

General

Review the process and develop new recruitment procedures

Draw up a handbook of steps to take for each appointment on: Advertisement placing and wording – Shortlisting – Interviewing – Appointment – Induction

Initiate a review of job descriptions

Prepare adequate and accurate background materials, copies of your equal opportunities policy, and monitoring forms

For Each Job

Draw up an accurate job description

Derive a realistic person specification with relevant standards

Prepare a fair application form

Advertise widely including women's press, black and ethnic minority press, lesbian and gay press, disabilities journals

Prepare the pack of written material, to include: – Job description – Person specification – Application form – Background to the project – Equal opportunities policy – Equal opportunities monitoring form – Covering letter

Develop a foolproof administrative system

Monitoring the process

Review the process and improve as necessary

This system allows those people born in the UK, but whose origins are not white European, to answer in such a way as to stress their colour and origins without any suggestion that they "belong" elsewhere. The purpose of keeping ethnic records is not a social survey, but to see whether some people are being treated less favourably than others on ground of race, colour or ethnic origins.

If you can demonstrate under-representation by comparing the ethnic origin of those employed with the local or national populations, positive action under the Sections 37 & 38 of the Race Relations Act can then be considered.

Covering Letter

The covering letter should remind applicants of the closing date, state the interview dates if you know them, tell applicants if receipt of their form will be automatically acknowledged or not, point out that the monitoring form and separate envelope for its return, and inform people when they can expect to hear if they are shortlisted for the job. You can also include details of when you would like people to start if there are any particular considerations.

SECTION:	**SELECTION AND RECRUITMENT**
TITLE:	
AUTHOR:	

PRACTICAL PREPARATIONS FOR INTERVIEW

What to Tell the Candidates

Tell the candidates beforehand:

- the format of the interview

- how many people will be interviewing and who they are

- the sort of questions to expect

- how long the interview will last

- information about childcare expenses, travel expenses etc.

Inform unsuccessful applicants that they have not been shortlisted.

Preparing the Venue/Arrangements on the Day

People coming for interview need to be welcomed and need to feel that there is a welcoming environment in the workplace. Try to have a spare person to act as receptionist, to open the door and get candidates a cup of coffee.

Interviews should not be accidentally interrupted. Put clear warnings on the rooms where they are taking place so that people not involved don't wander in.

Potential staff should also have the opportunity to see the workplace and to meet other members of staff, and to see any pieces of work that they will be expected to carry on with, for example the books for a finance worker, the hostel for hostel workers and so on. It needs to be made clear that any staff who are involved in showing people round and not on the interview panel will not have any say in who is appointed.

Preparing the Panel

There should be a clear plan of the shape of the interview, the scope of the questions, who should ask which ones, the beginning and ending.

SECTION:	**SELECTION AND RECRUITMENT**
TITLE:	**PRACTICALITIES FOR INTERVIEWS**
AUTHOR:	Adapted from Equal Opportunities in Recruitment and Selection

Clear roles

The panel should allocate roles amongst its members. Most important is the person who chairs the interview. Other roles could be timekeeping, getting expenses and seeing out.

The person chairing:

*   introduces everyone

*   explains the process of the interview

*   tells candidates if they can ask questions on the way through or at the end

*   moves the questioning on

*   keeps the flow going

*   keeps the interview to time

*   tells the candidate what will happen next

*   deals with problems or irrelevances

*   chairs the deciding discussion

Questions

The question areas should be divided up according to expertise among the panel members and certain common questions agreed beforehand.

Flexibility

Each candidate will have different skills and experience and therefore will need probing on different areas. These should be decided before each candidate is interviewed.

The panel also need to agree a formula for other interviewers interrupting the main questioner on a particular topic if they feel they need more information.

THE INTERVIEW

To avoid being unfair in the interview, you need to be:

- well prepared
- systematic
- objective

Asking the Questions

In the interview – which is a nerve racking situation for any candidate and for interviewers – care needs to be taken to put the candidate at their ease and to ask an easy introductory question to get things going.

An open and frank attitude should be taken towards any people with disabilities. Do not make assumptions about people's skills and abilities: ask them. If the candidate is to be offered the job, then arrangements can be made to make any modifications to the workplace necessary.

- Take care to speak clearly and directly and to explain.any questions that are not understood.

- All questions must be clearly related to job requirements (as described in the person specification).

- Questions about family commitments or marriage and family plans should not be asked since they are likely to discriminate against female applicants.

- Questions should not be asked to test ethnic minority candidates' understanding of UK customs or to check their fluency in English unless these are bona fide job requirements.

- Make sure that candidates have an opportunity to ask their own questions.

Listen and Take Notes

All members of the panel should be alert and listen carefully to the candidate's answers. They must keep notes in order to make fair comparisons between candidates when deciding. One person can be allocated as main notetaker, with others making their on notes after each interview has finished.

What to Tell the Candidates at the End

Before each candidate leaves:

- Tell them when they will be informed of the outcome.

- Make sure they get any expenses due.

SECTION:	SELECTION AND RECRUITMENT
TITLE:	PRACTICALITIES FOR INTERVIEWS
AUTHOR:	Adapted from Equal Opportunities in Recruitment and Selection

MAKING A DECISION

When the interviews have been completed it is good practice to make a decision immediately. It is very important in carrying out the equal opportunities policy not to let bias creep in at the very final stage. For example it is not acceptable to rank an able bodied person above a disabled person or a single parent with childcare needs over a non parent owing to the extra cost of meeting their needs when they are of equal rank in all other respects.

Principles

- Do not make any assumptions about the candidates on the basis of information not received. Stick to the answers they have given.

- Selection decisions must not be influenced either by the traditional sexual or racial profile of the post holder or else by any colleague's unwillingness to work with, for example a lesbian or black person.

- Where there is doubt about the suitability of a candidate because of the nature of their disability, further advice should be sought about the nature of the disability and the availability of aids to employment or the adaption of buildings before a decision to reject is taken.

- If any members of the interview panel feel that discrimination has occurred in the selection process, the matter must be reported direct to the management committee. No selection decision should be made until the issue is resolved.

Process

- Rank candidates according to the information on the written forms.

- Gradually eliminate people, then come up with a first and second choice.

- If doubt arises between two candidates, see them again.

- The panel should make a first and second choice in case the preferred candidate turns the job down or has unsatisfactory references.

- The panel must be clear about why people were not selected, and notes regarding this during the decision making process.

The panel may decide to appoint no-one. In the long run it is far better not to appoint than to appoint an unsuitable candidate. Failure to attract suitable candidates may mean that the advert, job description, application form or person specification were not well thought out or that the level or pay is too low for the level of responsibility held in the job.

SUMMARY OF ACTION IN SELECTION

Shortlisting

- Select a representative panel and arrange their training if required

- Draw up shortlisting criteria

- Shortlist on the basis or criteria not assumptions, making sure all applicants get equal treatment

Practical preparations

- Inform candidates of practical details and format of interview

- Prepare the venue

- Decide clear roles for the panel and prepare questions

Interviewing

- Have a clear structure for the interview

- Take notes throughout

- Treat interview candidates equally

Deciding

- Making your decision on information received not on assumptions

- Be clear about why candidates were not selected

SECTION:	**SELECTION AND RECRUITMENT**
TITLE:	**COMMUNITY WORKERS AND EMPLOYMENT**
AUTHOR:	Doug Nicholls

Community work is work, community workers are workers; they are employed to do a job. It is perhaps the historic denial of these facts that has resulted in the neglect of the employment conditions of community workers. A rather romantic attachment to the 'autonomy of the community group' has meant that within community work we have tended to drop our guard.

We would not accept that community workers should be subject in their workplace to being paid whatever the gaffer can afford, or thinks is the rate for the job. Yet it seems OK in some circles that community workers can be paid less than the going rate as determined by the Joint Negotiating Committee for Youth and Community Workers (JNC Report). Similarly if asked by a local resident for advice about dealing with their employer who had denied locally agreed procedures and employment law, we would advocate the toughest form of defence and support. Yet how often do community workers work somewhere without proper employment procedures in place?

It is perhaps the embarrassed confusion depicting the community worker as 'middle class' interloper in 'working class' impoverished neighbourhood, that leads community workers to neglect their own employment position. Is it fair to expect a management committee of unemployed local residents to approve my regrading claim for an extra £2,000 a year?

A determined trade union presence in the community work workplace, accompanied by clear employment procedures, helps to generate the highest quality community work. This is especially so, where that community work is related to the community action and 'liberating' traditions.

Many community work activists in the 60s and 70s came out of trade union activity at the workplace. The underlying values and objectives of community work are identical to those of the trade union movement. The affinity between trade unionism and community work is great, but often unrealised.

On this page is a straightforward checklist of employment procedures that should apply to any workplace situation.

- Staff Handbook.
- JNC Report.
- APT&C Report.
- Staff Contracts.
- Job Descriptions.
- Staff Development Policy.
- Pension Scheme that applies.
- Details of Employment Insurance.
- Equal Opportunities Policy.
- Recruitment and Selection Procedures.
- Redeployment Procedure.
- Redundancy Policy and Procedure.
- Part Time Worker Pay Rates.
- Health and Safety Procedures/Policies/Structures.
- Sexual Harassment Guidelines.
- Job Share Policies.
- Outdoor Activity Procedures/Guidelines.
- Hazardous Activity Guidelines.
- Staff – young people/adult ratios.
- Detached work policies.
- Guidelines on taking responsibilities during work – (e.g. Secretary of Association, leaseholder).
- Parental Leave Procedures
- Carers' Leave Procedure.
- Policies on Violence at Work.
- Employers Welfare support structures.
- Sick Pay Procedures/Policies.
- Financial Management Guidelines.

- Disciplinary Procedure.

- Grievance Procedure.

- Collective Disputes Procedure.

- Regrading Procedure.

- Facilities Agreement.

- Joint Negotiating Committee Agreement.

- Time Off in Lieu Arrangements.

- Residential Pay Arrangements.

- Travel and Subsistence Allowance Schemes.

- Complaints Procedure (how does your organisation respond if a member of the public complains about you?)

- Compassionate Leave Scheme.

- Policy on writing references.

- Child Abuse Guidelines.

- Probationary Year arrangements (if applicable).

- Authorised Establishment Figures for JNC posts.

- Lists of all full and part time JNC posts.

- Working alone policies.

- Official Conduct Guidelines.

- Important examples of Official Conduct Guidelines are:

  - Whole Time Service.

  - Interests of Officers.

  - Information concerning Officers.

  - Contact with the Press.

CYWU also provides model·procedures and contracts. Please do not hesitate to contact us for more support and backup:

The Community & Youth Workers' Union,
202a The Argent Centre,
60 Frederick Street,
Hockley,
Birmingham B1 3HS.
Tel: 0121 233 2815

EMPLOYMENT PROCEDURES

All community workers are advised by CYWU to have on file all of the employment policies and procedures which the employing organisation agrees apply to their post. Contact CYWU on 0121 233 2815 for help and advice.

You are entitled to all of this information as an employee and as member of a trade union Branch.. There may well be other rules and policies which your employers have.

SECTION 15

SUPERVISION

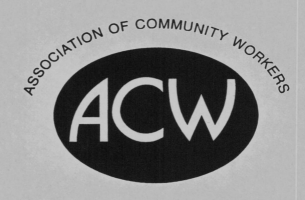

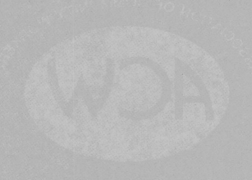

SECTION:	**SUPERVISION**
TITLE:	**SUPERVISION**
AUTHOR:	Peter Durrant

Introduction

Supervision is an unhelpful concept because it means, if you glance at your dictionary, inspection, control and overseeing. Perhaps community workers, with their healthy disrespect for authority and hierarchies, should be concerned with more reciprocal and shared relationships?

TECHNIQUES/GOOD IDEAS

Central to good community work practice is relating to people as people, consciously avoiding power issues which interfere with relationships and being prepared to admit that WE have problems too. But we too often find ourselves in 'supervisory' situations which fail to reflect these useful and helpful principles. This isn't to say some individuals haven't more experience, knowledge and ideas than others. It is to say that we've ALL got substantial amounts to learn from each other. Some golden rules might include:

a. Trying to consciously avoid the use of anything but open recording systems which should be agreed by all participants. This more explicit approach should enable people to know where they stand – and avoid hidden agendas.

b. Working at really reciprocal relationships by listening to each other and allowing mutually helpful communication skills to develop. Remember the co-counselling model before it became hopelessly professionalised. Ten minutes from each participant and then a useful, cooperative discussion which can, if you both do it well, mark out the boundaries in a constructive fashion, as well as achieving the benefits of dual satisfaction, honesty and growth, from which outcome measurements can then become possible.

Conclusions

We know from our 'practice wisdom' that working together, difficult though this often is, far outweighs insularity and individualism. 'Supervision', but perhaps we need to change the word and the concept to something like 'working partnerships' or 'working together', to make the theory work in practice. But only if we consciously avoid some of the subjective traps and hurdles we bump into at the moment.

Paul Henderson and David Thomas in 'Skills in Neighbourhood Work' NISW Library no 39 get it right (on pages 248/9) when they discuss support networks, support groups and the opportunity for the worker to have regular meetings with a consultant.

SECTION:	**SUPERVISION**
TITLE:	
AUTHOR:	

SECTION:	**SUPERVISION**
TITLE:	**THE USES OF SUPERVISION IN COMMUNITY WORK**
AUTHOR:	Camilla Tegg

Supervision has not always had a "good press" in community work, which is to do with notions that it is hierarchical, unsupportive, oppressive and negative. As the previous author in this section suggested, people do worry about and believe that the supervisory process and structure facilitates bad practices. However, if the process is made open, consultative, thorough and ordered, a very different and positive outcome can be had.

There's also the converse. Where nobody ever asks you what you're doing, you don't get a chance to reflect upon your work except informally, if trouble looms you are left strictly on your own to resolve it, nobody in your organisation ever tells you that you are doing good work or suggests that with a little training or reflection, there are some bits that you could do even better.

Supervision used properly can ensure that quality and quantity of work, support and enable, train and develop us.

There are several parts to this section which will try to introduce the basic structures and skills of supervision and to convince you that the process is worthwhile enough to investigate further and to instigate it, if it is not already present or seek to improve it if it is, but not working successfully.

THE PURPOSES OF SUPERVISION AND ROLES OF SUPERVISORS

Historically there has been a lot of confusion and differing expectations about the purposes of supervision. One of the first steps in the development of a supervision process is to ensure that all those involved come to an understanding of the meaning and purposes of supervision.

I would say that the two main purposes of supervision can be identified as follows:

a. To establish the accountability of the worker to the organisation (and in the case of the community worker to the community group).

b. To promote the worker's development as a professional person.

Since accountability is concerned not only with whether a task is performed but also with the quality or standard of the work, the two purposes of supervision are interwoven.

You could also identify the major purposes of supervision in the following way:

The MANAGING and ADMINISTRATION role
The TEACHING and LEARNING role
The SUPPORTING and ENABLING role.

The Managing Role

This is mainly to do with the planning, distribution and monitoring and evaluating of the work tasks. An essential part of this function will be to pass on the policies and values of the agency, and to give straight information about how the agency's practices and procedures work. The service to the community will be better if the worker knows her way around the agency and how to use the policies and procedures of the organisation to the benefit of the client. The supervisors will themselves need to understand policies if they are going to be able to interpret them to others. This element of the function is particularly important in relation to equal opportunities where the supervisor must be able to explain the implication of equal opportunities policies on the day to day work, help the worker integrate their practical application and monitor and evaluate whether they are being integrated successfully.

In addition the agreed allocation of work, prioritisation of work, involvement in some of the detailed planning of work would all be part of the managing and administrative role.

Monitoring and evaluating that work once it has started is an important element. Giving workers positive encouragements for their achievements, guidance to sustain their works to certain goals, and feedback on things they need to change or improve to work well.

Teaching and Learning Function

I have called this the teaching and learning role because I am sure that nobody ever embarks on this sort of process without learning a great deal in the process of imparting learning to others. However in supervision, it is important to remember that the learning of the supervisee is prime and that your role is to facilitate that learning in every way you can. Workers will have needs for a whole range of knowledge and skills to complete the task in hand. Sometimes your role will be as simple as giving straightforward information, e.g. how to fill in a grant application. At other times it may be a complex ad sensitive task to enable the worker to change attitudes or learn a new skill, for example helping and at the same time expecting a worker to develop anti-racist skills and awarenesses. The supervisors experience of learning for themselves will influence how they impart knowledge and understanding to others. It is important to make it relevant (the need to know), accessible (familiar elements), appropriate to the learner and as imaginative and interesting as possible – tell stories, act out a little scene, use a cut from a video, take them on a tour of the building.

The Enabling and Supporting Role

Support can cover a variety of activities such as backing up a workers's decision, providing time by helping a worker organise her work, or simply lending a sympathetic ear for when it all gets on top of people. Community work can be and often is a stressful occupation and supervision should attempt to reduce the impact of those stresses, which will impair a workers ability to offer an effective service. In order for that to happen it is important that the worker feels trustful of, and confidence in the supervisor/s. This is particularly relevant in relation to race and gender. Where a supervisor has the additional power of being white or male in addition to the power of the role of a supervisor it is important to acknowledge that power, and ensure that it does not inhibit the workers from seeking support from you, particularly in relation to such issues as racial or sexual harassment.

This is by no means an exhaustive list of the roles of supervision, though most of the other roles will probably come under these headings. And I am sure that each of you will, dependant upon your agency and your style wish to emphasise one role more than another. However you see the role of supervision, the most vital activity in establishing a good supervisory relationship is to make that view explicit, consult others involved in it and mutually agree what these roles should be – that's all good community work practice after all!

SECTION:	**SUPERVISION**
TITLE:	**TYPES OF SUPERVISION**
AUTHOR:	Camilla Tegg

I think that the word supervision often implies that it is always an activity that takes place between a manager and a worker, and although that is often the case it is not always the case. There follows a brief list of types of supervision that can be used.

TYPES OF SUPERVISION

a.   One to one managerial supervision

This is the more common type of supervision of a worker by a manager. It does not have to be directive or oppressive if it is carefully set up and agendas and boundaries are checked regularly as a matter of course. One of its major functions will be the accountability of the worker, and in community work where the worker also see themselves as accountable to community groups this may provide a tension between the community groups' and agencies' expectations. But this tension has always been there and is better addressed rather than left to be exposed by a crisis or conflict.

b.   Co-supervision

This type of supervision takes place mostly between peers. That is two workers of equal status. Sometimes it is between two workers on the same project, or in the same department doing different work. The essence of it is to offer each other mutual support and attention, though accountability should by no means be ruled out. From my experience it is quite difficult to give this sort of supervision enough structure and regularity, and although informal supervision, mentioned later, is useful it does not offer the same measured support, feedback and assessment. I think therefore that the most important thing is to mutually agree and properly sustain a proper time and structure for this type of supervision.

c.   Groups Supervision

This is supervision of a small group of workers with some common work or goals. I stress the smallness of the group, too large a group, say over 5 or 6 could result in nobody getting any real support or guidance from it. Again it has to be carefully structured to ensure that everybody gets a space and all the agreed topics are covered. Whoever constructs the agenda for such a group has to be quite skilled in establishing and prioritising it. This group can be led by a manager or an agreed member of the group. What I feel will not work is to have no leader or facilitator at all which will result in a free for all causing more stress rather than alleviating it.

d.   Informal Supervision

I suspect this type of supervision is what a lot of people get a lot of the time, you know, two minutes in the corridor or in passing during a discussion on something else. I have to say quite firmly that I think when it is undertaken solely in this way it is inadequate and unsatisfactory. It almost certainly doesn't meet the needs of the worker for support or proper feedback or evaluation or the needs of the organisation for a clear and ordered picture of what the worker is doing.

Clearly informal supervision is sometimes appropriate and necessary but it should be recognised as "an as well as and not an instead of". It should be as brief and to the point as possible, not drifting on to other subjects that can best dealt with sitting down with a note book and a cup of tea!

e.   Crisis Supervision

People often do have crises and they do need immediate help. What they don't need is someone who reflects back their feelings of anxiety or panic, or doesn't appear to be concerned at all. They need someone to help them to clear a space, physically and emotionally, to think about what has happened; to decide what can be done immediately and to help them to cope with the anxiety and worry that may ensue. Please don't panic with them, if you can possibly help it. Some physical serenity, like a quiet room, a cup of tea can help enormously, often with such a space it emerges that the crisis is not quite as bad as at first feared or if it is, then tea and quiet will help you to get to grips with planning the quick actions and strategies you need to undertake. Crisis response is a skill in itself, you can learn to develop those skills but if you feel at a loss or overwhelmed along with the worker don't hesitate to ask other people for help whose knowledge and skills you respect.

I constantly emphasise how important it is, for the sake of clarity, non oppressive practice and straightforward good practice that the processes of supervision are carefully agreed between the participants. Do try to cross as many of your bridges before you come to them as you can. That way you can often avoid that dawning sense of panic when someone being supervised says to you "You never said that we were going to use these discussions to write my annual evaluation, I don't agree with that" or "I don't see why I should tell you how many contacts I made this week" or "Well as this session is for my support I really would like to discuss with you a row I had with my partner" on and on...

There are a series of structures in supervision that can address these issues, these are:

The Beginning of Supervision

Contracts in Supervision

Agendas in Supervision

Evaluation in Supervision.

Beginning Supervision

1.   You must be clear for yourself what you think the purpose of supervision is and what you want to get out of it, either as a manager or a co-worker, before you start the first session.

2.   You must ensure that the first session is spent clarifying the purposes etc. of supervision rather than launching in to the issues that the worker is currently facing, that may be difficult for them, but will pay off in the end.

3.   The sorts of things that you need to sort out with the supervisee are:

a.   what you both want to get out of it.

b.   what does your agency expect you to do in it.

c.   what you can/can't talk about.

d.   confidentiality.

e.   whether it will be recorded by either of you.

f.   how frequent it will be/how long will it be/where will it be.

g.   recognising the "power bases" that you or they have e.g. supervisor being a manager and/or male and/or white, supervisee being white or male etc.

h.   what will happen, will you just talk or will one of you bring written work or reports etc.

i.   how are you going to check if supervision is going OK.

j.   how are you going to deal with racism or sexism etc., on the part of either of you.

Most importantly WHAT IS IT (SUPERVISION) FOR? e.g. accountability, support and education.

4.   One of the things that I have found most useful to do at the beginning of supervision, is to discuss both of your previous experiences of supervision. This will give you a real insight into what "luggage" people bring with them, do they view supervision as potentially destructive because of past experiences or really welcome it? It also gives you an opportunity to find ways of avoiding the negative experiences people have had previously.

Contracts in Supervision

Nearly all of the above can then be incorporated into a written document which forms the supervision contract between you. This may seem over elaborate, but even after all the above discussion it is possible for misunderstandings to remain and with so many powerful expectations hanging on this process it is important to be as clear as possible.

It also gives you a reference point to review the process of supervision and to check if you are doing all that you agreed or whether one or both of you feel that certain things could change.

Agendas in Supervision

The compiling of agendas at the beginning of each session are very central to ensuring an equalitative atmosphere in supervision. It is important that you both get a chance to indicate what your priorities are, whilst at the same time meeting any agency requirements. People hardly ever get through all the things they hope to get through in supervision, so when compiling an agenda you must be REAL ABOUT TIME.

The following are the basic guidelines for agendas:

1.   List items from both parties, including essential items.

2.   Agree some prioritisation of the list.

3.   Give items some approximate timing.

4.   Discuss what you are going to do about items you clearly won't have time for (be real!)

5.   Talk about methods for dealing with items – discussion, listing etc.

Evaluation in Supervision

Supervision is often used as a central part of a regular formal or informal assessment of a worker's performance. If so, it is absolutely essential that that is made clear to the worker when the process is instituted, and should be included in the contract. Because of some of the persistent discriminations that have taken place in the assessment of black workers and women it is particularly important to be explicit about that process of assessment. The criteria on which that assessment will be based should be made clear and will require you both to take a good look at the worker's job description – if there is a one! (How do you assess if a job is being done well if there is no thorough account of what that job is?) This sort of evaluation should be regular and ongoing. If there is a formal evaluation process, there should be no surprises for the worker, all of the work performance issues both positive and negative should have been shared with the worker as you go along. If this does not happen, then the worker is prevented from either gaining confidence in the work they are doing well or being able to change aspects of their work that need improving. This is where the skills of critical feedback, positive and negative come in. I cannot emphasise enough the effect of sitting on opinions of a worker's performance and not sharing it with them. It is also disempowering as it prevents the worker from giving an explanation of their actions.

SECTION:	**SUPERVISION**
TITLE:	**USES OF POWER IN SUPERVISION**
AUTHOR:	Camilla Tegg

As community workers you would be expected to have an understanding of the impact that power, be it institutional or personal; political, race or gender based, can have. Those innate or institutional power bases that we carry around with us as individuals, can and do have a considerable impact on the nature and quality of supervision that we are able to offer. If we are a manager or white or male etc., we carry the potential to oppress a range of people being supervised by us. We cannot divest ourselves of that power, but we can in establishing a supervisory relationship acknowledge that it is there and discuss with the worker some safeguards for them in relation to that potential.

The first and primary thing to do is to acknowledge its existence and then to discuss with the supervisee in what aspects of your relationship can you see that having an impact.

How will you deal with a situation where the supervisee experiences you as discriminatory, without them fearing that you might use your power as manager or a co-worker to suppress or dismiss that complaint.

How will you support them if they come to you with a complaint of sexism or racism from other members of staff or from people with whom they work, will you minimise it or dismiss it?

Can they be assured that you will not, because of your fears of being accused of racism or sexism, refrain from giving them proper critical feedback to enable them to develop as a professional worker.

All of these issues will be on their mind if on yours and acknowledging that and making some mutually acceptable agreement about how to act in these matters will facilitate their ability to trust in you considerably.

SECTION:	**SUPERVISION**
TITLE:	
AUTHOR:	

SECTION:	**SUPERVISION**
TITLE:	**SKILLS IN SUPERVISION**
AUTHOR:	Camilla Tegg

This section is an introduction to the skills you may need, then you can check whether you think you have them already, you could do with polishing them up or you need to learn them from scratch. You could go on a course, learn from your peers, watch a video – whatever works for you. Though I am bound to say that practice, with some good feedback from colleagues, is the best for me. It has proved to aid a sense of equity in all sorts of ways, reminding me of what it feels like to be on the end of critical feedback and giving me a chance to review my own skills.

The main purposes of supervision were identified under three main headings: Administration and Accountability, Teaching and Learning, and Support, and the following skills are all intended to contribute towards those functions.

Communications
Teaching and Learning
Constructive Critical Feedback
Workload Management
Dealing with issues of Race and Gender

There are in addition a whole range of other skills such as agenda building, evaluation, prioritisation of time, career development, which play a large part and which you should check in your skills inventory, another thing it is worth learning to do in supervision, i.e. getting the supervisee to take a detailed look at their skills, experience and knowledge base assessing their strengths and weaknesses and encouraging them to work at those areas that could be improved. That will work for you too!

COMMUNICATION SKILLS

Communication skills are, of course central to all our work. However there are some aspects of them that are particularly central to good supervision. I would say the ability to listen carefully, to check out what you think you heard, to agree with the supervisee what the nature of the issue is and then move on to finding solutions is the essence it. As a manager/supervisor the temptation often is to assume that you know what difficulties are, that you are clear about what the solutions are and consequently not to listen carefully to what the worker has to say. That will result in not paying attention, appearing not to be interested and probably interrupting before they have laid out before you the full extent of their achievements or problems.

There are even more basic elements of communications which I hesitate to mention but feel are still so often neglected and so often spoil any chance that we have of offering people some proper care and attention, that I am not going to risk it by leaving them out.

They are: a quite room, comfortable chairs, no interruptions, no telephone, sitting so that you are not craning to look at each other. You must also be aware of your non-verbal communications – a joke I know, but nonetheless important. It is difficult to concentrate on saying something difficult if the person opposite is constantly winding and unwinding their legs around a chair, or fiddling with a pen. If a supervisee has to break some unpleasant news to a manager an immediately fierce or apprehensive look will deter them. You will know from your own experience that looking interested and sympathetic will reassure and encourage concentration on the topic in hand.

The regularity and length of supervision also play an important in enabling supervision to be constructive and a building opportunity. I'm not sure whether that can be regarded as a communications element but it can certainly inhibit or facilitate them. Supervision should be regular and for a regular period of time otherwise it becomes a response to crisis, not allowing the positive and developmental elements to tale place. If you have not agreed how long it will be, how can you plan your agenda, ensure that you get everything in, leave time for feedback for you and them about the session?

SECTION:	**SUPERVISION**
TITLE:	
AUTHOR:	

SECTION:	**SUPERVISION**
TITLE:	**TEACHING AND LEARNING IN SUPERVISION**
AUTHOR:	Camilla Tegg

This can be such a positive and rewarding aspect of supervision, to be able to play a part in the development of another worker's skills and knowledge base is very exciting. In order to do this effectively you need first to have an understanding of the different ways that people learn. That people learn at different rates. How to facilitate people's learning. As a community worker this would play a part anyway in your everyday practice and developing these skills can only benefit you all round. You already have a pool of knowledge on this topic from your own experience of learning, when you have learned most easily, what has made most sense to you in learning, what catches and holds your attention.

Did you know that we remember:-

10% of what we read

20% of what we hear

30% of what we see

50% of what we see and hear together

80% of what we say

90% of what we say while we do it.

Adults have particular ways of learning and understanding these can help you "get your point across", some of those ways are as follows:

- The need to know – the more adults understand the need to learn a particular thing the more effective and positive will be the learning, if they don't resistance often follows.

- The need to be self directing – adults want to be self respecting, responsible for their actions and have a hand in designing their own learning activities. Self directed adult learners use networks and ask for help when needed.

- The use of experience – adults make good use of their own experience in learning, they will also readily learn from yours.

There are also some basic laws of learning:

1. People learn best in pleasant surroundings.

2. Unpleasantness or hostility inhibit learning – positive reinforcement enhances it.

3. People learn best by doing, "practice makes perfect" – so use case studies, roles plays. Check also that there is not any unlearning of previous inappropriate behaviour needed e.g. assumptions about woman or gay people.

4. Every new fact is best learned if we can relate it to already known information. Like building blocks we add each new piece.

5. People learn at different rates from each other, and learn at different times for themselves.

6. Learning is continuous experience – as supervisors we should be good role models of this – ready to learn and acknowledge our learning from our supervisees.

7.   Learning results from stimulation to the senses so sound, visual activity are important. We increase learning threefold by letting people see as well as hear and increase it some more by encouraging them to talk about it.

8.   Whole/part/whole learning is best – look at the whole picture first, discuss it and break it down into it's component parts, then put it all back together as a whole.

9.   Understand that people need to be in a safe learning environment, if there is a danger of them experiencing discrimination either from you directly on in the material you present them, they will be concerned with that and not with the learning that you are trying to facilitate.

The list above is necessarily crude and very brief, but nonetheless if you apply it your own experiences of learning both good and bad I think it will make sense, and in combination with your own experience enable you to apply it in supervision.

Having got some clarity about the process and conditions which enable people to learn, it then leads you to consider the ways in which you can apply that in supervision. For instance a brand new worker is starting work with a local group, and is very unsure of his first moves, how would you go about enabling him first to start and then practice successfully. By working alongside him so that he can model from your good practice. By referring him to others who have knowledge and experience of the local area and the community. By presenting information in a range of ways – previous records, written papers, role plays, watching videos, from discussing television programmes, from analysing a piece of the workers own practice written up in detail, or recorded on a tape. You will no doubt undertake a range of these techniques and have done up to now without really thinking that you are teaching, well you are and if you do so more consciously you may be able to enhance that teaching and make it more lively.

Some of these ways of teaching may seem more appropriate to groups but can still successfully be applied. Ensuring the integration of opportunities for you and your supervisees to learn together and from each other, makes sessions much more positive and often balances off the accountability aspects of work which necessarily need undertaking.

Throughout the three major aspects of supervision – support, accountability and teaching and learning, there is a need to give a worker feedback about the nature, quality and quantity of their work, both positive and negative. The assumption that workers mostly do not want to hear is incorrect, in a survey we undertook with workers about supervision, those not receiving any mostly said what they missed was some idea of how they were doing, people want to improve their practice, they are not always sure of themselves and their work and they want to hear.

It is therefore amazing how hard it is to convince people that constructive criticism is just that, a CONSTRUCTIVE activity and that not dealing with criticism in a direct and open way is often a very destructive activity. You have a right as a co-worker or manager to want and expect people to improve their performance, for their own good, for the good of the people with whom you work and for the good of the organisation for whom you work. Do not imagine that because criticism is not being undertaken in this constructive way, it is not being undertaken at all. Very often it is being pursued in very destructive ways. You will I am sure recognise the following scenarios:

AGGRESSIVE FEEDBACK

"I have to do it. I've been saving this up for weeks and I'm going to get it over as quickly and with as much impact as possible, she wont forget this in a hurry."

FEARFULLY

"Supposing they tell me to stuff it, or criticise me in return, or worse still burst into tears. Maybe I'll just hint at it and see how it goes, I can always back off if it looks sticky."

SARCASTICALLY/JOKILY

"Well of course if we were all as good as you are at losing files, where would the system be? Oh late again, what was it this time, the bus, the baby or your cultural norms?" (great potential for racism and sexism)

NOT AT ALL

"I'm sure that if I just wait he'll realise it for himself, and, if I wait long enough, maybe he'll do something so bad that I can refer it to my boss and she'll take out a disciplinary. Or I'll wait until I'm really wound up have a good shout and get it off my chest that way". (Surely a mode of feedback particularly familiar to black staff where white managers afraid of being accused of racism give black staff no feedback at all, inhibiting their development, ensuring that they cannot defend themselves and resulting in extreme forms of action.)

Supervision offers the best possible opportunity to offer others critical feedback in a constructive and positive way. In first setting the contract for supervision it can be agreed that feedback is an essential and necessary part of the workers development. You can discuss ways that the supervisee copes best with critical feedback and can make best use of it. You will of course also give the supervisee the opportunity to give you feedback about your work with them i.e. the quality of supervision, this will give you a further insight into just how useful and developmental criticism can be not only for others but you. It will also ensure that you understand from your own experience the good and the bad ways of doing it.

There are a range of basic rules and techniques for critical feedback, the most important of which are:

- be specific about your criticism, offer concrete examples of what your talking about, don't just say you are wonderful or you are terrible;

- criticise the behaviour not the person;

- offer a description of the behaviour not a judgement of it e.g. you have missed out several areas of work from your report – NOT your report writing is sloppy;

- be certain that the feedback is of value to the receiver and not just a way for you to vent your spleen;

- only criticise behaviour that you know people can change;

- focus on an amount of feedback that the receiver can usefully use at one time – don't fall into the "and another thing" trap;

- discuss the feedback with the recipient and come to some agreement about it as far as possible;

- talk about ways that the behaviour in question can be changed.

I know that this is a lot to take in but I'm sure that if you sit down with someone else and discuss good and bad feedback that you have experienced, you will recognise clearly all the guidelines listed above, and will begin to have a clear idea of how to apply them.

SECTION:	**SUPERVISION**
TITLE:	**WORKLOAD MANAGEMENT**
AUTHOR:	Camilla Tegg

Workload management for the individual and the agency are essential and should be embarked upon honestly and without embarrassment, it is not intrusive or oppressive to ask a worker to be accountable for their time and for you to ensure that they are giving the best possible service to the community and that they or their group are not being exploited or undermined in the process of doing that.

It is in this area in particular that the job description comes into it's own, though clearly it also has its applications in the areas discussed above. In my experience the major debates around workload management are:

1. Exactly what the worker is supposed to be doing/wants to do/has agreed to do with someone else.

2. How much time is to be spent on particular activities, can you agree on whether it is 1 day in that area or the other.

3. Can you accommodate the interests and inclinations of the worker, with the needs of the community group and the organisation.

4. At what speed should a worker accomplish the agreed tasks, there is so often a differing view of this between worker and supervisor.

In order to deal with these complex and difficult topics, it is essential at the beginning of any supervisory relationship to establish some clear agreement that all of the above questions are an appropriate part of supervision.

It will also be most useful to discuss in what form are these issues going to be reviewed.

Is the worker going to present you with a regular verbal or written report?

Are you going to get feedback from the groups with whom she is working?

Are you going to regularly review her time allocation to certain tasks?

On a regular basis (monthly perhaps) are you going to agree work targets for a specific period of time?

And so the list goes on, all of these things are best established before entering into the hurly burly of supervision and can give everyone some clear boundaries.

It is also most important to be clear that this is not just a policing mechanism, it is just as important to monitor whether a worker is undertaking too much work or too many responsibilities or that your expectations of them have been to high, that the worker is achieving a great deal and deserves recognition and confirmation of that fact (we're back to how am I doing?)

The clearer the agreement on these issues, the less likely the confusions and conflicts that so often arise when it comes to differing expectations of a worker. Though with all the planning and clarity in the world, these confusions do come about, most often I find from poor or inadequate information (regular supervision helps avoid that), so always check that first. Inevitably too, when a community worker is working to more than one set of expectations i.e. the agency's and the community group's there will be further conflict. It is important that this situation is reviewed at the beginning of a piece of work and that communications are maintained either through the worker or directly, so that the worker does not get torn limb from limb in the middle of all that.

SECTION:	**SUPERVISION**
TITLE:	**ISSUES OF RACE AND GENDER IN SUPERVISION**
AUTHOR:	Camilla Tegg

I am most hesitant about embarking upon such an important topic in such a limited way, but the alternative is not to mention it at all which is even more unacceptable. I therefore start by acknowledging that this is an extremely restricted account of this issue and urge everyone who reads this to ensure that continue to review their own practice in this area, learning from whatever sources are available to you but being as sure as I am that there is undoubtedly a great deal for you to understand and examine on this topic.

There are two main issues around race and gender in supervision, one is the supervisory relationship – whom it is between; and the other is how you monitor the anti-discriminatory practice of all workers in supervision. The key word in the supervisory relationship is power and who has it. What is your gender, what is your race, chances are if you are a community worker with some sort of supervisory responsibilities reading this article – you are white and male. Yes! I know that community work has come further than others but the above is nevertheless still true.

The role of supervisor even when undertaken with a co-worker and certainly when you are a manager, gives you undoubted power. Add to that the potential for power in your maleness or your whiteness and you begin to see the potential there is for abuse of this relationship. Even where the managerial power bases are reversed e.g. female manager, male supervisee, that abuse still takes place, references have been made to my shape in supervision and I have known white workers to imply all sorts of subtly racist things about a black manager. It is therefore of prime importance that these power bases and their potential for oppressiveness are acknowledged and discussed at the beginning of supervision. A black worker needs to know that they can challenge the racism of a white manager, without an immediately defensive response and even more importantly without the danger of jeopardising their job or promotion.

There are a range of issues which should be considered.

1. It is your responsibility to ensure a safe working environment for staff from discrimination against groups.

2. It is your responsibility to recognise that black staff and sometimes women staff, are asked to undertake many tasks outside their own arena "We need a black person on the interviewing panel" "Can you just look over this equal opportunities policy document", you should ensure that you are not overloaded or penalised any way for such commitments.

3. Do ensure that you ensure the proper career development opportunities for black people and women.

4. Do ensure that you give black people and women proper feedback about their work, do not let your own fear of being accused of racism or sexism stop you from enabling workers to look at their practice and develop their skills.

5. Do not assume that black staff will have a wider cultural knowledge than anyone else.

6. Do not be so anxious to further your own learning or demonstrate your right-on-ness that you dominate supervision with discussions of race and gender when the worker wants to discuss the technicalities of a funding application.

7. Do respect and value the knowledge and experience of those in oppressed groups

In order for you to ensure the integration of anti-discriminatory practice into your supervisees work, you will need to be clear about your own and that of your organisation. Too often this issue is expected to start at the bottom and permeate upward. Equal opportunities statements and policies, codes of practice, applied and detailed guidelines for all aspects of work are very important, I hesitate to say that they are essential, because as yet not all organisations could claim to have all of these in place. Consequently we must do the best we can until they are, as a supervisor you must monitor your own practice if no-one else does and also monitor that of the person you supervise.

Ensure that it regularly appears on the agenda for supervision, be specific about it, ask for exampled of peoples practice in this area, not "are you committed or doing anti-racist practice".

Look at the composition of your community and ensure that there is proper representation of all groups in the work undertaken by

SECTION:	**SUPERVISION**
TITLE:	**ISSUES OF RACE AND GENDER IN SUPERVISION**
AUTHOR:	Camilla Tegg

your agency and the worker.

Check that the worker does not sustain stereotypes of woman or black people, check that they do have an understanding of the impact of racism and sexism upon the individual and their communities.

Check that they do have respect for the strength that people from oppressed groups show in the face of these oppressions.

Where workers have not yet developed anti-discriminatory practice skills, ensure that they are given opportunities to do so, through supervisions or team discussions, external courses etc.

What is most needed to achieve anti-discrimination is a sustained commitment and an energetic vigilance. This is not only a highly emotive and inspiring issue but one that requires day to day grind and boring repetitiveness till it becomes an automatic part of our everyday work. Anti-discriminatory practice is good practice and vice versa.

SECTION:	**SUPERVISION**
TITLE:	**GOOD SUPERVISION AND HOW TO GET IT**
AUTHOR:	Camilla Tegg

This section is concerned with recognising that the receiver of supervision is not a passive figure and that there are things that she/he can do to influence that process and make it more responsive to their needs.

Often, when I run a training course on supervision, sooner or later the discussion comes round not to how to deliver good supervision, but how to get it. People quickly recognise that their ability to offer good supervision is partly dependant upon them receiving it as well.

The situations that course participants have found themselves in have been many and varied, no doubt you will recognise all or some of the following examples:-

"I just don't receive any supervision at all"

"We do occasionally meet but it always concentrates on checking up on me and my paperwork"

"We are supposed to meet regularly but they get cancelled more often than not, and when we do meet now neither of us know what to talk about"

Each one of you may be encountering different difficulties in relation to supervision but I guess the above will cover at least one aspect of that aspect of that experience, I therefore intend to take each one of the above as a sort of case study and look at what could be done to deal with them.

First of all, there are some basics which I think are important in all of these situations.

BASIC CHECKLIST

1. It is important for you to have in your mind a clear idea of what you want to get out of supervision, what it is that you feel that you are missing. For instance I would describe good supervision as a mixture of training, support and accountability. How does that strike you, is it what you want to ask for?

2. Be clear about how regular supervision will help you to do your job better. Yes I know that it seems an obvious question but if you are not currently receiving it then your line management is not necessarily au fait with the answer!

3. Any arguments, discussions, debates that you have on this topic, should be well thought out and prepared for in advance. Your best chance of getting what you want is to be clear and assertive. Maybe even get someone to go through with you the arguments you wish to put and the things you wish to ask for.

4. Please be clear in your own mind that like the groups and communities you serve, you are entitled to a good service from your line management too. In order to do your job well you need to be supported, encouraged and have structured way to review your own practice and service delivery. Supervision offers that and you should not be embarrassed to ask for it, IT DOES NOT IN ANY WAY IMPLY THAT THOSE WHO REQUIRE SUPERVISION ARE IN ANY WAY INADEQUATE.

"I DON'T RECEIVE ANY SUPERVISION AT ALL"

There could be a multitude of reasons for the above, but in any circumstances I would suggest that you first check whether there is anything in your terms or conditions employment, handbooks or whatever which indicates a commitment on the part of your agency to provide supervision. If that is so then at least you have written evidence to back you up.

If there is no such commitment, then I suggest you consult with fellow workers and see if you can put forward a collective case for the provision of supervision. If you are a single worker then I would do the same, but maybe consult with the workers in other similar agencies to check out the provision there, provision of supervision is common practice and should support your case.

If there is no-one to provide supervision "in house", then maybe your agency should consider using an outside consultant, who will at least be able to provide the support and training aspects of supervision.

Given the current state of funding in community work agencies, I can well believe that the above option is not going to a strong one for many, the final option then is to look around for another worker who is similarly isolated and see if you can negotiate co-supervision between you. I would suggest in the first instance that you make it for a limited number of sessions and negotiate the process and the content clearly and carefully, review it at the end of that time, give each other feedback about what worked or didn't work for you and decide whether to continue or not.

The last of the possible scenarios in this section, is a line manager who is supposed to provide supervision but doesn't. It is clearly important in putting your request for supervision to such a manager not to antagonise them, you do not want to embark on the process of supervision in an atmosphere of tension. I would refer you to the basics noted above and urge you to ensure that you have thought carefully about your request before you make it. Managers will often feel tentative about giving supervision because they feel it will reveal there own shortcomings, maybe some confirmation from you about the positive elements of their role as a manager will enable them to risk it. However, tentative or over worked a manager may feel, your supervision is important to the organisation, and your work and consequently their work will benefit from it, you should therefore be assertive about your request and not feel tentative or guilty about making it.

"WE DO OCCASIONALLY MEET BUT THE SESSIONS ALWAYS CONCENTRATE ON CHECKING ON MY WORK, AND ADMINISTRATIVE MATTERS"

I believe that good supervision always contains within it an element of the review of the process, so that it is possible to check out whether both parties are getting what they want out of it. I do this by leaving a space at the end of each session so that each of us can say what we feel worked well or not so well, and comment on the participation of the other if they wish to. So maybe that could be your first option if supervision is not working well for you, to suggest to your supervisor that you review it as a process either regularly or occasionally. You must then be sure to give your feedback about what is missing for you or wrong for you clearly and specifically.

The other strong option is to start at the other end of the process and request your supervisor to agree to the creation of an agenda at the beginning of each session, to which both of you can contribute. Because of the likelihood of there being more items than there is time for, you should always agree the order in which items are dealt with and ensure that order is not only skewed towards the needs of your supervisor.

Once again it is vital that you and your supervision have an agreed view of the purpose and process of supervision, if you have not discussed it before now please try and do so now.

I am aware of the issue of power in supervision and that some of you might be saying "It's all very well to direct us to put suggestions to our supervisors, but supposing they refuse to listen or listen but refuse to respond." I suppose my first assumption would be that community work supervisors should have an understanding of the function of power within their work, and if they haven't that they should! However I recognise that they might not be so. Perhaps it would help in that area if you referred them to the previous section, which discusses the role of power in supervision. Perhaps a further discussion about power and powerlessness needs to take place in a team meeting or a staff group so that you also feel empowered.

"OUR SUPERVISION SESSION GETS CANCELLED MORE OFTEN THAN NOT AND WHEN WE DO MEET NEITHER OF US HAVE MUCH WE WANT TO TALK ABOUT."

There are two wonderful articles on Games Supervisors Play and Games Supervisees Play, and the cancellation and avoidance of supervision plays a prominent part in both of them. I guess therefore the first thing to do in these circumstances is to ask yourself whether you are playing an active part in the series of cancellations, seizing upon excuses to postpone, being more than ready when asked tentatively if you would mind shifting supervision to agree to it, arriving so late that "it's not worth doing it" or just plain forgetting. If you are doing any or all of these things then maybe now is the time to ask yourself why? If you are not doing any of those things but your supervisor is then now is the time to ask them why? I suspect the answers would be very similar anyway – I'm not sure what we're doing, I don't get what I want out of it. The first response is often "it seems a waste of time, we have so many more important and pressing things to do" but you have to ask why supervision is not seen as a priority and the previous answers often follow. I think these responses indicate again a need to discuss with your supervisor what the purpose of supervision is, the best way that those purposes can be achieved for you. The most positive way to do that is think of a supervision session or a part of a supervision session which was helpful to you and to explain why it was helpful to you to your supervisor. Make sure the content of supervision is of interest and use to both of you.

As far as the problem about content is concerned in this example, as a supervisor I always feel very lost when a supervisee comes to a session with nothing to discuss. After the formal and administrative matters are dealt with where does that leave me to go? It certainly doesn't make me feel that my help or support is valued and I become more tentative about my skills. So come with topics for discussion, nobody's working week is so smooth that they don't have anything to talk about. Try to make it as vivid as possible, bring letters, minutes and/or records to supervision, it will help. One of the roles of good supervision is to help identify exactly what the problem is. So don't hesitate to bring an issue on which you are not entirely clear, hopefully discussion will help to bring that clarity and move you and your supervisor on to looking for a solution.

Throughout all of this example, the key word is feedback, the more you let your supervisor know about what your experience is of supervision, the more chance there is for them to respond to that and change.

I would not wish to give the impression that all elements of good supervision are entirely within the control of those being supervised. Ultimately it does depend on the willingness and openness of the supervisor, that they hear your feedback and respond to it. If they do not the routes open to you are much more formal and serious i.e. grievance procedures etc., which you may not wish to take.

But I think that there are a lot of things that can be done before that. A great deal of your work as community workers is about empowering people and although supervisors are of course people who have a degree of power already, you can use your skills as community workers to empower them in respect to their supervisory skills.

The longer these difficult and often collusive and unsatisfactory relationships continue, the more energy sapping and undermining they are. So please consider trying some of the suggestions I have made if they relate to your own experiences. Use friends and colleagues to test out strategies and feedback, get support and encouragement from members of your team but DO TRY!!

Conclusion

Well, I hope you have been convinced that supervision can be a very positive and powerful tool, enabling and empowering us all to the communities in which we work. Supervision does not require mystical, therapeutic or psycho-dynamic skills, just a measure of preparation, order, thoughtfulness, openness and good sense – all qualities that I would expect to find in a community worker anyway!

SECTION 16

SURVEYS

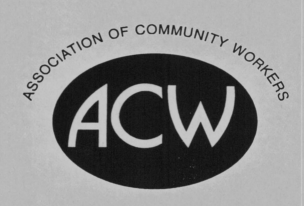

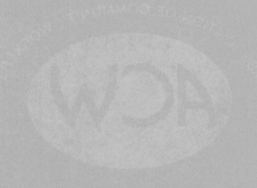

SECTION:	**SURVEYS**
TITLE:	**CARRYING OUT YOUR OWN RESEARCH**
AUTHOR:	Roger Green

WHAT IS RESEARCH?

Research is quite simply about asking questions, gathering information and finding out answers. We all collect information on a daily basis in our work, some of it we use and record, some of it we disregard, and probably never call it research. All the term research means is that information we collect and analysis is done so in a more systematic way. Anyone can do research within their own voluntary organisation, community project or group.

WHY IS IT NEEDED?

- to influence and challenge decision and policy makers

- to allow you to monitor and evaluate your project or group e.g. is it meeting its aims and objectives?

- to support an argument for additional or continued funding

- to check if policies are working in practice e.g. equal opportunities policies, user or client involvement, anti-discriminatory practice

- to examine whether the services a project or group provides/meets the needs of its users and/or the community are they responding to local demands?

- to provide more comprehensive information and details e.g. for grant purposes, informing others of a projects work

- for planning purposes and targeting resources more effectively

- to support a campaign for better services and/or a new service

- research creates knowledge. Knowledge is power

HOW DO YOU DO IT?

The method of research you choose will depend on, for example, what subject or issue you need to research, the type of voluntary organisation or community project or group and what services etc. it provides to the local community.

INTERVIEWS

You may intend undertaking some interviews with users or clients of a project to obtain their views of the service etc. they receive.

QUESTIONNAIRE

You ask people in the community to complete a questionnaire to find out whether there is adequate support for individuals with a heroin addiction in the community and if this support can be improved.

SURVEY/ACTION RESEARCH

You carry out a general needs survey of your community which examines such issues as poverty, needs of the elderly, racial harassment, local transport with the aim that it may enable local people to take action themselves.

COLLECT AND ANALYSE INFORMATION

A community group wishing to set up a carers network but needs to collect and analyse information on existing local and national carers networks so that it can consider this information before deciding how to establish their own network.

PARTICIPATORY RESEARCH

The users or clients of a project or group or members of the community define the research problem themselves, they choose the appropriate method or way of collecting the information and analyse and interpret the data or information themselves.

SECTION:	SURVEYS
TITLE:	CARRYING OUT YOUR OWN RESEARCH
AUTHOR:	Roger Green

WRITING UP THE RESULTS AND PRESENTING THE FINDINGS

As a point of principle research findings should be available to those individuals, groups and the community it affects.

- it should be disseminated or shared in a way which empowers people, for example, it supports change and/or action

- it should be written in laypersons language and available in appropriate community languages

- who the research findings are to be presented to, often known as its "audience", is important as this may well determine how you do this, for example, it may be an organisation which is external to your agency or project, such as the agency which funds your organisation (the local council or health authority). The findings may be just for internal use only, therefore it may be shared with staff, users or clients, volunteers or members of your management committee.

- it should be in a written form which is presented clearly and concisely i.e. sections or chapters clearly separated, appropriate diagrams and illustrations (tables, graphs, charts, photographs etc.)

- consider whether you should write up a draft report first so that it is a discussion document and get people to read it and comment on it before completing a final draft.

HELP WITH DOING RESEARCH

It maybe that you need some help with undertaking research in your organisation. Many community projects and groups enlist the support of researchers to help them. How to contact a researcher who may be interested can be a problem, however the following list is worth checking out.

Possible contacts

- local Council for Voluntary Service

- the social science or community studies department at your nearest university/college

- some of the larger voluntary organisations

- Association for Research in the Voluntary and Community Sector (ARVAC), 60 Highbury Grove, London N5 2AG

  Tel/Fax: 0171 704 2315

ARVAC is an excellent organisation to contact regarding undertaking any research within your own voluntary sector community project or group. Their aims are to "promote research into the voluntary sector; to disseminate research findings; to provide researchers with a supportive network; to link together researchers and practitioners and provide a forum for discussion".

An ARVAC publication: MAKING IT WORK: RESEARCHING IN THE VOLUNTARY SECTOR by Angela Everitt and Andy Gibson, Social Welfare Research Unit, University of Northumbria, is an easy step by step guide and will be essential reading for anyone undertaking research in the community.

SECTION:	**SURVEYS**
TITLE:	**DESIGNING A SURVEY QUESTIONNAIRE**
AUTHOR:	Greg Smith

If you are convinced you need to do a survey and have found the resources in people and money you are now ready to go ahead on a six to twelve month action programme. Much can be achieved by common sense and good planning but you will need some technical skill. The section which follows gives no more than hints but there are references to a number of useful resources which you may need to obtain.

STAGE 1: DESIGNING QUESTIONNAIRES

There is a tradeoff between asking all the questions you are interested in and making the questionnaire too long. No interview should normally take more than half an hour and it is better if you can complete it in ten minutes. So only include questions you really need.

Having said that do not forget to include basic demographic questions such as the age, gender, ethnic group, occupation, housing tenure, educational level, family situation of respondents so that you can break the results down by these groupings.

It is crucial to make all questions perfectly clear and unambiguous, and avoid questions which are loaded or leading and therefore liable to put answers into people's mouths.

Questions often need to be broken down into stages so that they are simple and clearly asking only one thing.

Some questions should only be asked if a respondent meets a particular condition e.g. IF YOU ARE A PENSIONER "Do you go to the Senior Citizen Club". IF NOT A PENSIONER GO TO NEXT QUESTION.

Multiple choice answers should be given wherever possible although some open ended questions or opportunities for free ranging comment are inevitable and useful. It should be clear whether the answers are mutually exclusive (only one answer can be given per person) or whether multiple replies are possible. Always include an "other; please give details" category to cope with the answers you hadn't thought possible. It is best to give each possible reply a code number and ask interviewers to put a circle round it (not a tick).

EXAMPLE QUESTIONNAIRE PAGE

1) DO YOU LIKE LIVING IN THIS NEIGHBOURHOOD?

1   very much   ☐

2   generally yes   ☐

3   not sure/mixed feelings   ☐

4   not much   ☐

5   not at all   ☐

2) WHAT ARE THE GOOD THINGS ABOUT THIS NEIGHBOURHOOD?

....

....

....

3) WOULD YOU OR A MEMBER OF YOUR HOUSEHOLD TAKE PART IN ANY OF THE FOLLOWING GROUPS IF THEY WERE SET UP AT THE REDEVELOPED PARISH CHURCH CENTRE?

Circle one answer in each row

	definitely	perhaps	not interested
under 5s	1	2	3
primary age children	1	2	3
teenagers	1	2	3
adults	1	2	3
senior citizens	1	2	3
the unemployed	1	2	3
the homeless	1	2	3
ethnic minority groups	1	2	3
disabled people	1	2	3
mental health problems	1	2	3
other	1	2	3

4) AGE

_____ years

5)   GENDER

male   1

female   2

6)   WHERE WERE YOU BORN & MAINLY BROUGHT UP?

1   locally (within 2 miles)

2   in London

3   S. England

4   N. England or Midlands

5   elsewhere in UK

6   overseas (please name country) ....

if not locally born WHEN DID YOU MOVE HERE? 19 ....

Be generous with the layout of the questionnaire form. Include instructions to interviewers if possible in a different type face. Print the questions themselves in a distinct bold type. You really need word processing facilities to design a decent questionnaire.

Further examples of questionnaires for community surveys are available from the author on hard copy or as ASCII text files.

Send a large SAE and/or blank formatted floppy PC/DOS disk to:

> Greg Smith CIU,
> Durning Hall,
> Earlham Grove,
> London E7 9AB

Before you use your questionnaire PILOT IT. That means test it out before you print the final version on at least half a dozen potential respondents to see if there are any major problems.

SECTION:	**SURVEYS**
TITLE:	
AUTHOR:	

Constructing a representative sample for a survey is a complex and mathematical process if you want to predict precisely the behaviour of the general public, (e.g. the outcome of an election, and even then as we have seen people lie to the opinion polls or change their minds at the last minute!)

HOWEVER

For the purposes of a neighbourhood or members survey, we can get away with a much less rigorous approach providing we remember a few basic rules.

1)   If you are gathering information from a small closed group of people such as the 105 members of congregation, or karate club, forget about sampling strategy just interview everybody who is willing. Simply note the number who refuse or are uncontactable and work out your percentage response rate.

2)   If you can only manage to interview a proportion of the population you are interested in the main thing is to avoid bias. For example in a general survey of residents it would be wrong for 75% of interviews to be with men rather than woman. If there are 30% Asians in your neighbourhood it would be wrong to have a sample which is 95% white. Other biases would be to miss out on interviewing council tenants, or to do all the interviewing in the day time and thus miss out working people. You may also need to think about which age groups are included.

The easiest way to avoid bias is to set up a quota system based on what you know about your local population.

e.g.

male	50%	female	50%		
whites	70%	Asians	20%	black	10%
council tenants	40%	owner occupiers	50%	others	10%
under 30s	20%	over 60s	20%		

Keep a record of who is being interviewed, and as the survey progresses instruct your interviewers to only interview the groups you are short of. This type of quota sampling is especially useful if you are approaching people for interview as you encounter them in a public place.

3)   Providing you avoid bias, for these sort of surveys there is usually no need to interview more than about 200 people unless you want to do detailed breakdowns for example of the views of Asian woman over 65 (there may be only 2 or 3 of them in a sample of 200). Generally speaking it is not the percentage of a large population interviewed that matters so much as the total number. Once you get into three figures you can be about 95% certain that the results reflect the population within a margin error of 10%.

4)   SELECTING HOUSEHOLDS

Despite what has been said above it is good practice and gives your research greater credibility if you have made a serious attempt to construct a systematic sample using some element of random choice. To do this you need to have an accurate and complete list of the population you are sampling. To sample household or individual adults in a neighbourhood the usual list employed is the register of electors (available in your local library or the town hall). You can also decide to use the post office's file of addresses in your area.

You could pick a true random sample using random number tables or a computer to choose say 200 names out of the 20,000 electors in your town's register. But they would be widely scattered and therefore hard to interview. A two stage clustered approach is easier to manage. First you choose say 5 council wards (either at random or deliberately chosen to get a particular social mix of housing types and ethnic group). Then within those wards you pick a random starting point and choose every 10th household in the streets until you have 40 addresses in each ward. There are many variations on this sort of sampling which you can read about in the reference books.

One further advantage of using electoral registers in sampling is that you can identify many members of particular ethnic minorities by looking at their names. This works particularly well for Sikhs, Hindus and Muslims. This technique can even be used for mapping the distribution of these groups within a neighbourhood.

5)   MAXIMISING RESPONSE RATES

Even the most scientific sampling strategy is little use if you fail to get back more than half the questionnaires. Usually non-response introduces a bias that distorts your results, as some groups are more likely than others to respond. This means you have to work hard to increase response rates.

By and large self completion and postal questionnaires are useless unless there is strong incentive such as £10 offered for each one returned. Failing that, you will normally be lucky to get 10% returned. However, a short self completion questionnaire may be appropriate for use in a group session, for example in a class room or as a ten minute exercise within a regular club or meeting.

A good team of interviewers can do much better, but persistence and persuasiveness are needed. In a household survey they may have to call round five times at different hours on different days before they find someone at home. In practice in a neighbourhood profile it is permissible to allow interviewers to move on to replacement addresses, for example by knocking next door to the address on the sample sheet, as long as this is recorded. Selling the questionnaire to busy people is an art, and you need to show how it is in the respondent's self interest to co-operate. An incentive such as a prize draw may help. The questionnaire should not be to long (taking more than 15 minutes is excessive) and interviewers need to be honest about the time required. It is important too to stress confidentiality, and that the whole of the data will be made anonymous in the reports.

People are most likely to respond to interviewers who they see as like themselves, but perhaps not so well known as to be part of local gossip networks. Thus this is a good idea for woman to interview woman, young interviewers to interview youth, Asians to speak to Asians etc. For some ethnic minority groups it is essential to have interviewers who speak the minority language. In a general survey it is not usually worth the trouble and expense to have a written translation in fifteen languages that may be spoken locally. But if you have more than one interviewer who will be using, say, Gujerati it is important to get them to meet, to work through the questionnaire and agree on a consistent way of translating each question.

TRAINING INTERVIEWERS AND FIELDWORK

If you are using interviewers it is essential to train and supervise them properly. A whole day or two long evenings is about right. They need a full briefing about the purpose and process of the survey, practical information about the mechanics of it and information on administrative procedures. However, practice is the most important element and should concentrate on two aspects. Firstly there should be listening skills exercises to make sure the interviewer hears and records what is actually being said. Secondly there should be extensive practice at using the questionnaire, in pairs with one person role playing a respondent and "changing ends" at half time.

You need to nominate a fieldwork supervisor who is responsible for collecting (and if possible checking through with the interviewers) the completed questionnaires. It is a good idea to number the questionnaires before they are issued and keep track of where they are, and what stage they have reached. The supervisor is also responsible for seeing that the whole selected sample is covered and that any quota system is maintained.

BASIC BOOKS ON SURVEY METHODS INCLUDE

Paul Nichols
Social Survey Methods: A Field Guide for Development Workers
1991
Oxfam Publications, (ISBN 0855981261)

David Phillips
Do-It-Yourself Social Surveys
1988
Faculty of Social Studies, Polytechnic of North London,

Hoinville, Jowell and Associates
Survey Research Practice
1978
Heinemann Educational Books, London

SECTION:	**SURVEYS**
TITLE:	
AUTHOR:	

SECTION:	SURVEYS
TITLE:	DATA INPUT AND ANALYSIS
AUTHOR:	Greg Smith

Once the survey is complete it is important to get on quickly with the data analysis. If you are working with a very small questionnaire you can get away with using tally sheets, perhaps using a blank questionnaire on which to mark off the number people giving each kind of answer. For most surveys however you will need a computer.

If you haven't got the hardware, software or skills to process the data it is worth while approaching a local college or school for help at the planning stage of the survey.

Some standard database packages maybe usable for analysing questionnaires but I have usually found it is better to enter the data as a spreadsheet with one row for each questionnaire and one column for each question. The data file (saved as ASCII) text can then usually be transferred quite easily into a statistical analysis package. A spreadsheet allows you to sort the data in whatever order you want and to print out all the (textual) replies to any open ended question listed in a single column.

The three packages I have used for statistical analysis are:

1) **SPSS** (Statistical Package for the Social Sciences) which is very powerful statistically and widely used in universities, but which costs a lot unless you are working as part of an academic institution.

2) **KWIKSTAT** is a shareware package running on IBM PC compatibles and does more than enough to analyse your data. It is cheap without being to cheerful.

3) **EPI INFO** is a public domain set of programs for the PC which are offered by the World Health Organisation. It has a brilliantly simple method of data entry based on a word processed version of your actual questionnaire. It can import and export files to spreadsheets, databases and SPSS.

PINPOINT from Longman Logotron is a product aimed at schools for use on Acorn Archimedes Machines and looks useful and attractive in presentation. Check if your local school uses it, or buy it for your Archimedes if you have one.

The author could let you have a copy of KWIKSTAT or EPI INFO if you send formatted floppy disks (with 2mb space)

Which ever program you use you will probably not want to do much more than extract basic frequency tables for each variable (i.e. how many people answered each question in each possible way), plus some simple cross tabulations for the major sub-groups of respondents (e.g. men v woman, age groups, ethnic groups, council tenants v owner occupiers).

SECTION:	**SURVEYS**
TITLE:	
AUTHOR:	

SECTION:	**SURVEYS**
TITLE:	**PRESENTING RESULTS**
AUTHOR:	Greg Smith

So your research is finished, and unlike many research reports is not going to gather dust on someone's top shelf is it?!

YOU NEED TO DISSEMINATE, PROMOTE, PUBLICISE.

SUMMARY REPORTS

Every researcher should consider doing a popular tabloid summary report of every piece of research. You can reach lots more people with 4 pages which are cheaper to print than 400, and more likely to be read. The golden rules are to write in a popular not academic style use catchy headlines and sub heads and to illustrate with graphs and photos or cartoons.

PRESS RELEASES

Prepare an interesting press release and send it to your local rag with a copy of the summary report. Unless there is a mass murderer at large, it will be news and you should be able to get a feature article in the local press.

PUBLIC PRESENTATIONS

Call a meeting or use existing regular groups to present your findings. It is well worthwhile producing some exhibition boards, OHP slides or a slide show, even a video to get the message across.

THE FULL OR REFERENCE REPORT

There needs to be a full version of your findings for the serious reader although these can be very expensive to produce, especially as not many copies will be needed. With our disability survey we have only 2 main copies, which are available as chapters or as a whole for photocopying for anyone who wants them.

The full report of a neighbourhood profile usually needs to contain:

MOVING TO ACTION

Now we have reached the (new) beginning of the story. You have the ammunition, now the action begins. Your can start reviewing your objectives on the basis of information rather than groping around in the dark on hunches. You can begin your new projects and apply for funding knowing that there is a substantial need which you can tackle. Or you can plunge afresh into specific issue campaigns knowing that information is power and you will be able to get the council or Government to do something!

Or you can of course think about all the unanswered research questions, and start all over again!.

- Contents page
- Summary of key findings
- Method: who, did what, when why (Questionnaires should be printed in an appendix).
- Background on your neighbourhood. (History/Map/Boundaries/Environment/Transport links)
- Statistical Data from the Census etc.
- Extensive results from your own surveys; including basic tables and graphs.
- Perceptions, opinions, stories gathered from your networking survey, or group discussions.
- Conclusions gathered around key themes
- Implications for your own work
- Addresses of other agencies serving your patch
- Acknowledgements

SECTION:	**SURVEYS**
TITLE:	
AUTHOR:	

SECTION 17

CAMPAIGNING

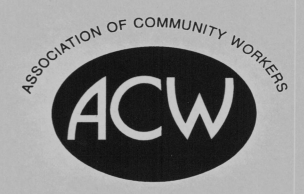

SECTION:	**CAMPAIGNING**
TITLE:	**TRAINING FOR OUTDOOR WORK**
AUTHOR:	Quaker Action for Peace and Justice

This material was developed by Quaker Action for Peace and Justice, for short training sessions intended for groups and individuals who had little or no experience of outdoor campaigning.

Such training is useful even for groups or individuals who are experienced in street campaigning. It provides an opportunity to clarify ideas, and guidance for those who are new to the group or new to street work.

Street campaigning isn't just a question of getting it together on a Saturday morning, going down to the shopping precinct, putting up a table with some literature on it, then standing around hoping that someone will come up and talk to you. It involves a whole lot more. Nor is it enough to get together a good exhibition, several interesting things for people to do, and then assume they are going to flock you.

Any street campaigning has to be seen as a whole, from beginning to end, in all its details, with a consciousness of what image is being presented to the world at large.

The whole process involves:

VISION – what do you want to achieve

ANALYSIS – who, what, where and how?

STRATEGY – preparation, what needs doing on the day, and evaluation and next steps.

VISION

The starting point for any action has to be a clear vision of what you hope to achieve by the end of the day. There are usually four broad possibilities:

- First, you can aim to be seen by thousands of people, but with little or no personal or individual contact. If this is what you want to achieve, you'll want some highly visual event.

- Second you can have minimal direct contact with two or three thousand people in a day, through saturation leafletting.

- Third, by using street theatre of some kind followed by selective leafletting of the audience, you can have closer contact and more impact.

- Fourth, you can aim to have direct one-to-one contact, through dialogue, with only a few individuals over a two or three hour period.

These four levels are not mutually exclusive but it helps to recognise that the more people you aim to impress in a day, the briefer the personal contact will be. Similarly, the more deeply you want to engage individuals in conversation, the less "spectacular" your event will probably be. All four levels have their place in street campaigning at some time, but it's important to choose the right action for your group.

Making that choice is the first step in planning your action. And since people – even within the same group – are likely to have different visions, it's important to involve as many people as possible. One way of releasing your groups imagination is to divide into two's and three's and ask each pair or small group to come up with some visions about what the action could achieve. The visions can be practical, imaginative, realistic or unlikely. At the end of five minutes or so, pool the thoughts of all the small groups. Reject the really unlikely unachievable ones, so you end up with a list of several possible visions, for example "we'll have 10 new members" or "we'll feel less scared of putting our case to strangers." These visions are now ready to become part of the analysis.

SECTION:	**CAMPAIGNING**
TITLE:	**TRAINING FOR OUTDOOR WORK**
AUTHOR:	Quaker Action for Peace and Justice

ANALYSIS

A very useful tool to use for this is a "Who What Where When and How" chart. Put up several long sheets of paper and move rapidly through the following questions, using brainstorm techniques.

WHO are you are aiming at? What specific group in the population i.e. teenagers, young couples, woman with children, everybody?

WHAT is the focus for action? Look at your visions and decide. WHAT are you hoping people will do as a result of your action?

WHERE are there sites available for you for a static event? WHICH roads or routes are most effective for a mobile campaign?

HOW are you going to get the message across? What are your groups resources and strengths? Do they include, for example, theatre, soapbox speaking, visual design, talking?

WHEN is the best date/day/time of the day for this work?

The point of this exercise is to assemble as many ideas as possible so that whatever you finally decide to do is underpinned by a thorough appreciation of all the factors involved. The specific action you take becomes a deliberate choice rather than something that happens because that's what another group did. Here are some points that might come out of this kind of chart, with some examples.

WHO

Usually a street campaign is aimed at "the general public" with little thought given to the infinite variety of individuals that go to make it up. Different groups of people are on the streets at different times of the day or on different days during the week. On a weekday in a village or a small town you might get a preponderance of young parents with toddlers delivering or collecting older children from school; in a large, busy city centre on a Saturday you'll get a broader cross-section of the population, possibly with a higher proportion of young adults.

WHAT

Among the many possibilities are, for example, a widespread leaflet distribution within the community to make people aware of your group's existence, a campaign on a specific day, a questionnaire campaign to find out how much is known about a specific local situation, a campaign to get signatures on a petition for a national campaign.

WHERE

Street campaigning can be mobile, or can be fixed or static. Mobile can mean on wheels (cars, motorbikes, bikes) or on foot. If a route is well chosen a mobile campaign can get maximum visual coverage, or can link several villages or areas.

Sometimes a local authority has designated spaces where groups can set up a fixed activity. In other places the whole shopping area will be open to use, Provided there is no obstruction to pedestrians or traffic. Some venues are available on a one-off basis, either by getting local authority permission (for example in a local park or carpark) or by getting private permission (for example to use the area outside a church or shop). If you have a choice, pick the site to match the action.

A blanket leaflet action simply to get a bit of information across to as many people as possible could make good use of a limited space where people are passing rapidly between, say, transport and shops. But a campaign to inform and mobilise people and get signatures on a particular issue might need space for people to browse, talk and actually sign. For that sort of action, you would look for a site which is not too busy, but where there are plenty of people around.

Street theatre needs more unobstructed space – an open space in a precinct, with plenty of people passing either side to side or approaching head-on and dividing to go past, or a broad patch of pavement.

If there is no designated space, do some research by going to potential places at the time of a possible campaign to see what is actually going on. It would be very useful to do the same with an offered site. It's a good idea also to keep an eye on other groups and where they are allowed to campaign, and see what effect their efforts seem to be having.

HOW

There are a variety of street activities including:

- A mobile event on wheels, driving a van in processions of cars and floats. These events were big, flamboyant and colourful, and got across a clear message about what was happening.

- Joining in ordinary marches, where it's important to have as many placards or banners as possible to create a clear identity for each group and a clear message for the public.

• Working with people in local areas to use the technique of a dramatic procession. Where half a dozen people, dressed in black cloaks and hoods with "skull" masks, are each partnered by an "ordinary" person. Each pair carried double-sided placards on short sticks making parallel opposing statements. A drummer led the way to attract attention, and a leafletter came behind to offer people information about the campaign.

For fixed events try to maximise visual impact by using banners or flags, by having an information desk, and by putting out poster boards for passers-by to read. One good idea is to have an information board relating to the locality.

The sorts of actions you might consider can include leafletting; collecting signatures on a petition or postcards; engaging in dialogue; selling or giving away badges, literature and/or balloons; games; questionnaires; music; street theatre; and street speaking.

After you've come up with a range of possibilities, you will have to decide which will best achieve your objective. But it may be necessary to defer this decision until you've collected some necessary information, for example about which sites are available.

When all the information is in, decide which part of the WWWWH analysis chart it's easiest to deal with. There aren't any hard and fast rules. There may be only one focus under the heading WHAT, because the group has decided to campaign because a particular event is coming up. Everything else then stems from how best to achieve that focus. Or the HOW might be the starting point – if there are just five of you with very limited resources and money it's not practical to think in terms of a busy general campaign, and you might choose to focus on letting a large number of people know of your existence. Or it could be that you have no choice of site, for one reason or the other, and this governs the HOW. For example, the only site available might be in the middle of a busy town centre with continuous traffic, with flow and access to the site controlled by zebra crossings. It might be very busy, but there's not much space and real danger of obstruction.

Another factor governing the WHAT and HOW will be your own experience and confidence. It's important not to try to do things like street theatre if you don't feel ready for them. Work from your strengths as individuals and as a group.

In general, It's often easiest to start with the WHAT first, rejecting any ideas that are obviously impractical or unsuitable and eliminating others by bearing in mind your vision and the information you've collected about when and where.

This is a long and difficult process, but going through it means the ensuing campaign will be well grounded. Wherever you start, a pattern should gradually emerge that will become the blue print for the forthcoming action. Write this up on a clean sheet of paper as a WWWWH chart. This is the basis on which the strategy is built.

STRATEGY PRACTICALITIES

There are two main strands to any strategy. One concerns all the practical details to do with the campaign, such as permissions, printing, etc. The other has to do with the preparation and training of the group as a well grounded team.

To deal with practicalities, start by listing every single job to be done, no matter how small. Apportion responsibility for specific broad areas of work. These broad areas are likely to include:

- Site
- Main leaflet
- Press and publicity
- Actions
- Equipment
- Rotas
- Refreshments
- Transport
- Facilitation (running the day)
- Personal support

SITE

Approach the police first; they will tell you if you need further permission from the council or a private owner. This process can take several weeks. When approaching officials be very precise about how the campaign is to be run – the time, space and actions.

Arrange parking space either for unloading or long-term. Arrange access to the site if it's not a public road.

Visit the site at the time of day and the same day of the week that you plan to work and just watch the patterns of pedestrian traffic and its quantity. Unless you take the trouble to check, you wont be able to take advantage of the distinct patterns of movement that every area has.

MAIN LEAFLET

Decide whether you are going to use an existing leaflet from a national or local group – in which case order in very good time – or design your own.

SECTION:	**CAMPAIGNING**
TITLE:	**TRAINING FOR OUTDOOR WORK**
AUTHOR:	Quaker Action for Peace and Justice

PRESS AND PUBLICITY

Finding out about local media and building up contacts is a long process, best done over months rather than days. Always prepare a press release for local newspapers and radio/TV. And don't forget to send publicity material to local organisations, making it clear whether you're asking for help and support or just publicising the event. It poses a problem if, having laid out your site on the day, someone from another group also arrives and expects to set up their stall and dish out their leaflets.

Decide who will be interviewed by press or radio if this is offered. Then practise, perhaps through roleplay, coping with different styles of interviewers – the antagonistic, the sympathetic, the patronising, the one who just lets you ramble on.

If you want to, you can insist on two people being present at interviews, even if only one actually does the talking. If things aren't going well, the second person can step in to stop the interview and re-do it.

ACTIONS

Plan carefully how any particular activity fits in with the whole. An activity which needs a large table, for example, might seriously impinge on the effect of the site as a whole.

If you're going to use balloons, will they be helium filled or just plain puff? For sale or give away? The best method we've seen of keeping the strings untangled was tying the balloons (close to the neck with a tail dangling) on to a small clothing rack.

For street theatre you'll need to know if the performing space is in front of or to the side of the main site. What happens to any other action during performances? Do you stop and concentrate everyone's attention on it or carry on? Everyone concerned will need to know the policy and be disciplined in it's observance.

What will you do if it pours with rain or blows a gale? Have alternative plans ready so that all your preparation is not wasted.

What will you do if there are any difficulties with passers-by or hecklers? We found that, difficult though it seems, it's easier to approach apparent trouble then wait for it to come to us. For example in a town where there had been recent trouble with the National Front at a public meeting, one of our supporters came onto the streets with us carrying a portable tape recorder. Had the NF appeared (which they didn't), she would have approached them to ask – and record – their views about what we were doing.

EQUIPMENT

If one person looks after all the equipment – Whether permanent or one-off for a specific action – there's a better chance of achieving unity of style and colour, and of having what you need with you when you suddenly want or need it.

ROTAS, REFRESHMENTS, TRANSPORT

According to the length and complexity of the event, rotas, refreshments and transport may be the responsibility of one person or divided among several.

Rotas are essential for a long day's work, or when there are a lot of people willing to help. Discourage workers from hanging around the site when they are not actually working; it's better to have 1½ hours on and half an hour off.

For the sake of your image, it's a good idea to try to keep all refuse and refreshments off the site area.

Speaking of image, you might want to give some thought to the way you present yourself as a group, and whether you want some sort of group identity. What about badges?

SECTION:	**CAMPAIGNING**
TITLE:	**TRAINING FOR OUTDOOR WORK**
AUTHOR:	Quaker Action for Peace and Justice

STRATEGY: NEEDS OF THE GROUP

Before the campaign, spend time building the confidence of group members. There are six important steps in this process.

- Hear from those without experience their worries and fears about being out on the street, and hear what the group as a whole can do to make things easier.

- Hear from those with experience what made it easier, what actually happened and how they coped with any problems.

- Imagine the public's response to you.

- Try out – perhaps through roleplay – ways to deal with problem people: the bores, the wafflers, the "that's all very well but-ers" and last but not least, the drunks.

- Agree a plan to cope with the worst that could happen; agree a "help" signal that can be picked up easily without being obvious to anyone else. Decide whether you want to buddy-up on the street, so you know one person is looking after you and so you're worrying about someone other than yourself.

- Learn more about each other as a people with an identity and life other than as a member of the group.

With this sort of preparation comes a sense of security and real trust in each other. This in turn has an effect on the general public, who are aware of the confidence shown by group members.

ON THE DAY

Perhaps the most important thing you're going to do is create an image which has an impact on people, even if they don't want to get into direct contact with you. So everything possible should be done to try to ensure that it's a good image. This includes:

- Arrive on time.

- Set up quickly and efficiently.

- Be ready to start up on time with all setting up finished.

- Everybody should work hard with energy and concentration for their agreed time.

- Keep up a good, positive atmosphere until the agreed time to stop.

- Pack away quickly and efficiently.

- Pick up any discarded leaflets or any other litter created by your presence. (This should be happening throughout the day anyway).

EVALUATION AND CELEBRATION

Evaluation and celebration can happen immediately after the action or a few days later. The temptation is to let it slide, especially if the group has recently been making heavy demands on everyone's time.

The main purpose of an evaluation is to look hard – and with pride – at the things you got right. If that's hard to do in a big group, break into pairs or groups of three or four.

An agenda for an evaluation and celebration might include:

- A shared meal

- Going round – "Something that surprised me" or "Something I hadn't expected during the day's campaigning."

- A formal evaluation – 3 large sheets of paper (old poster backs or newsprint) headed "Went well" "Went badly" and "Next time" or "Smiles" "Frowns" "Next time." Do this as a disciplined brainstorm and keep to a time limit.

- A discussion on the evaluation, comparing notes and responses. What next - make some notes or suggestions for the next action.

- Go round "I particularly enjoyed..." (It's important to finish on a positive note.)

Ask yourselves if you want press coverage at all. You will have no control over the quality or quantity of such coverage, and may find that all your work will culminate in a fraction of a column inch on page six. You should trade off the amount of work that may be required with the possibility of disappointment in the coverage obtained.

If the answer to the above question is yes, read on!!

TWO MONTHS BEFORE THE EVENT

It's helpful to appoint one person to act as press contact. This person should have time, a daytime and evening telephone number and the ability to communicate well verbally and through writing.

Put together a list of all the media in your area. The local library will help, and you can do a survey of local newsagents and talk to people about where they get their information about local events. There will usually be several TV stations, radio stations as well as morning and evening regional newspapers. There may also be other local newspapers with Sunday, urban and rural editions, community and "street press" papers, weekly magazines, student newspapers, free newspapers, hospital broadcasting services and local pressure groups' news-sheets. Include on your listing the names and the addresses of the editor(s). Larger media services may have separate news, features, church and women's editors who will need to be contacted separately.

ONE MONTH BEFORE THE EVENT

Send a press release to each name on your list, stating clearly the 5 W's and H: what is happening, why it's happening, who is doing it and who it's for, when and where it's happening and how it's happening. The press release should be typewritten, double-spaced on one side of the page only, and should end with the name of your contact person(s) and day and evening telephone numbers.

If you like, include a covering letter inviting them to send a reporter and/or photographer to the event.

ONE OR TWO WEEKS BEFORE THE EVENT

Telephone important media which haven't acknowledged your earlier press release. Ask if they received the press release, or if they would like you to send another copy.

IMMEDIATELY BEFORE THE EVENT

Confirm any final arrangements for reporters, photographers, television crew etc. to be at the event.

POINTS TO NOTE

The catchment areas for press, radio and TV don't follow tidy city, county or Monthly Meeting boundaries. Remember to include media from neighbouring areas on your list.

Whenever you speak to the press be careful. It's easy for what you say to be misinterpreted or misrepresented. On Q-PAC we only spoke with the press if at least two of us were present at the interview.

A useful book to read is "Using the Media" by Denis McShane, which is published by Pluto Press and costs £2.50. Highly recommended!

SECTION:	**CAMPAIGNING**
TITLE:	
AUTHOR:	

SECTION:	**CAMPAIGNING**
TITLE:	**A TRAINING SESSION ON CAMPAIGNING SKILLS**
AUTHOR:	Zbyszek Luczynski and Val Lunn

The method and process of campaigning can be introduced in a series of fairly artificial stages which flow into one another.

It is a dynamic process and the various aspects and stages occur at different points in this process. Often many happen all at the same time while other events/aspects/stages may be missed altogether.

What we wanted to obtain from participants in this session on campaigning was to use their own experience of campaigning to reach an overview of this dynamic process, its stages and all of its possibilities. In a three hour session we could not hope for any great depth, more of a check list, an "aide memoire" of campaigning technique – i.e. the skills behind a good campaign.

The session's aims

To consider:

a) How to start and set up a campaign. Ways of getting people involved.

b) Drawing up a plan of action.

c) Ways of checking out progress made by evaluation before moving on.

Method used

We split the participants into four campaign groups:

*   one campaigning for adaptation for people with physical disabilities at a Community Centre;

*   one campaigning against racial attacks on an estate;

*   one campaigning about women's safety on a local estate;

*   one campaigning on issues surrounding lesbians, gays, bisexuals coming out at a local youth club.

OUTLINE SESSION PLAN

INTRODUCTIONS

Names and what group/campaigning group you're from, introduce the aims of the session and timetable for the morning.

STARTING AND SETTING UP A CAMPAIGN (30 MINUTES)

What – to look at what kinds of issues you need to consider when starting a campaign.

How – brainstorm in large group.

*   Understand what your aim is.

*   Be clear what the group is there to do.

*   Who has the power/resources.

*   What is your target.

*   Who are your supporters.

*   How will you contact them.

*   How will you finance the campaign.

*   Who will the contact/ co-ordinator be.

*   Will you form an organising group.

*   How will you make decisions.

*   What guidelines will you agree for the way you work.

*   Give yourselves time to become a group.

*   Set up democratic structures to maximise involvement.

*   What will this campaign mean for different people, lesbians and gay people, people with disabilities.

*   Will everybody who wants to be able to get involved in the campaign e.g. is your campaign accessible.

STARTING AND SETTING UP A CAMPAIGN II (30 MINUTES)

What – work on case study.

How – in small group of 4/5, choose a situation and work out a plan for starting and setting up your campaign using the checklist drawn up.

BREAK

DEVELOPING A PLAN OF ACTION/TAKING ACTION (15 MINUTES)

What – what different types of action could you adopt in your campaign.

How – in large group brainstorm different actions.

- Contact making – door knocking/pubs, shopping centres.

- Survey, use information.

- Petitions.

- Public meeting.

- Press releases/radio.

- Negotiations.

- Lobby – power holders, councillors etc.

- Demonstration.

- Direct action.

TAKING YOUR CAMPAIGN FORWARD (30 MINUTES)

In small groups continue to develop your plans of action, prioritise your actions and give reasons for choosing these actions.

CHECKING YOUR CAMPAIGN'S PROGRESS (30 MINUTES)

What – what do you need to do in order to check your campaign's progress.

How – in large group, brainstorm ideas.

- Hold reflection/evaluation meeting.

- Ask what have we achieved?

- Have we achieved what we set out to do?

- Evaluate each action – what worked? What didn't work?

- Are people still involved?

- Do we need to re-evaluate the aims of the campaign?

- How can we learn from other campaigning groups?

- Are there any other campaigning groups doing the same as us?

WIND UP/EVALUATION (15 MINUTES)

Brainstorm in large group and say one thing you've learned from today's session that you will carry with you into any future campaigns. Complete Evaluation Questionnaire.

SOME CASE STUDY EXAMPLES

Your local community centre is not accessible for people in wheel chairs and with physical disability. A number of groups have complained as they have not been able to involve some people because of this. You are a member of one of these groups. How would you campaign for adaptations to the centre?

You work in a neighbourhood centre on an estate with a large Muslim community. You receive a visit from a very distressed Muslim woman who has just had her windows broken and been verbally abused by two white men who she thinks are members of the British Party, a racist and fascist political party. This is one of several recent racist attacks in the neighbourhood. Local people are feeling afraid and angry and want to organise resistance and opposition to these attacks.

There has been a number of street attacks on women in the local area. You are a community worker based at a Community Centre on the estate. How will you go about organising a campaign to publicise the attacks and to try to improve women's safety?

The word has got around that the local youth club is encouraging open discussion about sexuality and as a result some of its members are coming out as lesbian, gay and bisexual. This has led to physical attacks on the youth club leaders and some of the members and the threat of disciplinary proceedings against the youth club leaders. How will you go about starting a campaign knowing that lesbians, gay men and bisexual people are not specifically named in either the Council's Equal Opportunities Policy or its Anti-Harassment Policy?

SECTION:	**CAMPAIGNING**
TITLE:	
AUTHOR:	

SECTION:	**CAMPAIGNING**
TITLE:	**FIGHTING BACK – A CAMPAIGN PLANNING WORKSHOP**
AUTHOR:	Zbyszek Lucynski

The authors ran a day workshop on campaigning skills entitled "fighting back". During the workshop they used three large group brainstorms and their purpose and content are reproduced here. They also have adapted a campaigning checklist from Co-ordinate.

BRAINSTORMS AND CHECKLISTS

1. Starting and Setting up a campaign

What to look at, what kinds of issues you need to consider when starting a campaign.

How to brainstorm in a large group

- understand what your aim is
- be clear what your group is there to do
- who has the power/resources
- what is your target
- who are your supporters
- how will you contact them
- how will you finance the campaign
- who will the contact/co-ordinator be
- will you form an organising group
- how will you make decisions
- what guidelines will you agree for the way you work
- give yourself time to become a group
- set up democratic structures to maximise involvement
- what will this campaign mean for different groups of people e.g. for women, black people, lesbians and gay people, disabled people
- will everybody who wants to, be able to get involved in the campaign e.g. is your campaign accessible.

2. Developing a Plan of Action/Taking Action

What different kinds of action could you adopt in your campaign.

How – In large group brainstorm different actions

1. contact making door knocking/pubs, shopping centres
2. survey – use information
3. petitions
4. public meeting – leaflets
5. lobby – power holder, councillors etc.
6. press release/radio
7. demonstration
8. direct action
9. negotiation

3. Checking your Campaign's Progress

What do you need to do in order to check your campaign's progress.

How – in large group, brainstorm ideas.

- hold reflection/evaluation meeting
- ask what have we achieved
- have we achieved what we set out to do
- evaluate each action – what worked – what didn't work
- are people still involved
- do we need to re-evaluate the aims of the campaign
- how can we learn from other campaigning groups
- are there any other campaigning groups doing the same as us.

SECTION:	**CAMPAIGNING**
TITLE:	**FIGHTING BACK – A CAMPAIGN PLANNING WORKSHOP**
AUTHOR:	Zbyszek Lucynski

CAMPAIGNING CHECKLIST

- You need to know how the machinery operates if you want to put a spanner in the works – find out how your local council works and which committees make the decisions that affect you.

- Make sure you know who made the decision and why. Don't take it for granted that the public occasion when the decision was formally announced reveals who is really behind the proposals.

- On the basis of this information, decide who is to be the target of your campaign.

 Who is going to lead the campaign?

 Who are all the possible participants?

 Who has to take a back-seat, well out of site? (Local advisors may have invaluable advice, but cannot be seen to campaign against their own employers official policy.)

- You need to be able to show that you have support in all sections of the community. Never align your cause with any political party: it will be used to make party political points against you which will make it virtually impossible for any sympathisers in the opposing party to support you. You also need to be free to criticise the policies of any party.

- When do you need to go it alone and when do you need to act jointly? Where are your allies both locally and nationally? Only ever go it alone if your case is based on you being an exceptional e.g. the only project in the area catering for a specific group.

- Be well informed. Make sure that you get copies of all council committee papers, reports, press releases and so on.

- Plan your strategy, based on the vulnerable points – whether or not a councillor is committed to some aspect of your cause. They all care about votes so numbers always count. If one of the threatened services is in a marginal ward, this may be the one to feature in your campaign.

- Think very carefully about how you frame the issue. Go for positive messages – try to be for something rather than against – and make it very hard for people not to feel sympathetic.

SECTION:	**CAMPAIGNING**
TITLE:	**FIGHTING BACK – A CAMPAIGN PLANNING WORKSHOP**
AUTHOR:	Zbyszek Lucynski

- Don't let campaigning interfere with your constructive work – the better your track record of high profile local events, projects and activities, the harder it will be to cut your funding.

- Don't throw away any opportunities to make your case, such as consultations to which you can respond. You could use consultations on the local development plan, anything at all on job creation, employment and training, equal opportunities, and so on.

- Use every possible means to promote your campaign:

  Letter writing – with strategically distributed copies (media, officers, committee chairs and members – remembering to treat all parties even-handedly. MPs, local celebrities, leading academics)

  Agendas – get your issues onto the agenda of as many and at as many levels as possible. You may need to line up a committee members as your ally and, if all else fails, get them to raise it under any other business. Issue briefings in advance of the meeting to every member of the relevant committee, no matter how unsympathetic their party's official policy may be, setting out the key facts of your case and posing the crucial questions which need to be asked about the proposal. You never know which committee member will take it upon themselves to put one of your questions to the meeting.

  Lobbying – use every opportunity which is officially available to turn up and press your case. This includes councillors and MPs, surgeries, outside the town hall as members arrive for a meeting, in the public gallery at every meeting which might conceivably be relevant. The impact will be enhanced if someone makes sure that a photographer is present. Be sure that a clear banner is "in shot" so that the message doesn't get lost in a general crowd of people.

  Petitions etc. – use every other means allowed for democratic representation. Find out what standing orders cover public question time in council committees, the public presentation of petitions and so on.

  Publicity – there is plenty of published advice on how to issue press releases and so on. You could guarantee your own publicity by paying for space in the local papers and advertising your cause – not necessarily prohibitively expensive if a lot of groups are contributing. Local radio is often pleased to have a good local story. Remember to be positive in your approach, if you are not careful, you may win the battle but lose the war: in other words you may show what idiots the politicians are but then they will never be willing to back down. You must frame your case so that they can change their minds without "losing face".

Ubiquity – don't let them escape from you. Officers may begin to have doubts about any policy which is obviously going to mean endless hassle: politicians may have doubts about a course of action which is going to lead to bad publicity at every public occasion (and loss of votes) Be sure that you are highly visible (in some photogenic way, such as waving a banner or balloons, if possible) in the front row of the public gallery whenever the topic is on the agenda.

SECTION:	**CAMPAIGNING**
TITLE:	
AUTHOR:	

SECTION:	**CAMPAIGNING**
TITLE:	**SPEEDOMETER**
AUTHOR:	adapted from the original Skills Manual by Val Harris

The purpose of the technique is to analyse the "balance of forces" confronting a worker or organisation wishing to promote change or resist an actual or potential development.

STAGE 1

Write the issue under consideration at the top of a large sheet of paper or blackboard. The issue is either the objective/initiative the organisation wishes to achieve or the development the organisation wishes to resist.

Draw the diagram below:

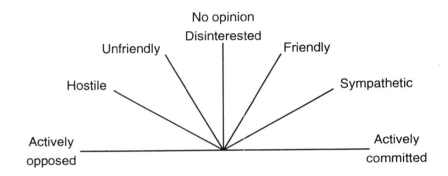

STAGE 2:

Identify those groups/categories/organisations occupying the various positions in the diagram on the specific issue under consideration.

STAGE 3:

Consider those actions/developments that the organisation may take which have the affect of causing another group or organisation to change their position or attitude.

STAGE 4:

Having considered the various options available, choose the strategy.

Ideally the second stage should be completed quickly to allow adequate time to be spent on the third and forth stages; however the second stage should not be glossed over. The diagram should be used as a reference point for discussion so that group members have a shared starting point and can consider the likely affect of a course of action.

The technique involves the labelling of groups/organisations as such; it is important that some effort should be made to test the group's perception by group members and that the evidence for the labelling is made explicit.

Finally organisations are not always consistent; check that the issue you are concerned about isn't going to be the exception that proves the rule. Many campaigns have strange companions.

SECTION:	CAMPAIGNING
TITLE:	LISTS OF TACTICS
AUTHOR:	adapted from the original Skills Manual by Val Harris

These lists can be used as a quick memory aid in suggesting tactics and responding quickly to a particular situation.

LIST 1: PROTEST AND PERSUASION

Formal statements

public speeches
letters of opposition
declarations by
organisations and
institutions
signed public statements
declarations of intention
group or mass petitions

Communication with a wider audience

slogans, caricatures and
symbols
banners, posters and
displays
leaflets, pamphlets and
books
newspapers and journals
records, radio and
television

Group representations

deputations
mock awards
group lobbying
picketing
mock elections

Symbolic public acts

displays of flags and
symbolic colours
wearing of symbols
prayer and worship
delivering symbolic
objects
protest disrobing
destruction of own
property
displays of portraits
paint as protest
new signs and names
symbolic sounds
symbolic reclamations
noise making

Pressure on individuals

"haunting" officials
taunting
befriending
vigils

Drama and music

humorous skits and
pranks.
performance of plays
and music
singing

Processions

marches
parades/pilgrimages
motorcades

Honouring the dead

political mourning
mock funerals
demonstrative funerals
homage at burial places

Public assemblies

assemblies of protest or
support
protest meetings
teach-ins

Withdrawal and renunciation

walkout
silence
renouncing honours
excommunication
suspension of social
activities
strike
social disobedience
stay-at-home
total personal non-co-
operation
collective disappearance

LIST 2: NON-VIOLENT

SECTION:	**CAMPAIGNING**
TITLE:	**LISTS OF TACTICS**
AUTHOR:	Adapted from the original Skills Manual

INTERVENTION

Physical intervention

sit-in
stand-in
ride-in
non-violent obstruction
non-violent occupation
sing-ins

Social intervention

establishing new social patterns
overloading of facilities
speak-in
alternative social institutions
alternative communication system

Economic intervention

reverse strike
stay-in strike
non-violent land seizures
defiance of blockades
seizure of assets
dumping
selective patronage
alternative markets
alternative transport systems
alternative economic institutions

Political intervention

overloading of administrative systems
seeking imprisonment

LIST 3: POLITICAL NON-COOPERATION

Rejection of authority

> witholding or withdrawing of allegiance
> refusal to publicly support
> literature and speeches advocating resistance

Citizen's non-cooperation with government

> boycott of legislative bodies
> boycott of elections
> boycott of government employment and positions
> boycott of government departments and other bodies
> withdrawal from government educational institutions
> boycott of government supported organisations
> refusal of assistance to enforcement agents
> refusal to accept appointed officials
> refusal to dissolve existing institutions

Citizens' alternative to obedience

> reluctant and slow compliance
> non-obedience in absence of direct supervision
> popular non-obedience
> disguised obedience
> refusal of an assemblage or meeting to disperse
> sitdown
> civil disobedience of "illegitimate" laws

Action by government personnel

> selective refusal of assistance by government aides
> blocking lines of command and information
> stalling and obstruction
> general administrative non-co-operation
> judicial non-co-operation
> deliberate inefficiency and selective non-co-operation by enforcement agents

Domestic governmental action

> quasi-legal evasions and delays
> non-co-operation by constituent governmental units

LIST 4: ECONOMIC NON-CO-OPERATION

Action by consumers

consumers' boycott
non-consumption of boycotted goods
policy of austerity
rent witholding
refusal to rent
national consumers' boycott
international consumers' boycott
buying shares and disrupting annual meetings

Action by workers and producers

workpeoples' boycott
producers' boycott

Action by holders of financial resources

withdrawal of bank deposits
refusal to pay fees, dues and assessments
refusal to pay debts and interest
severance of funds and credit
revenue refusal
refusal of a government's money

Symbolic strikes

protest strikes
quick walkout, lightning strike

Strikes by special groups

prisoners' strike
craft strike
professional strike

Ordinary industrial strikes

establishment strikes
industry strike

Restricted strikes

detailed strike
slowdown strike
working-to-rule strike
reporting "sick"
strike by resignation
selective strike

SECTION:	**CAMPAIGNING**
TITLE:	**POWER STRUCTURES**
AUTHOR:	Adapted from the original Skills Manual by Martin Wyatt

The purpose of the technique is to develop and apply one's own personal concepts of power structures. This is important because an understanding of power structures and information about them are necessary in order to bring about change.

THE TECHNIQUE

Theoretically this is a four-stage process:

1) Develop concepts relating to power structures.

2) Use them to collect information.

3) Relate different power blocks to each other.

4) Use the concepts, information and relationships to bring about change.

In practice, all four stages react on and modify each other.

Two lists are offered: a suggested list of concepts and insights, and a possible list of institutions to which they can be applied.

List of Concepts

What gives power?

- the right to make decisions
- money
- the ability to influence decisions
- hard work
- information/connections – control of resources etc.

Who gives power? – what is an individual's power base?

What gives community groups power?

Power fluctuates, it is dynamic, not static.

Organisations of the same theoretical type (e.g. local authorities) may have quite different power structures.

A distinction needs to be made between (elected) members and employed officers.

The relationships between (elected) members and employed officers.

Where do decisions get taken?

What influences decisions?

No large organisation (or department) is monolithic.

Any large organisation (or department) is likely to contain potential allies.

Cross-membership of organisations *

The larger the organisation, the broader its views.

Gatekeepers – people who can grant or deny access to people with power (can be receptionists or principal officers or somewhere in between).

What are the routes for bypassing obstructive gamekeepers.

How can we build up alternative sources of power.

*   The concept of "partnership" can mean that whether or not people have cross-membership of organisations, they can bring influence to bear.

SECTION:	**CAMPAIGNING**
TITLE:	**POWER STRUCTURES**
AUTHOR:	Adapted from the original Skills Manual by Martin Wyatt

List of Institutions

Local authorities

Institutions of central government

Political parties

Major firms

Influential or wealthy organisations

Churches

European Government

MPs

Trade Unions

Health Authorities

Housing Associations

"Community leaders"

Co-operatives / Collectives

Funding bodies

There may well be other powerful institutions which you want to add to this list and then apply the kind of analysis suggested in the first list.

To use the insights gained you must:

a)   Be able to convey them to others

b)   Get them to think about what they want to achieve.

Knowing your way round the system is no substitute for either:

a)   Getting the system to produce what disadvantaged people want, or

b)   Changing the system!

SECTION:	**CAMPAIGNING**
TITLE:	**GUIDELINES FOR PLANNING ACTION**
AUTHOR:	adapted from the original Skills Manual by Val Harris

These guidelines have been developed for tenant groups in their dealings with the local authority. They can be used as the basis for discussion by any campaigning group and amended/added to as the group reviews its progress in dealing with organisations.

GUIDELINES TO CONSIDER

1. Lower your sights/limit your targets

   - Don't take on the whole authority

   - Don't expect overnight changes because you ask for them

   - Choose smaller targets and win

2. Get your facts

   - Don't just attack

   - Collect information and facts

   - Put your argument together

3. Know your target(s)

   - Find out which authority or organisation is responsible

   - Find out which department or section is responsible

   - Find out which individuals control what you are concerned about

   - Make sure you find the right target(s)

4. Keep copies of all correspondence

   - Keep an original file for the group

   - Keep a copy of everything (dated and signed)

   - People come and go in groups, individuals lose pieces of paper, make sure someone in the group is keeping the originals on file on all issues

5. Get decisions in writing

   - Verbal statements can be misunderstood by the recipient

   - They can be forgotten by the giver

   - Written statements can't be ignored

6. Don't fight amongst yourselves

   - Use meetings to discuss, debate, criticise

   - Don't take your quarrels outside the meeting

   - Put your energies in one direction only

7. A constitution is a guideline

• Use constitutions and rules as guidelines, not gospels

• Being democratic is not the same as being a slave to a constitution

8. Always present a united front

• At meetings with "the opposition" don't appear fragmented or divided

• Always work out your line of approach before hand, don't do it at the meeting

9. Choose your tactics to suit the problem

• Use appropriate tactics

• What worked in one situation may not work in another

10. Use the existing machinery

• Even if you do not have a very high opinion of the existing political machinery use it to your advantage

• Don't ignore the help of an elected representative just because they belong to a party you don't like.

FOLLOWING UP A MEETING

The group writes back to the key people or person they have met with as follows:

> "We appreciate your meeting with us on ...... to clarify certain points about ...... To avoid any confusion we have put in writing the information you gave us on the ...... points brought up. If there is any misunderstanding please let us know. We are sharing this information with those unable to attend the meeting and want to give an accurate account of what was said".

An account of the outcome of the meeting is enclosed based on the groups understanding of what was agreed to. Copies can be circulated to the group's membership.

SECTION 18

FUNDING

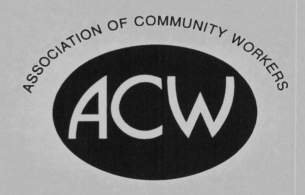

ASSOCIATION OF COMMUNITY WORKERS

ACW

SECTION:	**FUNDING**
TITLE:	**DEVELOPING A FUND-RAISING STRATEGY**
AUTHOR:	Steve Saddington

A fund-raising strategy is the backbone of good fund-raising. The purpose is to define where you are now, and where you want to be by answering the question how are you going to get there. In its initial stages it can be time consuming but it will save hours of fruitless activity in the longer term. It defines the needs of your organisation, the sources from which you can seek funds, the limitations in terms of time and resources that may constrain you. On that basis you will make choices that shape your strategy.

Fund-raising cannot function effectively in isolation. Discuss your ideas with staff, volunteers and committees of your organisation. Agree your fund-raising strategy, and stick to it, reviewing its course at 3 – 6 monthly intervals. If one part of your strategy is performing badly, review it urgently, ascertain the reasons and either adapt or abandon it.

WHAT SHOULD A FUND-RAISING STRATEGY CONTAIN?

A fund-raising strategy should contain the following:

- a description of your organisation

- an outline of its mission

- a list of its major achievements

- a summary of its strengths and weaknesses

- a description of your goals and major projects

- the barriers to effective fund-raising

- a financial plan to cover the funds your organisation will need in the next 2 – 3 years

- sources of income you can tap into

- the resources you will need

- how will you measure your success?

No fund-raising strategy is static, no fund-raising is static. New trends and ideas come and go and you must adapt your strategy to allow for this. However, do not make changes just for the sake of change but work your way through the following to help you decide what to do next:

- plot your income of the last 3 years

- chart sources that are increasing

- chart sources that are decreasing

- are there any obvious reasons for any perceptible change?

- is yes, can you capitalise on these?

- has any source of income peaked?

- if not, can you stimulate this source of income further?

- have you reached a dead-end? Why not try something new?

- have you been given a budget for expenditure set against projected income?

- can you cut your costs?

- set yourself realistic targets for each source of income and monitor the results

SECTION:	**FUNDING**
TITLE:	
AUTHOR:	

SECTION:	**FUNDING**
TITLE:	**WHERE SHALL WE LOOK FOR MONEY?**
AUTHOR:	Steve Saddington

No two organisations/ groups have exactly the same income profile. Organisations in similar fields of wok may tend to draw income from certain sources rather than others. A bit of research will help you decide which types of fund-raising are more appropriate for your organisation.

Ask yourself the following questions:

- what are you doing now?

- what do you want to do?

- what type of income do you need? (capital revenue, project linked or unearmarked)

- what sources of income have you tapped?

- what sources of income remain untapped?

- what are your priorities?

- what will you concentrate on in the next 12 months?

The following chart may help concentrate your thinking:

YOUR FUNDING MIX

	NOW	IN 5 YEARS
TOTAL INCOME	£.................	£.................

	NOW		IN 5 YEARS
100%		100%	
90%		90%	
80%		80%	
70%		70%	
60%		60%	
50%		50%	
40%		40%	
30%		30%	
20%		20%	
10%		10%	

What are your sources of income now, and what do you plan them to be in five years time?

Insert the income and percentages from each source to fill up the bar chart.

SECTION:	**FUNDING**
TITLE:	**WHERE SHALL WE LOOK FOR MONEY?**
AUTHOR:	Steve Saddington

The following action programme will help you keep on top of implementing your strategy:

Complete the diary on the basis of your knowledge of current applications that need to be made, and roll it forward into the next year adding additional information as you go.

Finding Sponsorship for Community Projects; a step by step guide. Caroline Gillies. ISBN 0 907164 54 4

Getting in on the act, A guide to Local Authorities powers to fund voluntary organisations. Clive Grace and Richard Gutch. ISBN 0 7199 1218 0.

ACTION PROGRAMME

199_ (Year One)

January

February

March

April

May

June

July

August

September

October

November

December

199_ (Year Two)

SECTION:	**FUNDING**
TITLE:	**FUNDRAISING: MONEY**
AUTHOR:	Jo Habib

Most organisations need resources of one kind or another.

Make a "shopping list". Some things on the list will be one-off things (capital), some will be on-going needs (revenue). Some of the resources might be supplied by the members of the group themselves (people to drive the minibus, for instance, or people to staff the creche), some in kind from other bodies (a room to meet in from the council, free paper for the playgroup from the high-street printshop) but probably some will require money.

Publications to look out for

There are a lot of directories and other books that give information about funders and advice about how to approach them. A large number of these are published by The Directory of Social Change, based at:

Radius Works,
Back Lane,
London NW3 1HL.
Telephone 0171 435 8171

It may be worth writing for a catalogue (and then finding copies in the library or an agency) because they bring out new titles quite often.

Directories

The main directories published by the Directory of Change include:

A Guide to the Major Trusts (published every two years, in the "odd" years) - gives details of about 400 wealthy grant-making trusts likely to respond to appeals from voluntary groups. Policies and past grants are given in greater detail than in the Directory of Grant-Making Trusts.

The Major Companies Guide - covers the top most generous 400 companies, with detailed information about their community giving.

A Guide to Company Giving - gives brief details of the top 1,300 companies and has useful guidelines on how to make an appeal.

The Central Government Grants Guide – lists grants available from government

There are three sorts of money to consider.

- Money from individuals (the car boot sale, the sponsored thing...)

Many funders will want to see evidence that the group is doing its own fundraising. This kind of fundraising can also publicise the group, provide opportunities for people to meet and work together and produce money with very few strings attached.

- Money from statutory sources (the council, central government schemes...)

Statutory sources are most likely to provide revenue funding and can sometimes fund workers or projects long-term. Some statutory schemes have annual grant cycles, so plan ahead. It is often necessary to get political support and officer support for an application, as well as filling in an application form.

- Money from private organisations – charitable trusts and companies (and student rags, trade unions, rotary clubs...)

Trusts and companies are more likely to provide grants for one-off things or projects. Trusts may meet only once or twice a year. They don't usually have application forms; you write a letter.

Companies are much happier being approached by telephone than trusts. High street companies often have policies of supporting local voluntary action with small donations or with goods – prizes for raffles, food for the pensioners' Christmas party.

It is easier to get grants from companies and charitable trusts if you're a registered charity; if you're not, arrange to have the grant paid through an agency that is one (like a Council for Voluntary Service – see below). Sort out all the arrangements with the CVS or other agency first. They will need to be able to prove (to the Inland Revenue if necessary) that all grant has been spent on something recognised as charitable in law. Then, when you write to a company or trust, say something like:

We are not ourselves registered with the Charity Commission but Voluntary Action Spotton (registered charity number 123456) has agreed to administer any charitable money we might receive.

If the funder decides to give you a grant, they will make the cheque out to the CVS, who in turn will make a cheque out to you.

SECTION:	**FUNDING**
TITLE:	**FUNDRAISING: MONEY**
AUTHOR:	Jo Habib

FUNDRAISING: WHERE TO GO FOR HELP AND INFORMATION

Agencies that can help you

- Councils for Voluntary Service (CVS's are often called Voluntary Action Somewhere) and Rural Community Councils (RCC's) should be able to give advice and information about local authority funding and may have other information – books and directories, possibly a newsletter with information about funding opportunities and deadlines, suggestions and experience of local do-it-yourself fundraising.

- Some local authorities provide information and advice about the funding they provide and may employ people (whether community workers or voluntary organisations liaison officers or community development staff) who are knowledgeable about sources of money.

- In some cases there are also specialist funding advice services. The CVS or RCC should be able to tell you if that's the case.

- There may be other resource centres of local government agencies in the area. National networks sometimes produce resource material for local branches. Community Matters, for instance (8-9 Upper Street, London N1 0PQ; 0171 226 0189) provides information to local groups. The Regional Arts Board is likely to have information about money for community arts activities (as well as providing money directly), the regional Sports Council may have information about money for local sports-based work, and so on.

- Books, magazines and directories may also be available in your local library.

Your own research

- Don't be afraid to phone the council and ask for information about grants.

- Phone local companies and ask the switchboard how their charitable giving system works.

- Look at the annual reports of other groups and see who they get money from.

- Look in the local newspaper to see who's handing over giant-sized cheques.

departments and from non-departmental statutory bodies (like the Countryside Commission) and "arms-length" government giving (like through the National Aids Trusts).

High Street Giving – handy guide to the policies and practices of high street shops at a local level.

Charities Aid Foundation publishes The Directory of Grant-Making Trusts every two years (also in the odd years). This is expensive and not very easy to use but is more comprehensive than the others. Borrow it and use it to check out local trusts; there are geographical indexes in the back.

There are three periodicals that try to keep groups up to date with news about grant-makers. These are:

Funding Digest published by RTI (18-20 Dean Street, Newcastle NE1 1PG. Telephone 0191 261 6581).

Trust Monitor published by the Directory of Social Change (address above).

Corporate Citizen (launched April 1992), also by the Directory of Social Change.

Look out also for Funderfinder, a computer program which helps identify the right charitable trusts for a particular project or activity. (Try your local CVS or Telephone 01924 382120).

Books to help you Do It Yourself

The Directory of Social Change also produces books and leaflets to help with fundraising through activities. There are a number of other publications that might be worth looking at, including:

Community Start Up – How to start a community group and keep it going; by Caroline Pinder, published by the National Extension College and the National Federation of Community Organisations; includes the Fund-Raising Alphabet produced by Community Matters.

Step by Step – a Guide to Volunteer Fundraising, published by the Volunteer Centre (29 Lower King's Road, Berkhampstead HP4 2 AB).

SECTION:	**FUNDING**
TITLE:	**FUNDRAISING: WHAT MIGHT GO IN AN APPLICATION FOR FUNDS**
AUTHOR:	Jo Habib

You might write a one-page letter asking for money. You might write an eight page proposal. It will depend on what you need, how much you want, and who you want it from. But these are some of the elements that might be in your application.

Summary – if it's a long proposal, you may need to start with a short summary paragraph. This will say:

*   who is applying
*   for how much (and what other funders, total cost of project)
*   to do what
*   in what way

The message of this section might be: We are business-like.

Introduction – some background to your organisation, which might include:

*   who you are
*   what you do
*   where you operate
*   when you were established
*   why you do what you do
*   your track record – what you've already achieved
*   your management
*   your current funding
*   what has led you to this particular proposal

The message of this section is: We have credibility.

What's the problem? – if there isn't a problem, why should anyone help?

Try and express your need in terms of a problem – out there in the real world, not "our problem is we haven't got any money". Try and show the problem is:

*   concrete, not abstract
*   to do with people's needs, not just lack of provision
*   there are some bad effects
*   it's urgent
*   it's solvable
*   there's a demand for a solution from the people affected

And then show why you're the organisation to tackle the problem.

This is often the hardest part of an application to write. The message you're trying to get across to funders is: Here's something that should concern or interest you.

As an example, imagine a group trying to find funding for a sandpit for a playgroup. It would be very easy to come across as saying: "We haven't got a sandpit, other playgroups have sandpits, we know that you're interested in funding play equipment so can we have a sandpit please." It's a much more powerful appeal if expressed in terms of a problem out there, experienced by children, along the lines of: "The children have very little equipment altogether, and nothing that encourages imaginative play or helps them with co-ordination and motor skills. The parents are worried that lack of opportunity for creative and co-operative play is hampering their children's development.

Programme and Methods – here's what can be done

- what you're going to do about it (objectives)
- how you're going to do it (methods)

In the example above, the objective would be to improve the children's opportunities for creative play and motor development. The method would be by providing a sandpit.

Evaluation and/or Monitoring

Depending on the size and nature of the work you want to do, you may need to say how you'll know whether you are managing to solve the problem you've outlined. You may need to state:

- whether you're doing one or the other or both
- whether it's self-evaluation or outside "experts" or both

It's easy to be panicked into going over the top. The message you want to give is: We care about the problem, we care about spending money effectively.

The Budget

Make sure:

- it's clear
- it's comprehensive
- it adds up
- it's enough
- it's not too much
- it shows any other funders involved
- it shows other (not money) support if appropriate.

The message in this part is: We care about spending money efficiently.

Future Funding

- will the project go on and on?
- will you need more money later?
- will someone else pick up the bill in due course?

If you possibly can, try to convey the message: We won't bother you for ever

WHAT MAKES A GOOD APPLICATION?

Put yourself in the funder's shoes. What are they going to want to know?

Be clear:

> Who are you, how much do you want, what for, why?

Be concise:

> One or two sides of A4 unless it's a really major proposal.

Be business-like:

> Show you've thought things through and know what to do if you get the money. Attach or include figures – budgets, accounts, costings.

Be relevant:

> Why should **they** fund you?

WHAT ELSE SHOULD YOU DO?

Plan ahead

> Work out who's doing what, when.

Above all, keep records.

> Who did you write to, when, for what? What was the result. It's easier to get money out of organisations that have given you money before, so cultivate your donors – say thank you, send them reports, or photographs, or invitations to visit.

SECTION:	**FUNDING**
TITLE:	**CONTRACTING**
AUTHOR:	Ann Hindley

We may not like it but the system of financing for the voluntary sector is changing. Funding authorities are moving away from giving grants towards a system of service agreements or contracts whereby service provision will be tightly defined.

There are a number of reasons for this shift:

- public sector spending cuts are increasing the pressure for cheaper services,

- there is greater pressure on voluntary groups to be more accountable and to give value for money,

- most local authority services are now subject to Compulsory Competitive Tendering,

- the NHS and Community Care Act is moving Social Services Departments away from their role as providers of services towards one of purchaser.

These factors have led to the establishment of the "contract culture".

Services are to be "contracted out" to the independent sector, which is a mixture of voluntary, private and not for profit organisations. Funding arrangements with the voluntary sector will start to take the form of service agreements or contracting.

Contracting is viewed in a variety of different ways by different organisations. It is having a good effect in that it is forcing the voluntary sector to be more efficient and more effective, setting clear objectives and becoming better organised. However, contracts may stifle innovation and creativity and might kill off some small organisations.

Differences between grants and contracts:

- a contract is legally binding where a grant isn't necessarily so,

- grants are not subject to tax and VAT,

- grants are not a payment for service; there is no expectation of a return for a giver,

- contracts involve unconditional offer and acceptance,

- contracts involve a legally binding relationship.

There may be legal implications of entering into a contract:

- taxes may have to be paid on profits or surpluses made on the contract,

- both parties have a legal obligation to do what they have agreed,

- members of the management committee could find themselves legally responsible.

Service agreements generally specify the level of service to be provided as well as the quality expected and arrangements for monitoring and evaluation. The legal status of service agreements is not quite so clear as that of contracts.

In a quickly changing area the most definitive books currently available are:

Getting Ready for Contracts: a Guide for Voluntary Organisations: Sandy Adirondack and Richard MacFarlane, Directory of Social Change. £8.95.

Getting to Yes, Negotiating an Agreement without giving in: Roger Fisher, William Ury and Bruce Paton. Business Books. £5.99.

SECTION:	**FUNDING**
TITLE:	
AUTHOR:	

SECTION 19

ORGANISING CONFERENCES AND EVENTS

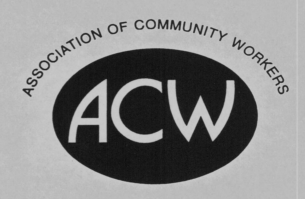

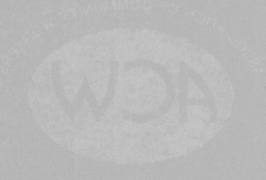

SECTION:	ORGANISING CONFERENCES AND EVENTS
TITLE:	GROUND RULES FOR A CONFERENCE
AUTHOR:	A.C.W.

To make sure that all participants get the best from the conference some organisations have developed a set of ground rules which are given out to all those attending. Here are those used by ACW for its annual conference. You may wish to adapt them for your workshop/conference.

We want the conference to be welcoming and enjoyable for everybody. Some people may not be at all used to working with others in this kind of event. Others may be only too familiar with the problems that can arise during an event like this!

We would like everybody to agree a "contract for working together on the day. We would like to include the following items, and will give people a chance at the beginning of the day to make comments and additions to these "ground rules".

Equal opportunity

We would ask everyone to respect the rights of other, and participate in the day's proceedings as equals.

Please avoid language which patronises others or puts down their experience. We ask people not to use language which could be constituted as racist, sexist, or which discriminates or offends people on the grounds of their ability/disability, sexuality, age, or any other grounds.

We also ask that participants don't interrupt, talk over or try to dominate other people.

People should feel free to challenge what they feel is offensive or discriminatory language or behaviour. Sometimes we can offend without meaning to, and we would ask that people challenge each other in a constructive and supportive way if this seems to be the case.

Co-operation and Support

We ask everyone to work together in a spirit of co-operation and support. We ask that people respect and value differences in ways of working and contributing. Please do not act on "hidden agendas" (i.e. things you may want to get out of the day which you cannot be honest about and share with others). Please do not go on "power trips" (where you seem to have more status than other people, and you use that to "pull rank" over them or make them feel less important).

Everybody is equally important, and should co-operate with, and support, everyone else. We want all those who come to enjoy themselves and not to feel excluded by the actions or words of others.

Participation

Everyone should be able to contribute what they want, when they want and how they want. We should not put pressure on people to participate when they don't want to, in ways they don't want to; we should encourage people to participate.

We ask that people should avoid the use of jargon, or unexplained initials (SCCD = Standing Conference for Community Development etc.) or "long words" where short ones will do. Anything other than "plain language" discourages the participation of many people – i.e., most of us. If you need to ask, you have a right to support in getting the information you need.

Confidentiality

Some of the day will be spent in workshops, smaller groups discussing different issues and experiences. If anyone wants to say anything which they feel is confidential, they should make this clear, and then this confidentiality should be respected within the meeting and outside.

People should feel free to join the workshops they want to within reasonable constraints of the group size.

Time out and Timekeeping

We have tried to make space in the schedule for people to have time out when they need it, for a glass of water or a change of scene. If at any time people feel physically or mentally that they need time out, they should not feel pressurised to stay.

Please help us with keeping to our timetable – there's a lot of work to do!

Smoking

Smoking will not be allowed in the dining room, alcohol free room, main conference room and workshops. Smoking areas will be signed – i.e. reception area, lounge, the bar, and in the ballroom during the social only.

Problems

If anyone feels at any time that there is a problem with something that is happening, please feel free to raise it with other people, or with the organisers, whichever is appropriate.

There will be time at the end of the day to make any comments during the evaluation session.

The purpose of this technique is to work out how to deliver a message.

Community workers spend a lot of time verbally communicating with others. Effective communication means more than the content of what is being passed on. It also requires an awareness of how to present what one wants to say. Included in this is a knowledge of who one is communicating with, how others are receiving and hearing what you are saying, and so on.

Use the following points to prepare and then deliver your speech.

Preparation

1. Decide the purpose

- consider what is to achieved by your talk e.g. is it to stimulate discussion, explain a course of action, give information, or gain support for a cause.

2. Determine the type of audience

- what information do they have?

- are they sympathetic/apathetic?

- will they understand your jargon.

3. List your material

- jot down headings for the material you want to cover

- do it as it occurs to you, in any order.

4. Edit your material

- eliminate from your list what is not relevant to your purpose or necessary for your audience.

5. Prepare headings

- arrange your material under heading e.g. background, current thinking, conclusion, plan of action, how to involve others.

6. Writing the talk

- consider what visual aids you can use e.g. graphs, sketch plans, OHP/slides, photographs, models, posters.

- write out your talk following certain rules e.g.

   a) no sentences longer than 20 words
   b) use short rather than long words
   c) use concrete rather than abstract words
   d) use the active rather than the passive tense.

7. Revise

- read your speech aloud and time it (and allow half as much time again for real!)

- revise and shorten as necessary

- repeat until your message is clear and your talk the right length

- ask a friend to listen and to criticise you.

8. Prepare notes

* rather than read your talk it is preferable to speak from a few main headings written on small cards.

Delivery

1. Variety

* the more variety in the talk the less monotonous it is

* vary volume and tone of your voice

* use your hands, look from side to side across the audience – keeping eye contact with the whole group.

2. Enthusiasm

* an unenthusiastic speaker bores the audience whatever the subject

* enthusiasm is communicated by looks and tone of voice.

3. Visual aids

* almost any visual aid is useful when used in moderation provided it is relevant and clear.

4. Break up content

* the content of a talk should vary from generalisation to specific illustrations, from abstract to concrete, from serious to light. Heavy information parts are broken up by lighter interludes.

5. Be explicit

* tell the listeners what you are going to say, say it, tell them what you have said (remember that 70% will have been forgotten unless you reinforce your message).

6. Break up long talks

* if a talk is long or complex, summarise and review at intervals in the talk; this shows the progress of the talk.

7. Set the tone

* the tone of the talk is set in the first few remarks

* during this time the audience are weighing up the speaker and are particularly open to impressions.

8. Look for feedback

- watch 2 or 3 people in the audience for signs of puzzlement or boredom

- skilled public speaking involves knowing when you "lose" your audience

- modify what you are saying to regain attention.

9. Be clear about your ending

- the final parts of the talk are the ones most remembered. Questions usually follow the concluding part

- end with a punch if possible, don't slowly fade away, restate and emphasise the most important points.

10. Don't irritate

- avoid irritating mannerisms, speak slowly and clearly, project your voice to the back of the room

- use words economically

- choose the right words as the clearest formulations of the points

- don't restate endlessly.

11. Questions

- anticipate the most obvious questions and prepare answers

- if you don't know the answer, say so.

SECTION:	**ORGANISING CONFERENCES AND EVENTS**
TITLE:	
AUTHOR:	

SECTION:	ORGANISING CONFERENCES AND EVENTS
TITLE:	ORGANISING AN EVENT
AUTHOR:	Val Harris

Community workers are often involved in planning and organising an event. This is a checklist of some ideas to think about.

- Decide what kind of event you want to create and what you want to achieve e.g. formal/informal, practical sessions, speeches, how many people?

- Draw up an invitation list, always invite more people than you actually want to attend – one third at least usually refuse. It is useful to have a reserve list, as many of those invited will be unable to attend.

- Work out the costings.

- Design and print the invitations.

- Send out invitations preferably six weeks in advance. Reserve list invitations can be sent out 4 weeks before the event. Ask people to R.S.V.P. to a specific person and keep a record of replies.

- Advertise the event - posters, leaflets, local radio – consider translations.

- Design programme and decide who is going to meet the guest(s) and who is going to make introductions and start the event off.

- Are you going to have any speakers/workshop facilitators? Who should they be? Brief them well in advance. Book signers/translators.

- Decide on a venue – will it comfortably hold the number of people you are proposing to invite? Is it accessible? Does it have a loop system?

- Arrange to see the venue in advance and check all the details and arrangements and that it is fully accessible; that there is a kitchen available, space for a creche, are there enough seats, where are the power points, who has the keys?

- Arrange refreshments in advance – decide what is needed; coffee, tea, juice as people arrive. Will you ask people to bring something for a shared meal?

- Are exhibition materials needed which will explain your groups work and activities.

- Will transport be needed? Will you need to make special parking arrangements especially for disabled drivers.

- VIPs – if an MP/or other celebrity is involved you will need to obtain their approval of the draft programme and send brief details of all the people they are to meet, a copy of the final programme and a map about a week before the event.

- Do you want your guests to wear name badges? Prepare these in advance and lay them out in alphabetical order in readiness for guests to arrive.

- Would you like to present each guest with an information folder? What do you think it should contain e.g. typed programme, Annual Review, leaflet about your group.

- Think about the need for PA equipment and arrange if necessary.

- Do you need to provide a creche for children? – arrange if necessary. Have you budgeted for carers' costs to be reimbursed?

- Make sure everyone in the group knows what they are doing.

- Have fun!

- Organise a clean and tidy up afterwards.

- Review it at an agreed date after the event.

SECTION 20

HANDLING INFORMATION

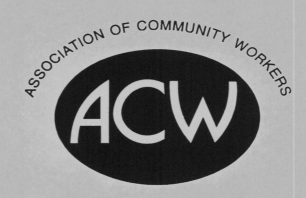

SECTION:	**HANDLING INFORMATION**
TITLE:	**GUIDELINES ON FILING**
AUTHOR:	Adapted from the original Skills Manual by Val Harris

The purpose of this technique is to assist community groups and community workers to store information effectively.

The simpler the filing system, the easier the system will be to operate, so aim to eradicate any necessary complications.

1. Obtain agreement as to which files should be kept centrally and those to be kept by individuals. Beware of files kept by individuals. There is a tendency for only one person to have access to the files. Arguments for individuals to keep files such "I am the only person who uses/need file XYZ" are not solely arguments about personal convenience, decisions will affect who has access to what information. Keep files centrally whenever possible with open access.

2. Filing cabinets should not be prisons – with access only through the warder.

    Ensure easy access, allow files to be borrowed but ensure that there is a system for keeping track of files when loaned out e.g. signing files in and out.

    Remember that other people will have to understand and work the system. If an individual or small group are the only ones who understand the filing system they are the only ones able to use it. Scrap it and start again.

    No one individual should be the owner or warder of the central files but it is advisable to ensure that periodic checks are made so that files do not get lost and to check that papers are filed correctly; if that means making someone responsible so be it.

3. It may be sufficient merely to arrange files in alphabetical order but if not consider what different sections you will require e.g. internal files – finance, fundraising, wages, insurance, minutes, other organisations and campaigns.

    Don't sub-divide subjects unless you have to. The more you sub-divide subjects the more likely it is you will have to copy letters etc., because you need to file the letter on more than one file. Ideally any one item should only need to be filed on one file.

4. Don't underestimate the number of files you will need – paperwork has a tendency to grow and not diminish as organisations grow. Allow for growth.

5.   If the issue of confidentiality arises consider

- Why do you think you need to keep the information?

- Whether you really need the information or is it merely information for information's sake.

- Who are you seeking to protect? Confidentiality usually protects others apart from the person or persons in whose name it is invoked.

If you need confidential information store it separately. The existence of confidential information should not be used to restrict access to non-confidential information.

6.   All papers don't necessarily need to be kept indefinitely. Weed your files periodically and throw out any useless papers.

7.   Once the filing system has been agreed and established circulate a list of the files and any necessary instructions to all those likely to use the filing system. UPDATE as necessary.

8.   Within files, work strictly by date, either date order or reverse date order. Reverse date order is the most popular choice as the most recent papers are readily available (on top of file).

9.   Store spare copies of reports etc. separately. (Wallet folders are good for this purpose). Don't keep duplicate files unless absolutely necessary.

10.   Don't let filing build up: set aside regular filing sessions if necessary. Papers should be on the files not on the desks.

11.   If you are involved in circulating papers to numerous different groups it may be useful to maintain a file of the documents/ circulars sent to particular groups.

12.   THE WASTE PAPER BASKET IS AN ESSENTIAL PART OF ANY FILING SYSTEM.

The purpose of the technique is to provide a guide to resources, facilities, equipment, suppliers etc. that are available to local groups. The preparation of lists is particularly useful where groups may have only occasional needs for the resources or facilities.

STEP 1

Decide the subject of the resource list or lists you wish to compile and who the list is aimed at i.e. who are you seeking to provide with information and are they likely to need the information; if not why bother? Possible subjects for resource lists include: local information/advice services, local meeting places, halls for hire, printing services, where equipment may be used borrowed or hired (video, printing, projectors, etc.), or resource centres where you can get access to computers: local entertainers, companies prepared to donate waste materials for use in playgroups, summer projects, sports equipment, groups prepared to enclose circulars in regular mailings, local trusts or other sources of finances etc.

STEP 2

Identify those who have the information you want, there are likely to be two categories – the providers/owners of resource and those local organisations who have already used the service or resource. Decide whether you need to approach both categories, and how you wish to collect the information (personal visiting, telephone or postal survey).

STEP 3

Decide what information you require – usually:

a.   what is available and where it is available

b.   conditions upon which resource available

c.   cost/charges

d.   Who to contact to arrange use, include name, address and telephone numbers

e.   any comments (optional)

f.   RECORD THE DATE THE INFORMATION WAS CORRECT

These are the probable minimum requirements, see example for a longer list. Draw up a checklist of the information you require for each entry on the list.

STEP 4

Decide when you will reach a point of decreasing return, i.e. when further efforts to identify further resources is not warranted. Lists don't need to be fully comprehensive to be useful.

STEP 5

Decide how you are going to produce and distribute the information once it has been collected.

STEP 6

Review steps 1–5. CHECK YOUR PLANS CAREFULLY. Ideally test your checklist on one or two providers and potential users of the resource. If you fail to include a point by this stage it will involve double the time to include it later.

STEP 7

Duplicate your checklist of the information you require for each entry on the list.

STEP 8

Collect and collate information.

STEP 9

Before PRINTING lists, information should be checked with the owners or providers of the resource if the information was not obtained from them originally CHECK FINAL DRAFT AND ARTWORK FOR ANY INACCURACIES, small details are important; wrong addresses or telephone numbers will not please anyone. Finally ensure that the date when the information contained in the list was correct is prominently displayed.

STEP 10

Produce and distribute lists.

Comments: While it is possible for a single individual to prepare a resource list, the more people involved the less work is required from individuals or many hands make light work. Secondly the experience should be shared to develop the skill in the community, if the skill is not shared the groups will be dependant on the provider. It is important that others are able to prepare resource lists when and as the need arises.

SO INVOLVE OTHERS

EXAMPLE

**Checklist for resource list:
local meeting places**

- Name & address of Meeting place

- Owners

- Person responsible for hiring/booking

- Type of premises

- No of rooms and capacity (number of people) of each room

- Chargers per hour for each room

- Can disabled people obtain easy access/are there suitable toilets

- Is there a creche/playgroup

- Any restrictions on the use of the premises (no music, bingo, alcohol)

- Hours available

- Is the meeting place already heavily booked

- How much notice is required for booking

- Facilities list

  - Parking
  - Charges
  - Cooking facilities/ refreshments
  - P.A. System
  - Toilets
  - Number of tables and chairs
  - Stage
  - Black out
  - Storage space
  - Cleaning

SECTION:	HANDLING INFORMATION
TITLE:	INFORMATION TIME LAG
AUTHOR:	Adapted from the original Skills Manual by Val Harris

Community projects abound with pieces of paper, books, journals and it is not always clear how up to date the material is.

The purpose of the technique is to assist an individual to assess how up to date information in different forms is likely to be.

Once information has been collected there is inevitably a time lag while the form of information e.g. book, is prepared and distributed. The table below gives an indication of the minimum time lag for different forms of information, in most cases the time lag will be longer. The time lag should be taken from the date of publication to calculate the date when the work was completed; e.g. a book published in 1994; take a time lag of a minimum of one year. The book is unlikely to consider any events after 1993. (A quick check of any references used will give you a clue.)

- Computerised systems: for all practical purposes instantaneous (on-line and real time). Check database updating frequency.

- Radio, Television and News Wires: from a few minutes to about 12 hours depending on source. (Documentaries usually take between a few months and a year to prepare.)

- Newspapers: from 6 – 12 hours for news articles, from a few days to a few weeks for features and background articles.

- Local papers: minimum is usually 24 hours but the majority of the paper is usually two or three days old at least.

- Periodicals: from under a week for review (news) articles, for the rest allow between a fortnight and a month at least.

- Pamphlets: minimum is usually several months depending on the subject.

- Books: usually take about a year once the manuscript is handed over thus authors will have been collecting their information at least two or more years before publication. The ideas contained within a book are usually even older.

- Directories: usually take a few months to put together and publish.

SECTION:	**HANDLING INFORMATION**
TITLE:	
AUTHOR:	

SECTION:	HANDLING INFORMATION
TITLE:	INFORMATION CHECKLIST
AUTHOR:	Adapted from the original Skills Manual by Val Harris

There is a lot of printed material being targeted at the community sector and it is not always easy to decide if it is worth acquiring or following up.

The purpose of this technique is to assist an individual or groups to evaluate a piece of written information, and to assess whether a reference is worth pursuing.

Checklist of questions to ask yourselves:

- What is the document's relevance to your present interests?

- Does it say anything new? Will it add to what you already know?

- Is the document purely descriptive or "factual"? If it includes analysis, is the analysis useful, sound or merely opinion masquerading as facts? Are the facts relevant or important?

- What authority does the document claim? Is it entitled to its claim?

- What is the author's bias, do you share this bias or perspective? Is the perspective or bias relevant to your context?

- What is the source/publisher of the document and who is the author? What is your relationship to the source? Do you need to monitor the activities of the source?

- Does the document claim to be objective? (BEWARE)

- What is the physical form of the document? Can you handle the form if you wish to store the document?

- What limits does the document admit to; can you identify any further limitations? Are the limitations important?

- Is the document clearly written, or is it full of jargon?

- Is the document dated? Is it up to date? Will it be updated, if so when? Does the date matter anyway?

- Will the document be useful to others?

- What is the future availability of the document likely to be? Where is it available from?

- Why was the document produced?

- Does the document include any references or further reading?

- If you want to obtain a copy of the document you should record the following information where appropriate:

  - Title:
  - Author: (organisations and groups can be authors)
  - Publisher: (address if given)
  - Date published:
  - Cost: (+ any postage and packing charges)

The technique implies a rational approach to the use of information.

While this will allow a more efficient and probably effective use of information there are occasions when it is necessary to speculate and trust your intuition.

Care should however be taken when speculating if you do not wish to turn your filing cabinet into a wastepaper bin.

If your speculation fails or your intuition is wrong throw the document out.

A document does not have to justify itself against all the question in the list for there to be sufficient grounds for obtaining and reading the document.

SECTION:	**HANDLING INFORMATION**
TITLE:	
AUTHOR:	

SECTION:	HANDLING INFORMATION
TITLE:	PROJECT JOURNAL
AUTHOR:	Adapted from the original Skills Manual by Val Harris

Many projects are run with part-time staff and volunteers who need to find a way to keep in touch with each other and know what is happening in the project.

The purpose of this technique is to establish a means of communication between the users/workers of a project/centre or office. The Journal should become a central reference point to which any person can refer and should also provide a record of the project/organisation's development.

In principle the Journal is of value to any organisation but there are a number of contexts where the Journal will be of more use than others; these include: direct action campaigns, campaigns in general, large buildings with no collecting points, common areas or congregating area, and offices used by a number of people at different times.

Organisations are dependent on the flow of information, the power of individuals within organisations is linked to the information available to them.

If individuals are not prepared to share information the organisation will suffer and members of the organisation will be unable to participate in the decision making process.

This technique provides a method of seeking to ensure that all members of an organisation have the opportunity to communicate information and receive/obtain information without numerous pieces of paper flying round the office.

Obtain the agreement from all those using the office and or likely to make entries in the proposed Journal. Without the agreement of all concerned, forget it.

Agree the type of information to be recorded in the Journal. The essential information for each entry is the name of the person making the entry, date of entry (time optional) and the entry. Possible types of entry include: telephone messages, signing in and out, when next in, people expected to be coming in, meetings, conclusions and minutes of meetings, notices, reports of events that are likely to affect the organisations, relevant press cuttings etc. Do not swamp the Journal, be selective. Someone answering the phone won't want to wade through press cuttings and reports of meetings to find out if someone is in the building.

Select the most convenient place for the Journal to be located. Hanging it on a wall in a passage is unlikely to encourage people to make entries.

Equipment:

Notebook of some sort preferably with movable marker, pen/pencil and a table/ ledge at a convenient height and place for writing.

If a loose-leaf form is used the Journal may be used as a day file as well.

Do not throw the Journal away. Its purpose is not just an immediate one. It can be used for evaluation and monitoring purposes.

Conditions for the technique to work:

a.   There must be a need to share information otherwise the Journal will become conversation by proxy.

b.   People must be prepared to co-operate and place a high priority on maintaining the Journal. This is only likely if the benefits from the Journal accrue to many and that people don't seek to use it as a management tool i.e. for control purposes.

SECTION:	**HANDLING INFORMATION**
TITLE:	
AUTHOR:	

SECTION 21

PUBLICATIONS

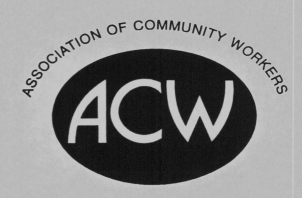

SECTION:	**PUBLICATIONS**
TITLE:	**EVALUATING A LEAFLET OR NEWSLETTER**
AUTHOR:	Adapted from the original Skills Manual by Val Harris

People usually have a lot of circulars and printed handouts put through their letter boxes. A newssheet from a local organisation can easily get thrown in the bin. In order to stand a chance of being read a newssheet will need maximum appeal.

This checklist can be used as a basis for evaluating the newssheet. An example of a checklist is given here. If the questions seem inappropriate to a particular local situation, then use this checklist as a basis for a group to compile its own.

EXAMPLE:

Front Page   YES   NO

1. Does it contain the name of the organisation?
2. Does it have the date of issue?
3. Does it contain something of importance?
4. Does it make the newssheet look interesting?
5. Is the layout attractive and uncluttered?

General Appearance   SCALE 1 to 5

1. Does the newssheet look neat and attractive?
2. Do headings and layout of stories reflect their comparative importance?
3. Is the type clear?
4. Are the layout and illustrations effective?

Content   YES   NO

1. Is it aimed at the general public?
2. Does it say who is doing what in the newssheet?
3. Does it say what is happening over the next month?
4. Does it show the scope of the organisation's activities?
5. Does it have other local news?
6. Is the space well used?
7. Does it say who is responsible for compiling the newssheet?

Style   YES   NO

1. Is it readable and to the point?
2. Will the language be understood and appeal to the general reader?
3. Are the headings pertinent?
4. Is there repetition or monotony?

Tone   YES   NO

1. Does the newssheet give a good impression of the organisation?
2. Does it indicate a membership actively working towards the objectives of the organisation?
3. Does it show an organisation that is wanting to involve all sections of the community?

SECTION:	**PUBLICATIONS**
TITLE:	
AUTHOR:	

SECTION:	**PUBLICATIONS**
TITLE:	**PUTTING AN ANNUAL REPORT TOGETHER**
AUTHOR:	Ann Hindley

Most groups and organisations need to produce a yearly report on their activities to satisfy their constitution or their funders. Many groups choose to use their annual report to account to their members and to publicise their existence.

Before putting pen to paper, it is important to ask yourself two questions:

a.   What do you want your annual report to do?

- publicise your activities?

- present your organisation in an acceptable way to potential funders?

- recruit volunteers?

- acknowledge the efforts of people who have been involved over the past year?

b.   Who do you want to see it?

- funders?

- local people?

- just your members?

The easiest and quickest way to produce an annual report is for the director/organiser/co-ordinator to sit down and write it. A broader and richer view of the organisation will be given if each member of the organisation makes their own contribution. It also gives more people the chance to participate in an important annual event of the organisation.

The best annual report is one that is interesting, easy to read, and is broken up by headings and by graphics. Think about the format that you want. Some very good annual reports are produced in simple A4 or A5 booklets, but you might want to be more imaginative and produce an eye catching design. Examples include a single sheet that folds out into a wall poster. This way you could have pictures of your activities or your telephone numbers pinned in offices or homes throughout the year. How about a folder with a transparent corner containing a collection of leaflets, each in a different colour describing a different aspect of your group's work. Look at other annual reports and see what others have done.

SECTION:	**PUBLICATIONS**
TITLE:	**PUTTING AN ANNUAL REPORT TOGETHER**
AUTHOR:	Ann Hindley

PRACTICAL MATTERS

Photography

Get black and white photographs of your activities taken. They print better.

Printing

Make sure that you get some quotes in writing from a number of places. Work out before you go to the printer, how many copies you'll need, how many pages there are likely to be, what size the report will be.

You'll need to decide on a budget before you can go ahead so that you know whether you can afford a glossy cover or for the printers to collate and staple for you. Local schools or community organisations may have offset litho printers which produce very good, cheap copies.

Distribution lists

Think about this early as you'll need to take numbers into account when budgeting. Do you want to send copies to the following:

*   press and radio
*   councillors
*   management committee members
*   past, present and potential funders
*   other voluntary organisations
*   statutory agencies
*   groups that you work with
*   members and volunteers
*   your local M.P./M.E.P.

Will the report go out on its own or do you want to put a covering letter in with it or a compliments slip? A covering letter takes a little more time and money for photocopying. Do you have a sufficient supply of compliment slips?

THE CONTENTS

*   accounts of what the organisation has done over the past year
*   figures and statistics if appropriate
*   pictures, graphs, pie charts, cartoons and other graphics
*   acknowledgements to paid and unpaid workers
*   a list of management committee members
*   audited accounts
*   your constitution and equal opportunities policy
*   your address and telephone number (easily forgotten)

SECTION:	**PUBLICATIONS**
TITLE:	**REPORT WRITING**
AUTHOR:	Adapted from the original Skills Manual by Val Harris

The need to write reports is becoming increasingly important in community work, whether it be to obtain resources or to account to funders, or to raise issues such as emerging needs.

The purpose of this technique is to bring together concise, logical and well thought out information, ideas and arguments in a written form. Further purposes can be:

- to keep people informed

- to gain publicity

- to focus attention on a situation.

The Technique includes listing the stages involved in producing the report, work out tasks associated with each stage. Use this in turn to set the time scale for each stage and allocate tasks among those involved.

1. Initial thinking

- Why is a report needed?

- Is a report the best way of dealing with the issue, what are the alternatives?

- Who would a report be aimed at? How does this affect the information needed, length and style of presentation? Is it aimed at technical experts, councillors and politicians, the general public, funders?

2. Content

- Establish the right mixture of facts, arguments, opinions, references elsewhere.

- Consider opinion surveys, reprints of important letters, legal references, press statements, statements or reports from official meetings etc.

- Ensure the changes being recommended or requested are clearly and unambiguously stated.

- Consider holding back certain arguments and information which may best be imparted verbally and/or used to follow up the report.

- Consider further options that you could agree to and which might be suggested. Consider arguments against options you could not support.

- Clarify further information and further options in relation to the actual content of the report. e.g. should the report be amended in light of these?

- Establish beyond doubt the accuracy of facts you state.

3. Compiling the report

- Who is going to put the report together? Bear in mind that whoever puts it together, it will bear the stamp of their thinking. Will it be done by a few individuals on behalf of a group or will it be a group enterprise?

- Clarify who is taking responsibility for writing what and when.

- Ensure the technical facilities exist to support writing of the report e.g. typing, photocopying, word-processing etc.

- Clarify the stages with participants e.g. amending first drafts, deciding final layout.

4. Layout

- Reports should be clearly laid out and easy to follow.

- Put a summary sheet at the front followed by a list of recommendations. People will read this rather than the whole report initially. They will read the rest if you've caught their attention.

- Break the report up into sections, consider sub-headings, diagrams, pictures, tables, cartoons, reproductions of press articles, different coloured pages etc., as a means of making the report easier to read.

- Consider using numbered paragraphs to make it easier to refer to parts of the report when it is being discussed e.g. 1.00, 1.01, 1.10 etc.

- Consider the kind of cover to put on the report.

- Consider where to put further references and notes. Consider using appendices for lengthy items which don't fit easily into the main body of the report.

- Consider an index for lengthy reports.

- Use of Desk Top Publishing, to give a consistent look.

5. Publishing the report

- Make a list to whom the report will be sent. Is it a public report?

- Consider whether or not to leak the contents beforehand.

- Clarify relations with the press: e.g.

  - is a press conference to be arranged?

  - are certain reporters to receive copies?

  - is a press release to be used?

  - how are the press likely to distort the report?

  - does distortion by the press matter, to whom, what can be done if it happens?

  - can the press be used to clarify the opposition response?

  - know the TV, radio, newspaper's deadline and work with it in mind.

  - clarify follow-up action after the report is published.

- Consider likely reactions to your report and be prepared to defend your conclusions.

SECTION:	**PUBLICATIONS**
TITLE:	**GUIDELINES FOR COMPILING A DIRECTORY**
AUTHOR:	Adapted from the original Skills Directory by Martin Wyatt

Directories of information are invaluable to community workers and activists: you may choose to compile a directory of what is happening in your neighbourhood to advertise the range of groups and services available for instance.

The purpose of this technique is to provide some guidelines on the gathering and handling of information when compiling a directory of organisations.

PRELIMINARIES

1.   Clarify your purpose in preparing a directory. Traditionally a directory is a reference document providing a limited amount of detailed information on a large number of organisations. The prime purpose of the directory usually being the same as a telephone directory namely to enable people/organisations to contact communicate with each other. Recently directories have tended to include reference information about the area or subject area also.

You need to answer these questions:

*   Why do we want/need to produce the directory?

*   Who are we seeking to inform?

2.   Define the information you wish to include in the directory. What range of organisations do you wish to include? – all voluntary organisations or more limited categories such as local political organisations, sports, cultural, education, leisure, youth, religious, community, campaigns, branches of national organisations, advice, the local authority, local industry etc.

What geographical area is the directory going to cover? Neighbourhood, town/city, borough, county etc.

3.   Check that a directory does not already exist or that others are not already compiling the same directory. Try to obtain a copy of any relevant directory/list whether current or out of date. These will provide a starting point when collecting information later. It is also useful to obtain and/or study some examples of directories for different areas or subjects. These may provide some useful ideas for designing the directory particularly on the question of layout.

DESIGNING THE DIRECTORY

This should be done before any attempt is made to collect the information, except for 3 above. Failure to design and plan adequately will inevitably lead to considerable waste of time and effort.

1.   Review steps one and two, redefine and expand if necessary.

2.   Decide the form of presentation of the directory. It will then be possible to store the information in the required form. Three variables are usually used; namely alphabetical order, subject order, and geographical area. In the case of the last two these are usually combined with alphabetical order within the subject or geographical division. If alphabetical order is adopted a subject index ought to be included; a geographical index could be optional depending on the purpose and size of the area covered by the directory.

3.   Decide the organisational details to be included in each entry. The following details might be included in each entry for each organisations:

*   Title of organisation

*   Objects of organisation

*   Activities

*   Number of members

*   Types of membership

*   Regular meeting (times and place)

*   Address and telephone number of office/contact

*   Name of contact

*   Means of financial support

*   Status of organisation – charity, friendly society etc.

Avoid personal names addresses and telephone numbers wherever possible as these will be the details which will change most frequently. (It is worth checking that information you wish to include is readily available).

4.   Decide on the form of publication and layout you wish to use. When collecting the information on the organisations it will save a considerable amount of time if you use a form using the chosen layout, maybe one set up on a computer. (It will enable you to check easily if you have all the required information and be far easier to transcribe).

5.   Decide on any additional reference information you wish to include. It is advisable to collect and prepare ready for printing any reference information before the information on organisations is collected.

6.   Because information goes out of date so quickly you must consider the problem of updating even before you collect the information. Basically you have two choices:

i.   Produce a cheap booklet which will serve your purpose for the time being, or can be replaced every two or three years. This option is preferable for directories which cover a narrow band of information and those which are aimed at the general public.

ii.   Produce a directory in loose leaf format for which updating sheets will be provided. This option is preferable for limited circulation directories mainly used by key people.

PLANNING

Compiling a directory involves a considerable amount of work and should be undertaken by a group and not an individual wherever possible.

1.   Identify those likely to have the information required and those who are in contact with the types of organisations you wish to include in the directory.

Likely sources of information on organisations:

a.   Local Authority Sources: The local authority is required to maintain a register of local charities by law. The information is supplied by the Registrar of charities. The register is open to the public and is likely to be kept in either the Chief Executive Department or Legal and Administration Department.

Libraries usually maintain various indices/lists of organisations, and frequently produce forthcoming events sheets.

Education Departments: Youth and Community service sections will usually know of most, if not all, local youth organisations.

Parent/Teacher Associations.

Leisure/Community Divisions of Councils.

Social Services (Under 8's Sections) are required to maintain registers of childminders, playgroups and nurseries, they are also likely to have a reasonable knowledge of groups of users.

Public Relations Departments may also be helpful.

b.   Co-ordinating bodies usually know about organisations within their own subject area – Councils of Voluntary Service, Trades Councils, Community Relations Councils, Play Councils, Age Concerns etc.

c.   Local directories: don't forget the Telephone directory and yellow pages. Try the local reference library for both.

d.   Some likely individuals include: local activists, community workers, trade union officials, newspaper reporters, religious leaders. Ask who is likely to know and then ask them.

Do not overlook the caretakers of local meeting places and local publicans.

e.   Local newspapers: both news stories and the diary column – the further you go back the more likely the organisations are to have folded.

f.   Other sources: it may be necessary to trace an organisation through its national or regional body.

Generally there is no shortage of information, it just takes a lot of hard slog.

2.   Decide how information is to be stored during compilation. If it can be put onto a computer, it will make updating much easier.

3.   Allocate tasks and responsibility for contacting each identified source. Do not duplicate effort, compiling a directory is time consuming enough without wasting effort. It will help if a central register is maintained.

4.   Once all the design and planning is complete, set a time limit for collecting the information on organisations. Try and ensure that the directory is printed and distributed as soon as possible after the time limit. If you need to raise money, raise it before you collect your information. Directories inevitably include inaccuracies as soon as they are printed but compilers should make every effort to keep inaccuracies to a minimum.

5.   Pay attention to physical appearance. Something attractive and easy to read is more likely to be used.

Check all plans/designs very carefully; mistakes and omissions at the planning stage can lead to a lot of wasted time, effort and paper. Test your plans/designs before it's too late.

Some Final Points

1.   When collecting information on organisations you should always confirm or check the information with the organisation concerned. You should also check that the organisation doesn't object to an entry being included in the directory.

Even when the directory is seeking to expose the activities of particular organisations care should be taken to ensure that the information is accurate.

2.   When the directory is sent to and returned by the printer check details carefully for any inaccuracies – wrong telephone numbers etc. can be very frustrating – issue an 'erratum' and 'stop press' if necessary.

3.   Few directories can be fully comprehensive. Do not try to achieve the impossible. Omissions can always be included in an update, supplement or new edition.

4.   If you intend updating the directory ask organisations to inform you of any inaccuracies, changes and omissions. It is helpful to maintain an original copy on which all changes are recorded between updates and supplements. This can save a lot of time.

5.   State prominently when the information in the directory was collected and was correct.

6.   Do not overlook the distribution of the directory – it won't get up and walk to the people you want to use it by itself. As much effort should be put into the distribution as the compilation.

Any directory is only useful if it is used.

SECTION:	**PUBLICATIONS**
TITLE:	**PREPARATION OF A LEAFLET**
AUTHOR:	Adapted from the original Skills Manual by Val Harris

One of the most useful ways of passing on information is through a leaflet. In this section we look at the purposes of a leaflet and how to compile one.

There are numerous purposes in leafletting for example:

- to inform or educate the public about an issue

- to clarify your position on an issue

- to announce or publicise an event

- to dramatise and generate enthusiasm for an event

- to affect public opinion

- to encourage participation

1. **Compiling the leaflet**

- think through the focus of the leaflet before beginning to write e.g. to what kind of audience is it directed, what are the purposes of the leaflet, is it for one occasion or general use?

- use simple language and limit the amount of information included. Quality not quantity. People only absorb very few words before throwing it away.

- watch out for the tone created by the language. What are the emotional effects of the words used (polite, annoying, dramatic etc.).

2. **Content of the leaflet**

- check facts thoroughly and use them carefully

- identify the sponsoring group on the leaflet, give people a contact.

3. **Design and layout**

- arrange the content for simplicity and clarity

- vary the material e.g. different size print, boxes, indent, diagonals, cartoons, pictures; but don't make it messy.

- choose the size of paper which fits the amount of information. Note possibilities which arise from different ways of folding the leaflet.

- evaluate the final product before going to print.

SECTION:	**PUBLICATIONS**
TITLE:	
AUTHOR:	

SECTION:	**PUBLICATIONS**
TITLE:	**THE ART OF LEAFLETTING**
AUTHOR:	Quaker Action Peace and Justice

When you're out leafletting, you're there because you want to be there. It's important. So ...

DISTRIBUTING

- Choose your site and time with care – check if any permission is needed.

- Prepare influential people in the area, give sample leaflet, indicate aims of group etc.

- Prepare leafleters, use roleplay, learn to approach people, handle indifference, hostility, interest, have answers to obvious questions etc.

- Don't hide in a doorway with knees knocking. Do ease in gently by working alongside someone more accustomed to leafletting.

- Do choose who you leaflet don't just blanket everyone in sight, or the person who hasn't got a hand to spare.

- Do choose an individual and make direct contact.

- Do consider the image you're generating. Is it going to help or hinder your communication?

- Don't stand talking to a friend, ignoring potential customers, perhaps causing an obstruction.

- Don't leave your possessions around for others to fall over.

- Do give yourself a break, even if you're enjoying it.

- Do think about your expression. The fixed grin doesn't help – nor does the miserable, bored or aggressive look, or the "if someone asks me a question again I'll scream" look.

- Do hold you're leaflet so its bold front can be seen at a glance.

- Don't get disheartened if you're refused.

- Do have a sentence or two ready for starters: "Can I give you a leaflet?" "We're campaigning for..."

- Do keep to your pitch, to your specific area, and leaflet in one direction only. This helps to avoid people being leafletted twice.

- Don't panic. There are plenty of people around to help, and someone watching for the "help" signal. See Campaigning Section.

Above all - enjoy yourself!

SECTION:	**PUBLICATIONS**
TITLE:	
AUTHOR:	

SECTION:	**PUBLICATIONS**
TITLE:	**WRITING UP RESEARCH**
AUTHOR:	Ann Hindley

The most important thing about writing up research is that it gets done. So many pieces of research have vast amounts of time, effort and money spent on them and then the energy or money runs out before the results get written up. The second most important thing is that it gets disseminated. No research will be worthwhile if it just sits on a shelf and gathers dust. With regards to both writing it up and dissemination, remember to build both into your budget and time plan.

1.   Plan the headings under which you are going to arrange your material early on in the process of the research, but be prepared to come back and revise them as the work progresses.

2.   Allow plenty of time. Writing up might seem like the easy bit but it can, in fact, take a long time.

3.   Think about your audience. Are you planning for it to be read by academics, by your funders, or by the community? The audience that it's aimed at will determine the way in which you present it. Your funders may be impressed by lots of flow charts and diagrams. Local people will want something that they can read and digest easily. Will it need translating or putting into some more accessible form? Again, think about this when drawing up your budget.

4.   Presentation. In these days of desk top publishing, there is no excuse for poor presentation, but remember to budget for it early in the process. However you decide to present the information be consistent throughout with headings, paragraphs, etc.

5.   Get it proof read before the final copy is produced. A final version that hasn't been proof read is always so obvious.

Dissemination

How widely you can disseminate your results depends very much on your budget. A list of people and organisations you want to distribute needs to be drawn up fairly early in the process, so that you have time to add to it as other opportunities come to mind. This list could include:

*   participants in the research

*   the funder(s) of the research

*   the bodies that are going to have recommendations directed at them

*   other people doing similar work in the same field.

Think also about the journals that exist in the field that you've been researching. Try sending them an abstract of your research to see if they will publish it. It's surprising how much response you get from readers of those journals.

SECTION:	**PUBLICATIONS**
TITLE:	
AUTHOR:	

SECTION:	**PUBLICATIONS**
TITLE:	**LAYOUT AND DESIGN**
AUTHOR:	Pauline Dorey

This checklist is designed to help you make your leaflets and other written material as accessible and effective as possible, so that you can get your message across to the widest number and range of people.

1.   Choose what information you want to put over, be as precise, concise and exacting as possible; use only the essentials as peoples attention is very limited. The fewer words, no jargon, the easier it is to read, catch the eye, take in the important points.

2.   Layout leaflets, and posters with plenty of space round the words so they can be picked out easier.

3.   Leave a border of 1.5cm all round as duplicators and printers can't always print up to the edge.

4.   Non joined up writing can be easier for people with learning disabilities or people with visual impairments (partially sighted) to read.

5.   Lower case (not capitals) writing can be easier to read for some people with learning disabilities or with visual impairments.

6.   Think carefully about the "style" of the writing if done on a computer, typewriter, with letraset or with headliner. Italics or more fancier styles can be harder to read for people with visual impairments.

7.   Think carefully about how thick or thin the print is. Sometimes thick print appears "to run together" or it is harder to distinguish the letters. Some very thin print is hard to see as there is not enough contrast with the paper.

8.   Make sure you have a good quality original copy as this will ensure quality reproduction. Make sure that the original copy ("artwork") is clear and not blotchy, that it has dark print so that there is strong contrast against the paper. Try and make sure that when publicity is photocopied, duplicated, printed that the copies are clear, not blotchy, not uneven, not faint (with good contrast). This can be difficult, I know, if you don't have access to good equipment.

9.   Enlarged copies. Try and ensure that you produce some copies that have been enlarged, advertise enlarged copies available. In order to enlarge the print i.e. an A4 or A5 size original up to A3 size (these are all sizes of paper) use a photocopier. This will enlarge the print for people with visual impairments. Ideally you should try and get things enlarged by a large print machine. As the type of print and thickness of it will be better. Obviously as each individuals level of impairment will be different, they will find different sizes, ways of presentation will suit them better. Ask people who have had experience with the Coalition of Disabled People, Centres of Integrated Living. For example as well as having large print publicity information available, advertise that you have

SECTION:	**PUBLICATIONS**
TITLE:	**LAYOUT AND DESIGN**
AUTHOR:	Pauline Dorey

it on the smaller print leaflets, or why not produce all of your information/publicity in a large print form (if this is possible).

10.   Contrast. It is helpful to have a good contrast by having by having "bold" or dark print. Think of the colours of paper you are using. Which colours give good contrast and which bad? Pastel and lighter colours are better i.e. white, yellow, cream, beige; red, purple, dark blue, dark green are more difficult to see. How else can you get good contrast? Colour of the print. Pale colour or red or green do not give such good contrast as blue or black. Some people may have different colours they can not distinguish or find it hard to. What colour felt tip pens do you use on posters or flip chart paper?

11.   Medium. So far we have mainly related to printed word, but how about other ways of putting your message across more directly, simply and not just for people who have difficulties reading?

Cartoons – anti-oppressive humour catches your attention.

Pictures – positive images can put over messages about your activity.

Signs and symbols – you can put over your message using signs and symbols for example.

12.   Format. Consider other forms of presenting material for those who have severe visual impairments or find other mediums more accessible. Any materials can be presented in Braille, on tape and on video.

Obviously this checklist does not only apply to publicity but to:

* any information
* displays
* letters
* newsletters
* handouts
* community newspapers
* leaflets
* minutes etc.

This applies to whatever you are involved in, whether it be a parent and toddlers group, black women's group, community centre association, volunteer project, voluntary organisations, large agencies.

In reality most of these points can be achieved: it often takes a little more thought and in some cases more time. Occasionally it will need equipment, finances or energy which will limit how much you can do. If you are not sure the best way you can present things, where you can get things put into Braille or access to better equipment contact local resource centres, volunteer bureaux, CVSs, community workers, action resource centres, disabled people's organisations etc.

Once you have decided on the content of your leaflet you need to consider what equipment you can use to help with layout, and then what methods to use for printing. This will partly be determined by your budget and access to equipment, but many community and resource centres have a variety of machines for groups to use.

118 Workshop explain the main kinds of equipment that are likely to be available to you.

SOME MACHINERY EXPLAINED

Computer

A relatively new resource which is rapidly becoming used by groups, extremely versatile. If used with word-processor program and daisywheel printer, enables very simple alterations and adjustments of text and simplifies layout work. Disc drives enable work to be stored indefinitely.

Duplicator

Basic printing machine in which the ink is forced directly through a stencil to produce a print. Simple work can be cheaply produced by typing copy directly onto tissue stencil for shorter runs. More complex work can be achieved by making a vinyl stencil on a stencil cutter.

Electric Typewriter

An electric typewriter with a carbon ribbon is essential for good quality reprographic work. Golfball and daisywheel machines usually offer a choice of typefaces.

Headliner

Electric or manual headliners produce continual strips of self-adhesive tape printed with a variety of sizes and styles of numbering or lettering to form headings or big print for artwork. Less versatile than dry-transfer lettering, but far simpler and quicker.

Offset Litho

Printing machine in which the image is transferred (or "offset") from the original to a rubber blanket to achieve the print. Produces higher quality work than a duplicator and with a metal plate can produce much longer runs. Paper originals produced on a photocopier are sufficient for shorter runs of 1–3000 copies. Requires more skill to use than a duplicator.

Photocopier

A modern plain paper photocopier will instantly perform a high quality transfer of image onto another sheet of paper. Many have enlargement and reduction facilities, will handle A3, A4 or card, process paper masters for offset litho printing, and some now have a choice of colours.

SECTION:	**PUBLICATIONS**
TITLE:	**PRINTING OPTIONS**
AUTHOR:	118 Workshop Nottingham

Process Camera

Large, fixed machine for darkroom work, will produce same-size, reductions, enlargements, dot screening etc. for art work. In conjunction with the plate-maker will produce long lasting, good-quality metal plates for offset litho printing.

Silk-screening

For printing bold colours and designs on large posters, t-shirts, etc. Slow, messy, and laborious, but very effective.

Stencil Cutter

A machine that scans more complex artwork and transfers the image electronically onto a vinyl stencil for duplication.

Strip Printer

Older machine for producing headlines, big print etc., using a photographic process.

Thermal Image Fixer

Machine designed to apply a controllable quantity or heat to the surface of paper-masters after preparation on the photocopier and before use on the offset litho. Ensures bold headlines and other large areas of solids do not break up while in the press.

SECTION 22

EVALUATION

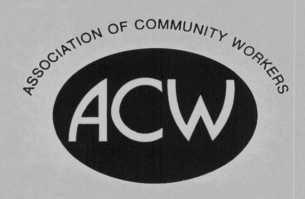

SECTION:	**EVALUATION**
TITLE:	**EVALUATION IN COMMUNITY WORK**
AUTHOR:	Alison Gilchrist

Community work is about change; personal, social and political. The role of the worker is as an agent of change.

What changes are we working towards in any particular situation? How do we measure whether we have succeeded in this purpose? How can we understand why we sometimes succeed and sometimes fail in our endeavours?

What are the factors that influence the strategies we choose and whether or not these are effective?

A POSSIBLE STAGED-APPROACH MODEL FOR PLANNING AND EVALUATING WORK

Use this to continually plan, review and reflect on your work.

ASSESSMENT OF THE SITUATION

Getting to know the area, identifying issues concerning local people, gathering evidence and opinions about particular needs and what resources and facilities already exist.

Checking out findings with members of the community.

Deciding to revise, change, or abandon previous goals and strategies.

EVALUATION

PRIORITISING AND PLANNING

Review in consultation with those involved in and affected by developments.

Consultation with those involved about strategies, methods and respective roles.

Analysing practice.

Setting goals and targets.

Monitoring progress against agreed criteria.

DOING THE WORK

Encouraging maximum participation in activities and decision-making.

Evaluation is looking at how effective a worker or agency has been in changing things according to agreed goals, i.e. in achieving those aims and objectives set out at the planning stage. These can usefully be divided into goals (concrete changes) and processes (psychological changes).

SECTION:	**EVALUATION**
TITLE:	
AUTHOR:	

SECTION:	**EVALUATION**
TITLE:	**A STAGED APPROACH TO EVALUATION**
AUTHOR:	Alison Gilchrist

The process of evaluation should be built into all stages of the work. Evaluation is fundamental to "good practice" in community work, and to the promotion of equality of opportunity.

It is important because it enables you to:

a) learn from experiences and to share them with others

b) adapt your strategy according to changes in the situation

c) monitor the effectiveness of anti-discriminatory measures

d) be accountable to relevant users and funding bodies

e) communicate to others the aims and values of your work

f) develop conscious decision-making in your practice

g) involve users in critically reflecting on your work.

h) see what you have achieved

i) to see if the effort was effective - what difference has it made?

j) improve your management

k) to identify strengths and weaknesses and so improve your programme

STAGE 1 – DECIDING ON GENERAL AIMS AND OBJECTIVES OF WORK.

These might include goals such as "the provision of holiday activities for children" or "the creation of an independent refuge for Asian women" or "gaining equal treatment for disabled people in employment opportunities". You may want to look at part of your project for example how the administration system works, or are you making the most of your volunteers' skills. The aims should also include some reference to the processes which will be used, for example "by encouraging strong participation by children and their parents" or "by supporting campaigning and self-advocacy by disabled peoples themselves", etc.

STAGE 2 – AGREEING THE TARGETS OR CRITERIA BY WHICH PROGRESS TOWARDS THESE AIMS WILL BE MEASURED.

This will set specific targets, such as "the play scheme will provide places for twenty children for two weeks in the summer holidays at minimum cost to the parents", "the membership of the playscheme will reflect the racial balance of children in the local community" or "at least five courses in disability equality and Equal Opportunities selection and recruitment will be run for employers in the next twelve months" or "by the beginning of next year, there will be a safe and supportive group for Asian women who experience domestic violence, which will begin to look at possibilities of long-term funding for a refuge in the region."

STAGE 3 – GATHERING INFORMATION (MONITORING AND FEEDBACK).

There are several methods for collecting information, including monitoring of who uses the project and for what purposes, (you may be already collecting some information but not fully using it) a comments and suggestions book, structured interviews with staff and users, self-evaluation perhaps using an outside consultant.

STAGE 4 – ORGANISING, CHECKING AND ASSESSING THE INFORMATION.

This might involve statistical analysis of figures, such as calculating the proportion of Black people using the project compared to the ethnic make-up of the local population, or it may involve sorting the qualitative feedback into categories relating to the original criteria such as the level of participation of users in decision-making, the effectiveness of social education methods, etc.

STAGE 5 – REFERRING BACK TO ORIGINAL AIMS AND DRAWING SOME CONCLUSIONS ON THE EXTENT TO WHICH THESE HAVE BEEN ACHIEVED.

This could be done through discussion, perhaps at a special workshop, with an emphasis on honest and constructive criticism which draws out the value of what has been achieved as well as learning the lessons from mistakes or wrong decisions.

STAGE 6 – CRITICAL REFLECTION AND ANALYSIS OF WORK SO FAR.

This involves thinking about and discussing with others the effects that the work has had on the situation, identifying significant changes and improvements and exploring areas where there has not been much progress. It is crucial to identify possible explanations for all the successes and failures, and to be alert to the possibilities of unforeseen but important developments and to understand the reasons for these.

STAGE 7 – THINKING THROUGH THE IMPLICATIONS OF FUTURE WORK.

This is the time for learning from mistakes and making adjustments to your programme or strategy. You may realise that your original goals were misguided or unrealistic. It may be that there have been unexpected, but highly significant changes in the situation, which need you to reassess the resources available or the priority given to different processes or goals. This is often the most difficult and painful stage as it is easy to be defensive about your past work, clinging to personal excuses and justifications when these are no longer appropriate.

STAGE 8 – DECIDING ON GOALS AND STRATEGY FOR THE NEXT PHASE.

This informs the next round of assessment and planning. It should be an open and regular process, involving as many people as possible in informal discussion or more formal consultation. It is vital to be clear about the outcome of this stage, so that criteria and targets can be set which everyone understands and agrees to (see Stage 2 above).

There is no simple formula which organisations wishing to evaluate themselves can follow. Organisations have different personnel, tasks, philosophies and resources. Each of these influences the evaluation process. So we cannot offer a blue print but we have set out a checklist of issues which you will need to address. This is not a step by step guide, discussion of one issue inevitably raises others.

Ideally the process of evaluation should happen continuously, not as a one off event.

Evaluating is part of the process of managing an organisation. Consider it in relation to other aspects of that process.

It is helpful to start planning the evaluation process early - when you start an initiative or set up a system.

A checklist of issues for you to address:

1. are we clear what the words mean

   - evaluating

   - monitoring

   - the evaluation process

   - the evaluation

2. are we clear why we want to evaluate?

3. are we clear what we want to use the findings for?

4. are we clear what we want to evaluate?

5. are we clear when we will be evaluating?

6. are we clear about the criteria or indicators we will use in evaluating?

7. are we clear who needs to be involved

   - in planning the process

   - in implementing the process

   - in gathering information

   - in evaluating

   - in implementing changes

8. are we clear about the style of the evaluation; will it be objective; interactive; quantitative; qualitative

9. are we clear about how we will carry it out

10. are we clear whose co-operation we need for each of the above; have we got it?

11. are we clear what resources we will need?

    - time

    - money

    - skills and knowledge

    - are they available

12. are we clear about the possible effect on relationships of evaluating?

13. are we clear what will happen once the findings are reported?

SECTION:	**EVALUATION**
TITLE:	
AUTHOR:	

SECTION:	**EVALUATION**
TITLE:	**A MODEL FOR NEIGHBOURHOOD COMMUNITY DEVELOPMENT WORK**
AUTHOR:	Neil McLellan and Christine Flecknoe

CRITERIA

EXAMPLES OF POSSIBLE OUTCOMES

INCREASED OPPORTUNITIES FOR SOCIAL INTERACTION AND COLLECTIVE ACTIVITY; leading to the development of more caring, co-operative and vocal community networks.

a) self-help groups e.g. parent and toddlers, credit union
b) caring groups – using the skills and talents of local people to help other local people e.g. youth clubs, senior citizens groups, holiday playschemes.
c) informal skill sharing arrangements e.g. baby-sitting circles, gardening and decorating schemes.
d) resource sharing e.g. second hand furniture store, community cafe.
e) campaigning activities e.g. for better housing conditions, or for funding for an advice worker in the neighbourhood

IMPROVED INFORMATION AND EDUCATIONAL OPPORTUNITIES WITHIN THE NEIGHBOURHOOD – the mobilisation of skills and capacities within local people.

a) community education classes
b) informal educational opportunities for learning and personal development
c) resource and information banks
d) activities organised and led by local people
e) surveys carried out

IMPROVED MATERIAL RESOURCES – which local people have created or negotiated for themselves.

a) establishment of community building
b) increased take up of welfare benefits
c) improved play facilities
d) environmental improvements
e) acquisition of grants for housing improvements

EVIDENCE THAT LOCAL PEOPLE ARE TAKING GREATER INDIVIDUAL AND COLLECTIVE CONTROL OVER THEIR LIVES AND THAT THEY ARE INFLUENCING EXTERNAL DECISION-MAKERS.

a) individual personal 'success' stories of change and growth
b) evidence of increased involvement of local people in social and political issues
c) links established with statutory and voluntary agencies and with community organisations in other neighbourhoods
d) growth of local democratic political structures which represent and 'speak for' the neighbourhood e.g. community association, tenants association.
e) raised pride in the neighbourhood.

This is an extract from 'Neighbourhood Community Development' by Neil McLellan and Christine Flecknoe; available from Windhill Community Centre, Church Street, Windhill, Shipley, BD18 2NR tel 0274 588831. £1.50 plus p&p.

SECTION:	**EVALUATION**
TITLE:	
AUTHOR:	

SECTION:	**EVALUATION**
TITLE:	**MONITORING**
AUTHOR:	Val Harris

Monitoring – are we doing what we planned to do?

To monitor an organisation means to collect information in order to see how it functions.

Monitoring means keeping in touch with what you are doing, It means that information is collected about the effects of your work. This information can be used to make appropriate changes. It is only by systematically noting what work is done, and comparing this with your aims and gaols, can you know that your work is worthwhile

You need to be able to review who is, or is not, making use of your services, how the services are provided and what needs are not being met. What information is to be collected, how, by whom and for how long will depend on the type of work and the nature of the goals that have been established.

Funders often require details of your work but any record keeping and collection of information should be clearly linked to a review in some form of the organisations gaols and working methods as well. Record keeping, statistics, log books or whatever are all means to check that an organisations activities are on target. This is crucial to effective management.

Information is the raw material for any type of monitoring. What are the facts? What have people involved in the project been doing?

Take note of unsolicited feedback from people who come into contact with your organisation. Do users frequently complain that you are never around when they need you? Do referral agencies complain that you are not doing anything for their users? Do funders turn you down because they do not understand what you want? Listen to what people tell you.

Before starting deliberately to collect any information ask yourselves:

purpose of monitoring;

- what do you want to find out

- why do you want to monitor

- what question is the monitoring to answer

- how precise does the answer have to be

- who is the information for

- when will its results be used

procedure for monitoring;

- precisely what information do you need to collect

- who will it come from

- how will it be collected

- are the methods appropriate

- have you tested them to make sure they work, i.e. is the wording on a questionnaire understandable

- when will the information be collected

- who is responsible for collecting which pieces of information

- who will be responsible for storing it once it is collected

- who will analyse and summarise it

- how you obtained all possible specialist advice and practical help

- when will you review the methods you have used

Setting up a monitoring programme is best carried out by a small group of people who will decide which of the organisation's goals it wants to monitor and then to answer the questions about the purpose of this monitoring.

The group should consider each proposal by asking:

a)   is it clear, detailed and consistent with the organisations goals

b)   is the task manageable, is the information needed available without too much trouble

c)   will the information lead to changes to the organisation

The group can decide the most appropriate means of collecting the information using the procedures checklist.

SECTION 23

MANAGEMENT COMMITTEES

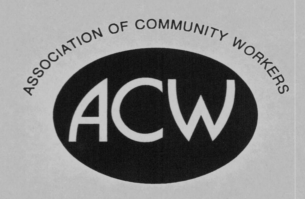

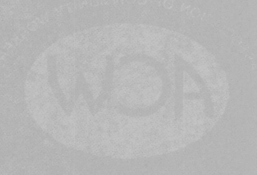

SECTION:	**MANAGEMENT COMMITTEES**
TITLE:	**WORKING WITH MANAGEMENT COMMITTEES**
AUTHOR:	Roger Green and Ann Hindley

One of the key tasks for the community worker is both to develop and support new and existing management committees of community groups and organisations.

This can mean enabling people to meet together to set up a management committee, to working with long established committees. However helping people to meet does not guarantee that it will be effective for the people involved or that issues will be discussed or that decisions will be made. Similarly working with existing committees does not equally guarantee that they are both aware and responsive to their wider membership and the needs of the community as a whole.

Intervention by the community worker using a range of skills, knowledge and awareness can help committees to become more effective as a representative group.

WHAT IS A MANAGEMENT COMMITTEE; SOME DEFINITIONS.

'The primary policy making body within the organisation ... elections and nominations take place annually, and the committee meets monthly' Tyneside Open College Federation 1993

'The management of community centres, village halls, tenant halls and other community buildings by autonomous community organisations is an important way by which people develop skills and confidence, and learn to participate more actively in their local communities. It can also help to ensure that the activities in a community building are responsive to local needs'. Local Authorities and Community development: A strategic opportunity for the 1990's, Association of Metropolitan Authorities, 1993.

'In a community work setting, committees refer to groups of people who have responsibility for organising activities which involve the community' – Kate Sapin and Geraldine Watters, Learning from each other. A handbook for participative learning and community work programmes, William Temple Foundation, 1990.

WHAT IS THE ROLE OF THE MANAGEMENT COMMITTEE?

1. to manage the community group or organisation

2. to ensure the group or organisation works to its aims and objectives; often called its constitution

3. to formulate policy

4. to promote the involvement of the group or organisations members or users and the wider community

5. to monitor and review its own role and functions

6. to be a 'good employer' e.g. support its paid workers and volunteers; have general employer responsibilities within the framework of a sound equal opportunities policy

7. to provide a resource management role e.g. funding, financial control, and decisions, buildings and equipment

8. maintains and develops the group or organisations 'service' to meet the changing needs of its membership/users and the community

NB different management committees will have different legal responsibilities depending upon the type of organisation, e.g. registered charity, companies limited by guarantee etc.

SECTION:	**MANAGEMENT COMMITTEES**
TITLE:	**WORKING WITH MANAGEMENT COMMITTEES**
AUTHOR:	Roger Green and Ann Hindley

DIFFERENT WAYS OF ORGANISING MANAGEMENT COMMITTEES – GIVING PEOPLE A CHOICE

The formal chair centred management committee structure is often the model that most people expect and may have already experienced. However this may not necessarily mean that it is the most appropriate for the management committee you work with or are helping to et up. The collective or co-operative model could as easily be as or more suitable. Choice should be the aim; as these 2 models often overlap they should be considered together;

formal	**collective/co-operative**
chair centred	member centred
officer posts (e.g. chair, secretary, treasurer)	rotating posts
formal processes (e.g. agenda)	informal processes (e.g. brainstorming issues)
formal constitution	flexible aims / objectives
limited participation (e.g. members/users)	participation encouraged

another way of working that could help to involve more people is to establish sub or working groups.

Each model gets as many members of the committee involved by using the technique of forming sub-committee or working groups. This way, members who find it hard to contribute in the larger gathering may feel able to take part in a smaller grouping which has a specific task. sub-committees may form around issues such as personnel, premises or a particular project for example.

MEMBERSHIP OF MANAGEMENT COMMITTEES

The aim here should be to encourage both membership / user and community participation

membership might include;

- community representatives; e.g. local people who reflect the diversity of the community

- representatives from community agencies and projects, e.g. local authority departments, such as Social Services, Housing; voluntary sector projects. These can be useful allies particularly on funding issues and grant applications.

- paid workers and volunteers representatives; a must except for registered charities who cannot have paid workers on their management committee

- professional advisors. People with special skills, knowledge and expertise who can be useful to the group/organisation. The downside of advisors is that they can sometimes inhibit discussion because of who they are. This can also apply to representatives of community agencies

- users of the service; is a service providing group/organisation – a priority!

- co-opted members; really anyone else who might be useful on the committee

POSSIBLE PROBLEMS AND ISSUES WITH MANAGEMENT COMMITTEES

Working with established and new committees can often present the community worker with problems and issues which really have to be tackled if the committee is to be both democratic and representative of the community.

Recognising such problems and issues can allow the community worker to help the committee take the first step towards being a truly participatory and accountable body and/or to reassess its overall workings.

Such problems or issues could be

- unrepresentative of the wider membership/users and the community e.g. does not reflect the cultural and ethnic composition of the community

- run by a small clique of people e.g. the same people are always re-elected for officer posts; apathy is rife

- minutes of meetings are difficult to get hold of and not circulated widely. The committee operates as the equivalent of a community Freemasons lodge – secrecy is paramount

- limited participation from members/users (particularly service led organisations)

- the work of the committee is never evaluated e.g. how decisions are made or not made

- 'English only' spoken here. The unchallenged and hidden presumption that the committee does and always will conduct it business in English irrespective of whether English is everyone's first language, and this can include speaking in jargon.

- men run the meetings whether the chairperson is a man or not

- user empowerment becomes workers disempowerment

- expectation of paid workers e.g. paid workers have continually to justify their existence and prove their worth

- lack of equal opportunities in practice, e.g. in the recruitment of paid workers and volunteers

- agendas seem to be 'fixed' e.g. that decisions feel as if they have been already decided prior to the meetings and that the meeting is merely going through the motions and is simply putting the rubber stamp on them. Similarly, getting items on the agenda is difficult if not impossible.

A CHECKLIST FOR CREATING A CLIMATE OF CHANGE

Where does the committee meet?

- is it a central location

- is the meeting adequately advertised

- is the time of the meeting convenient for everyone

- is there transport to and from the meeting

- what childcare arrangements are there, e.g. is a crèche available, are childminding costs covered

- are other dependants costs covered

- is there access for people with disabilities

- are refreshments provided

- is there access to a telephone if needed

- are interpreters/signers available.

Why are we here

It is useful to discuss this periodically as it gets people to focus on, for example, why they are on the committee, what they are achieving, their motivation, their specific interests.

TRAINING

what training needs does the committee have? has this question ever been asked?

check if committee members received and/or need any training for their role on the committee, e.g.

- members responsibilities
- how to chair a meeting
- how to take minutes
- the role of the treasurer
- induction for new members

other training needs might be:

- how to improve user participation
- how decision making occurs
- putting equal opportunities into practice
- communicating the committees decisions
- how to make priorities

Joint training with management committees from other groups and organisations might be considered as it allows people to network, to share experiences and ideas, to consider joint action to tackle a common community issue.

GETTING SUPPORT FROM YOUR MANAGEMENT COMMITTEE

A priority if the committee is your employer!

- ensure you have a clear job description / job specification
- regular supervision is a must, from someone on the committee, a worker from another project or from a support group formed by workers from projects in the community
- try and get a slot on the committee meetings agenda which gives you the opportunity to present a written and a verbal report on your work. This helps keep the committee informed of what's happening and is useful in dispelling myths and fantasies about your work.

Useful books and articles on most aspects of management committees.

Sandy Adirondack, Just about managing? A guide to effective management for voluntary organisations and community groups. London Voluntary Service Council 1995

Duncan Forbes and others; Voluntary but not amateur; a guide to the law for voluntary community organisations and community groups. London Voluntary Service Council 1995

Steve Clarke, Seeing it through; how to be effective on a committee, Bedford Square Press 1989

Michael Locke, How to run committees and meetings, Macmillan 1980

Malcom Payne, Linkages; Effective networking in social care; especially Being effective in committee, chapter 11; Committees and meetings strategy, Chapter 12; Whiting and Birch/ Social Care Association 1993

Caroline Pinder, Community Start Up, how to start a group and keep it going; especially Making meetings work, chapter 5; National Federation of Community Organisations (now Community Matters)/ National Extension College 1985.

SECTION 24

LOCAL GOVERNMENT

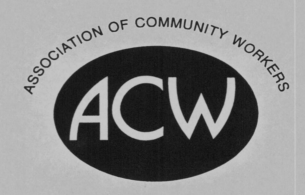

SECTION:	**LOCAL GOVERNMENT**
TITLE:	**FINDING OUT ABOUT YOUR LOCAL COUNCIL**
AUTHOR:	Roger Green

Local Government is important for community work – for its decisions on funding, resources, services and tackling problems, all affect local communities, to successfully challenge policies, obtain resources, get action taken on problems requires understanding of how to influence it. Recent changes to local government included the creation of Unitary Authorities, some of whom will not be fully independent until 1998. So this section can only outline the basics and suggest ways of making contact with key officers or councillors.

WHERE TO FIND THEM

Most councils have a town hall which is the centre or headquarters building of the council. Some councils now have decentralised offices called neighbourhood centres or offices. Council departments are also located in most communities.

WHAT IT DOES

Depending on what "type" of council it is they provide a range of services to local communities, for example, refuse collection, education (school and youth clubs), housing, social services, planning, environmental health, libraries, and recreation and leisure.

WHO RUNS THE COUNCIL

Councillors:

Who are elected at local government elections. They decide on councils policies and are responsible for the council services provided. Councillors are paid expenses only.

Officers:

People employed by local councils are called local government officers. They are responsible for implementing the councils policies by providing and administering services to the community.

WHO FUNDS THE COUNCIL

Councils receive their income from a mixture of direct grants from central government and locally raised taxes, for example, the council tax. Some councils also receive grants from the European Union.

WHAT POWERS DO THEY HAVE

Depends on whether your council is a County Council, City or District Council, London Borough, Parish Council or a Metropolitan District Council. Most councils powers and responsibilities are defined by Parliament.

COUNCIL MEETING AND COMMITTEE MEETINGS

Each council has council meetings and committees to deal with the council's business. Most of these council meetings and committee meetings are open to the public.

SECTION:	**LOCAL GOVERNMENT**
TITLE:	**FINDING OUT ABOUT YOUR LOCAL COUNCIL**
AUTHOR:	Roger Green

HOW TO CONTACT YOUR COUNCIL IF YOU HAVE AN ISSUE OR PROBLEM

- Contact the relevant council department.

- Find out who your local councillor is.

- Contact them. Council offices, particularly libraries, have their addresses and telephone. Most have "surgeries" where you can see your councillor.

- Lobby a council meeting or committee meeting.

- Raise issues at a "neighbourhood forum", or use area panels if your council has them.

- If no success contact your local newspaper and/or local radio. Get your local Member of Parliament involved.

INFORMATION ON LOCAL COUNCILS

Tony Byrnes book, Local Government in Britain, 1992 (5th. Edition) is a good guide to local government and how it works.

Some councils now have council newspapers as well as leaflets explaining the services councils provide and how to complain about them.

SECTION:	**LOCAL GOVERNMENT**
TITLE:	**DEVELOPING PARTNERSHIPS**
AUTHOR:	Ann Hindley

Partnerships involving local government, local businesses and local communities are springing up in wide variety of fields. The aim is to involve all the key actors in a joint venture leading to innovation and change. Reactions to proposed partnerships are mixed.

Examples of partnership arrangements can be found in Community Development Trusts, Housing Action Trusts, Estate Management Boards, Community Regeneration Schemes, School Governing Boards, SRB Partnership Boards, amongst others.

Many volunteer agencies are being asked to participate in such partnerships arrangement: the checklist is intended to help you in deciding whether to become involved in a partnership by considering the following points:

Important points to be borne in mind:

*   ownership of a partnership should be local,

*   users should be involved in development and evaluation,

*   there must be flexibility in programme and project development,

*   there must be both entrance and exit strategies,

*   the project must be allowed sufficient time to mature.

Reference:

A useful checklist on partnership formation and development has been produced for the Barnsley Partnerships. £5 from John Grayson at Northern College, Wentworth Castle, Stainborough, Barnsley, S. Yorks.

The likely benefits of partnership arrangements:

*   partnerships may provide local groups with a means of tackling larger projects,

*   they give councils a way of structuring community involvement and sometimes a way of securing new money.

*   they give the private sector a vehicle through which to contribute to local initiatives,

*   they involve a multi agency, multi faceted approach that involves tenants/users in defining the problems and suggesting solutions, together with an opportunity to integrate those views into major policies affecting the area,

*   increased confidence among user/tenants,

*   a new understanding of partnership based on a vision of several groups working to a new set of objectives which are beneficial to all concerned.

Concerns about partnership arrangements:

*   will there be partnership or will there be conflict?

*   will the focus be on joint and co-ordinated meeting of needs?

*   is there a real commitment to collaboration?

*   are the partners committed to mutual benefit, shared decision making and a readiness to learn new ways of working?

*   how is the common language created, shared goals identified, and partners provided with an equal say?

*   is control going to be weighted towards those holding the purse strings?

*   the partnership might be used as a way of excluding key players,

*   participation and consultation can mean different things to different people,

*   difficult issues may be deliberately avoided in order to make progress and meet a tight timetable.

SECTION:	**LOCAL GOVERNMENT**
TITLE:	
AUTHOR:	

BOOKLIST & ORGANISATIONS

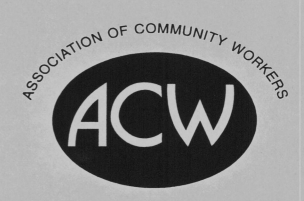

SELECTED BIBLIOGRAPHY OF USEFUL BOOKS

Saul Alinsky.

Reveille for Radicals.1969. Random House

Sandy Adirondeck and Richard McFarlane.

Getting Ready for Contracts; a guide for voluntary organisations. Directory of Social Change. 1990 ISBN 0-907164-64-1

Association of Community Workers.

Monthly Talking Points

You're Learning All The Time, women, education and community work. 1986. Spokesman Press. ISBN 0-85124-448-3

Association of Metropolitan Authorities (AMA)

Local Authorities and Community development; a strategic opportunity for the 1990's. 1993. 185677-063-X

Karl Atkin and Janet Rollings

Community Care in a Multi-Racial Britain. a critical review of the literature. HMSO 1993 ISBN 0-11-701758-2

Barclay Report. Towards Community Social Work. 1982

Mog Ball.

Evaluation in the voluntary sector. Forbes Trust 1988. ISBN 0-9513352-0-0. Forbes House, 9 Artillery Lane, London. E1 7LP

Paul Ballard (ed)

Issues in Church Related Community Work. University of Cardiff. 1990

A. Baptiste.

A Credit To You. 1992. Clarendon College, Pelham Ave. Nottingham.

James G. Barber.

Beyond Casework. BASW/Macmillan 1991

Sue Beardon.

The contract culture; a view from West Yorkshire. 1993. Voluntary Action Leeds. ISBN 0-9521100-8

Peter Bereford and Suzy Croft.

Citizen Involvement; a practical guide for change. BASW/Macmillan. 1992

Margaret Bond and Graham Benfield.

Towards Shared Aims; a good practice guide for Local Authorities and Voluntary Organisations. WCVA 1993. ISBN 1-871094-22-4

Ray Braithwaite.

Violence. Understanding, Intervention and Prevention. Radcliffe Press. ISBN 1-870905-92-X. 1992

Tony Byrne.

Local Government in Britain, Harmondsworth; Penguin 1992.

John Callaghan.

Costings for Contracts. Directory of Social Change and NCVO. ISBN 0-907164-81-1

Sally Capper et al.

Starting and running a voluntary group. Bedford Square Press. 1989.

Sam Clarke.

The Fundraising Handbook. Directory of Social Change. 1993 ISBN 1-873860-21-8

Steve Clarke

Seeing It Through; how to be effective on a committee. Bedford Square Press and CPF. ISBN 0-7199-1261-X 1989

Community Education Training Unit; (CETU)

Assertion and how to train ourselves; ISBN 0-9515122-1-8

Training and how to enjoy it; ISBN 0-9515122-0-X

Training and how not to panic.ISBN 0-9515122-3-4

Community Accountancy Project.

How to handle your money, if you have any. An accountancy handbook for community organisations. 3rd Edition

Community Links.

Ideas Annual.

Community Matters.

Managing your community building. 1994.

Emphasise the positive; a guide to positive action for racial equality 1989

Community Participation Group

UK Health for All Network. Community Participation for Health for All. 1991. from UK Health For All Network; PO Box 101 Liverpool L69 5BB tel 051-231-1009

Anne Connor.

Monitoring Ourselves. Charities Evaluation Services. 1993. ISBN 1-897963-00-9

Gary Craig et al.

Community Work and the State. 1982. ISBN 0-7100 9305-5

Community Work Studies. ACW

A. Curno et al.

Women and Collective Action. 1982 ACW

P. Curno.

Political Issues in Community Work. 1982. RKP. ISBN 0-7100-8975-9

John Daines and Brian Graham.

Adult Learning, Adult Teaching. Dept of Adult Ed, University of Nottingham. 1988 ISBN 1-85041-022-4.

Giles Darvill.

The impact of contracts on volunteers. Volunteer Centre 1990

Annie Davies and Ken Edwards.

Twelve Charity Contracts. 1990 Directory of Aocial Change. ISBN 0-707164-52-5.

Peter Dawson and Wendy Palmer.

Taking Self-Advocacy Seriously. 1993. EMFEC. Robin Wood House, Robin Wood Road, Aspley, Nottingham. NG8 3NH; tel 0602 293291. ISBN 1-85258-226-X.

Lena Dominelli.

Women and Collective Action. 1990. Venture Press. ISBN 0-900102-77-2

Jean Ellis.

Breaking New Ground. Community Development with Asian Communities. Bedford Square Press and CDF. 1989. ISBN 0-7199-1238-5

Angela Everitt and Andy Gibson.

Making it work; researching in the voluntary sector. ARVAC

Willem Van Der Eyken.

Managing Evaluation. Charities Evaluation Services. 1993. ISBN 1-897963-017

Federation of Community Work Training Groups

Setting up a Community Work Skills Course

Learning for Action; Community Work and Participative Training. AMA 1990. ISBN 0-902052-93-4

F.E.U.

The assessment of prior learning and learner services. 1992

Warren Feek.

Working Effectively; a guide to evaluation techniques. Bedford Square Press. 1988 ISBN 0-7199-1177-X

Roger Fisher, William Ury, Bruce Paton.

Getting to Yes, negotiating an agreement without giving in. Business Books.

Nic Fine and Fiona Macbeth.

Playing with fire; training for the creative use of conflict. Youth Work Press. 1992. ISBN 0-86155-141-9

Susan Forrester.

Environmental Grants. Directory of Social Change. 1989. ISBN 0-907164-47-1

David Francis and Paul Henderson.

Working with rural communities. BASW/Macmiullan. 1992.

Carien Fritze.

Because I speak Cockney, They think I'm stupid. 1982. ACW. ISBN 0-907413-08-0

Marie-Therese Feuerstein.

Partners in Evaluation. Macmillan. ISBN 0-333-42261-9. 1986

George Gawlinski and Lois Graessle.

Planning Together; the art of effective teamwork. ISBN 0-7199-1202-4 1989. Bedford Square Press

Caroline Gillies.

Finding sponsorship for community projects; a step by step guide. 1990. ISBN 0907164544

Clive Grace and Richard Gutch.

Getting in on the act; a guide to Local Authorities powers to fund voluntary organisations. ISBN 07199 12180.

G. Goetschius.

Working with Community groups. 1969

Gulbenkian Report.

Community Work and Social Change. 1968. Longmans

Christine Hallett.

Critical Issues in Participation. ACW. 1987

Margaret Harris.

Management Committees in Practice; a study in local voluntary leadership.. 1989. Centre for Voluntary Organisations. LSE, Houghton Street, London, WC2A 2AE.

Brian Harvey.

Networking in Europe; a guide to European Voluntary Organisations. NCVO/CDF 1992

Murray Hawkin, Geraint Hughes, Janie Peray Smith.

Community Profiling – Auditing Social Needs. OUP 1994. ISBN 0 335 19113 4

Paul Henderson (ed).

Working with Communities. Childrens Society 1988

Paul Henderson and David Francis.

Rural Action. CDF and ACRE. 1993 ISBN 0-7453-0732-0

Paul Henderson and David Thomas.

Skills in Neighbourhood Work. 1987 Allen and Unwin

Hoinville, Jowell and associates.

Survey Research Practice. Heinemann Educational Books. 1978

Christine Holloway and Shirley Otto.

Getting Organised; a handbook for non-statutory organisations. NCVO. 1985.

Anne Hope and Sally Timmel.

Training for Transformation. Mambo Press. 1984. Mambo Press Harare PO Box UA 320; Gweru PO Box 779. ISBN 0-86922-261-9

Gaie Houston.

The Red Book of Groups, and how to lead them better. 1990. ISBN 095-10323-3-X

Jane Hutt.

Opening the Town Hall Door. ISBN 0-7199-1201-6

Sidney Jacobs and Keith Popple.

Community Work in the 1990's. Spokesman Books 1994. ISBN 0-85124-569-2

Kirklees Met Council.

Housing Services. Tenants Consultation Charter 1993.

M. Langan and P. Lee

Radical Social Work Today. 1989

Alan Lawrie.

Quality of Service; measuring performance for voluntary organisations. NCVO/ Directory of Social Change. ISBN 0-907164-82-X

Local Government Information Unit.

Local Govt Finance; prepared in association with NALGO 1993. ISBN 0-9522-4569-X

London to Edinburgh Weekend Return Group.

In and Against the State. 1979.

London Voluntary Service Council.

Voluntary but not Amateur; a guide to the law for voluntary organisations and community groups: by Fobes, Hayes & Redson. ISBN 0-901171-95-6

Just about managing by S. Adirondeck.

Tackling Training, ed Simon Fuchs.

Jo Woolf. Beginners Guide to Contracts. ISBN 1-872582-55-9 1992

LVSC. 68 Cheelton Street, London, NW1 1JR

Martin Loney.

Community Against Government. The British Development Project 1968-78. Heinemann 1983. ISBN 0-435-82545-3

Neil McLellan and Christine Flecknoe.

Neighbourhood Community Development. Bluebell Publications (21 West Lane Baildon West Yorks BD17 5AG) 1992.

Denis McShane.

Using the media. Pluto Press.

Fred Milson.

An Introduction to Community Work. 1974 RKP

NCVO

Finding Funds; general information of funding for voluntary groups. 1993. ISBN 0-7199-1392-6

Fundraising Books and Pamphlets; a selected bibliography. 1992. NCVO reading list 6.

Getting into Training; guidelines for people organising training for voluntary groups. 1993. ISBN 0-7199-1280-6

How do we evaluate ourselves; good practice guidelines to evaluation for Local development Agencies. 1992.

Evaluating Training Programmes; guidelines for Voluntary Sector Training Organisers. 1992. ISBN 0-7199-1369-1

Paul Nichols.

Social Survey Methods; a field guide for development workers. Oxfam Publications. 1991. ISBN.0-855981261.

David Northmore.

Publicity for Free. Bloomsbury. 1993 ISBN 0-7475-0833-X

Michael Norton.

A guide to the benefits of charitable status. Directory of Social Change. ISBN 0-907164-26-9. 1988

Raising money from trusts. Directory of Social Change 1989. ISBN 0-907164-48-X

Ashok Ohri and Basil Manning.

Community Work and Racism. 1982 ACW

Jan O'Malley.

The Politics of Community Action. 1977 ISBN 0-85124-183-2

Organisation and Social development Consultants.

Anti-racist ways of working within raining - a guide for trainers. 355, Fulwood, Sheffield S10 3BQ

Sarah Passingham.

Organising Local events. Directory of Social Change

David Phillips.

Do it yourself social surveys. Faculty of Social Studies, Polytechnic of North London. 1988

Caroline Pinder.

Community Start Up - how to start a community group and keep it going. National Extension College/ National Federation of Community Organisations. 1985

Keith Popple.

Analysing Community Work – Its Theory and Practice. OUP 1995. ISBN 0 335 19408 7

Quaker Peace Action.

Street Campaigning. '1988 Quaker Peace and Justice. ISBN 0-901689-33-5.

Charles Ritchie.

Community Works – 26 case studies showing community operational research in action. PAULC Publications 1994. ISBN 0 86339 4574

Rick Rogers.

Managing Consultancy; a guide for arts and voluntary organisations. NCVO/ Arts Council. 1990. ISBN 0-7199-1295-4

Kate Sapin and Geraldine Watters.

Learning from Each Other. William TempleFoundation. ISBN 1-870733-30-4 1990. William Temple Foundation. Manchester Business School, Manchester M15 6PB

Save The Children.

Toolkits. Save The Children 1995. ISBN 1 870322 93 2

Scottish Council for Voluntary Organisations.

Committees; a training workpack. ISBN 0-903589-88-5.

Community development; a training workpack. ISBN 1-870904-26-5 1992

Swindon Community Work Training Group.

Building Portfolios; a training manual. Available form TVSC, 1 St John Street, Swindon, SN1 1RT

Gill Taylor.

Equal Opportunities in Recruitment and Employment; a basic guide. Nottingham Task Force; available from NCVS 33 Mansfield Road, Nottingham NG1 3FB. 1991. 0-9518176-1-2

Marilyn Taylor.

Signposts to Community development. 1992. Community Development Foundation

Telford FE College

APL project. Accreditation of Prior Learning. 1990. SCOTVEC

Tenants Participation Advisory Service (TPAS)

Participation; a tenants handbook. ISBN 1-871796091. 1990.

David Thomas.

The making of Community Work, 1983 Allen and Unwin

Neil Thompson.

Anti-discriminatory Practice. BASW.

Alan Twelvetrees.

Community Work, 1990, Macmillan ISBN 0-333-49506-3

Volunteer Centre UK.

Understanding Management Committees; a look at volunteer management committee members. 1992. ISBN 0-904-647-846

Step by Step - a guide to volunteer fundraising.

Sue Ward.

Getting the message across. Journeymen. 1992. ISBN 1-85172-043-X

Peter Willmott.

Community Initiatives; patterns and prospects. Policy Studies Institute. 1989

Anne Woodrow.

Building your portfolio. A basic Guide. 1990. F.E.U.

On line services available to community groups.

Poptel

the electronic network for the not-for-profit sector; developed by Soft Solutions who have also developed the HOST systems in Manchester and parts of West Yorkshire.

Soft Solutions

25 Downham Road London N1 5AA tel 0171 249 2948; fax 0171 254 1102

VOLNET UK

Data base service providing information for social change; gives access to other Databases e.g. Directory of Voluntary Action Research. Volunteer Centre UK 29 Lower King's Road, Berkhamstead, Herts HP4 2AB tel; 01442 873311, fax; 01442 870852 and Community Projects Foundation 60 Highbury Grove, London, N5 2AG tel; 0171-226 5375, fax; 0171-704 0313.

Video Suppliers.

Albany Video Distribution

Battersea Studios, Television Centre, Thackeray Road, London SW8 3TW. tel; 0171-498 6811. fax; 0171-498 1494

Mental Health Media Council produce lists of available videos on:

Cultural Identity and Racism

Women and Well-being

Coping with Bereavement

Managing Stress

Addiction

Ability and Disability

They also produce updates lists on other topics within their quarterly magazine

The Mental Health Media Council, 380-384 Harrow Road, London W9 2HU. Tel; 0171-286 2346

Small World Media

produce videos on public protest in Britain today. Their current videos look at the M11 campaign, the Public Order Bill, and Media coverage of direct action. Small World Media Ltd 3, Ashbrook Road, London, N19 3DF tel; 0171 267 1886. fax; 0171 267 6563. E-Mail Smallworld gn.@pc.org.

ORGANISATIONS

Association of Community Technical Aid Centre
64 Mount Plesant, Liverpool, L3 5SD.

ACRE - The Rural Communities Charity;
Somerford House, Somerford Road, Cirencester, Glos. GL7 1TW. 01285 653477

Association of Community Workers
Stephenson Building, Elswick Road, Newcastle upon Tyne, NE4 6SQ. 0191 272 4341.

ARVAC
60 Highbury Grove, London N5 2AG. 0171 704 2315

Access to Assessment Service
North Lincs. College, Cathedral Street, Lincs. LN2 SHQ

BASSAC
The Association of Settlements and Social Action Centres, 13 Stockwell Road, London SW9 9AU
0171-733 7428

Black European Community Development Foundation
150 Townmead Road, London, SW6 2RA.

Black Volunteering Resource Unit
First Floor 102 Park Village East, London NW1 3SP. 0171 388 8542

B.C.O.D.P. British Council of Disabled People
Litchurch Plaza, Litchurch Lane, Derby DE24 8AA. Tel 01332 295551; fax 01332 295580

Charities Evaluation Service
No 1 Motley Ave, Christina Street, London EC2A 4SU.

Child Poverty Action Group
4th Floor, 1-5 Bath Street, London EC1B V9PY. 0171 253 3406

Churches Community Work Alliance
Room 17-18 Mary Burnie House, Westhill College, Weoley Park Road, Birmingham, B29 6LL
0121 414 0104

Combat Poverty Agency
8 Charlemont Street, Dublin 2. Tel 01 4783355; Fax 01 4783731

Committee on the Administration of Justice (CAJ)
45 Donegall Street, Belfast BT1 2KG. 01232 232394

Commission for Racial Equality
Elliot House, 10-12 Allington Street, London, SW1E 5EH. 0171-828-7022

Community Computing Network
c/o UNET 45b Blythe Street, London, E2 6LN

Community Development Foundation

60 Highbury Grove, London, N5 2AG. Tel 0171 226 5375; Fax 0171 704 0313

Community Education Resource Unit

Ruskin Hall, Dunstan Road, Old Headington, Oxford, OX3 9DZ.

Community Links

237 London Road, Sheffield, S2 4NF 0114 258 8822

Community Matters (NFCO)

8-9 Upper Street London N1 0PQ 0171-226 0189

Community Workers Co-op

Pavee Point Centre, North Great Charles Street, off Mountjoy Square, Dublin. 01 8732802

Community and Youth Workers Union

202a The Argent Centre, 60 Frederick Street, Hockley, Birmingham B1 3HS. 0121 233 2815

Development Trusts Association

20 Conduit Place, London, W2 1HZ

Directory of Social Change

24 Stephenson Way, London, NW1 2DP. 0171 209 5151

European Anti-Poverty Network - Ireland

8 Charlemont Street, Dublin 2

European Contact Group

48 Peveril Crescent, Manchester, M21 1WS

Equal Opportunities Commission

Overseas House, Quay Street, Manchester M3 3HN 0161 833 9244

Federation of Community Work Training Groups

4th Floor, Furnival House,48 Furnival Gate, Sheffield, S1 4QP. 0114 273 9391

Institute of Race Relations

247-249 Pentonville Road, London. N1 9NG

Internation Federation of Settlements

The Derwent Centre, Clarke Street, Derby, DE1 2BU

Kids Club Network

279 - 291 Whitechapel Road, London. E1 1BY

Law Centres Federation

Duchess House, 18 Warren Street, London W1P 5DB 0171-387-8570

Learning from Experience Trust

6 Buckingham Gate, London, SW1E 6JP.

Local Government Association

26 Chapter Street, London SW1P 4ND. tel 0171 834 2222; fax 0171 834 2263

London Voluntary Service Council

356 Holloway Road, London, N7 6PA. 0171 700 8107

NACVS -National Association of Councils of Voluntary Service

3rd Floor, Arundel Court, 177 Arundel Street, Sheffield, S1 2NU. 0114 278 6636

NAVB National Association of Volunteer Bureaux

St Peters College, College Road, Satley, Birmingham B8 3TE. 0121-327 0265

NCVO National Council for Voluntary Organisations

Regents Wharf, 8 All Saints Street, London N1 9RL. Tel 0171 713 6161; Fax 0171 713 6300

National Federation of City Farms

AMF House, Whitby Road, Brislington, Bristol, BS4 3QF

National Playbus Association

AMF House, Whitby Road, Brislington, Bristol, BS4 3QF

Northern Ireland Council for Voluntary Action

127 Ormeau Road, Belfast, BT7 1SH. 01232 321224

Quaker Action for Peace and Service

Friends House, Euston road, London NW1 2BJ

Refugee Council

3 Broadway, London, SW8 1SJ. Tel 0171 582 6922; Fax 0171 582 0929

Runneymede Trust

178 North Gower Street, London NW1 2NO. 0171-387-8943

Scottish Community Education Council

West Coates House, 90 Haymarket Terrace, Edinburgh, EH1 5LQ

Scottish Council for Voluntary Organisations

18/19 Claremont Crescent, Edinburgh, EH7 4QD

SCCD; Standing Conference on Community Development

4th Floor, Furnival House, Furnival Gate, Sheffield, S1 4QP. 0114 270 1718

Sia

High Holborn House, 49-51 Bedford Square, London, WC1V 6DJ

Standing Conference of West Indian Organisations

5 Westminster Bridge Road, London SE1 7XW.

Tenant Participation Advisory Service (TPAS)

48 The Crescent, Salford, M5 4NY. 0161-745-7903

The Federation of Black Housing Organisations

374 Grays Inn Road, London WC1 8BB. 0171 837 8288

The National Federation of Tenants and Residents Association

Room 41/42, Estate Buildings, Railway Street, Huddersfield HD1 1JY. 01484 434943

Volunteer Centre UK

29 Lower Kings Road, Berkhamsted, Hertfordshire HP4 2AB. Tel 01442 873311; Fax 01422 870852

Wales Council for Voluntary Action

Llys Ifor, Crescent Road, Caerphilly, Mid Glamorgan, CF8 1XL
Tel 01222 869224/869111; Fax 01222 860627